The Practi... CORONARY D... PREVENTION

Michael Miller, M.D.
Robert A. Vogel, M.D.

The Practice of CORONARY DISEASE PREVENTION

Michael Miller, M.D., F.A.C.C.

Assistant Professor of Medicine
Director, Center for Preventive Cardiology
University of Maryland School of Medicine
Assistant Professor of Medicine
Johns Hopkins University School of Medicine
Baltimore, Maryland

Robert A. Vogel, M.D., F.A.C.C.

Herbert Berger Professor of Medicine
Chief, Cardiovascular Division
University of Maryland School of Medicine
Baltimore, Maryland

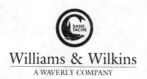

Williams & Wilkins

A WAVERLY COMPANY

BALTIMORE • PHILADELPHIA • LONDON • PARIS • BANGKOK
BUENOS AIRES • HONG KONG • MUNICH • SYDNEY • TOKYO • WROCLAW

Editor: David C. Retford
Managing Editor: Leah Ann Kiehne Hayes
Production Coordinator: Linda Carlson
Designer: Wilma E. Rosenberger
Illustration Planner: Lorraine Wrzosek
Composition: Mario Fernández
Printer: Victor Graphics

Accurate indications, adverse reactions, and dosage schedules for drugs are provided in this book, but it is possible that they may change. The reader is urged to review
the package information data of the manufacturers of the medications mentioned.

Printed in the United States of America

Library of Congress Cataloging in Publication Data

Miller, Michael, 1957 June 19-
    The practice of coronary disease prevention / Michael Miller, Robert A. Vogel.
    p. cm.
    Includes bibliographical references and index.
    ISBN 0-683-18045-2
    1. Coronary heart disease–Prevention. 2. Coronary heart disease–Risk factors.
    I. Vogel, Robert A., 1943- . II. Title.
    [DNLM: 1. Coronary Disease–prevention & control. 2. Coronary Disease–
    etiology. 3. Risk Factors. WG 300 M648p 1996]
    RA645.C68M55 1996
    616.1'2305–dc20
    DNLM/DLC
    for Library of Congress   95-45490
                                                         CIP

The Publishers have made every effort to trace the copyright holders for borrowed
material. If they have inadvertently overlooked any, they will be pleased to make the
necessary arrangements at the first opportunity.

96 97 98 99 00
1 2 3 4 5 6 7 8 9 10

For Avery

Foreword

Most medical books published today are multiauthored. Typically, one or two editors gather a group of investigators together and each of the latter produce a chapter. The usual result is that the quality of the chapters is highly variable. The present book is different. It is written in its entirety by the two authors. It contains 14 chapters and each is of high quality. Indeed, this is an outstanding book, and the best I have encountered so far on preventive cardiology. It is packed full of facts, figures, tables and references, and it reads easily. I heartily congratulate the authors, and highly recommend this book to all physicians encountering patients with cardiovascular disease.

—*William C. Roberts, M.D.*
Director, Baylor Cardiovascular Institute
Baylor University Medical Center
Dallas, Texas

Preface

Recent studies have demonstrated remarkable improvement in the clinical course of "high-risk" patients following aggressive modification of coronary risk factors. Nevertheless, most physicians *do not* incorporate this important form of medical treatment. These concepts have been recently emphasized by the American College of Cardiology, which currently recommends that all cardiovascular trainees develop expertise "in the primary and secondary prevention of cardiovascular diseases." To this end, we have detailed the major advancements in this rapidly growing field. In addition to cardiovascular trainees, all practicing physicians, nurses, dietitians, and other health care personnel involved in the day-to-day care of heart disease patients will hopefully find the information contained herein stimulating and applicable. Every attempt has been made to provide a succinct summation of major topics in prevention, which all too often are neglected in didactic classroom and hospital ward teachings.

We are greatly indebted to the many people who have contributed altruistically in facilitating publication of this edition. They include Ms. Esther Getz and Ms. Kate McWilliams for manuscript typing and revision, Ms. Christina Dolinar, Ms. Rachel Burgan and Ms. Gina Friel for journal searches and Ms. Myra Carpenter and Mr. Rick Angello of FCG International, Inc. for editing.

—*Michael Miller, M.D., F.A.C.C.*
Robert A. Vogel, M.D., F.A.C.C.

Contents

1/ Introduction

Most cardiovascular diseases, including coronary artery disease (CAD), are both highly prevalent and preventable. Currently in the U.S., more than 10 million individuals have symptomatic CAD. This results in approximately 1.5 million myocardial infarctions (MIs), 975,000 deaths, and a total economic burden of $120 billion annually. Asymptomatic CAD is even more prevalent. Autopsy studies of trauma victims demonstrated the presence of histologic coronary atherosclerosis in 50–75% of young men, with high-grade stenoses in 5–10%. By age 90, more than 75% of individuals have high-grade stenoses. Increasing evidence suggests that the atherosclerotic process can be greatly slowed and its consequences markedly reduced with both lifestyle changes and drugs. This handbook focuses on the evidence supporting the efficacy of preventive measures, identifies areas of continued scientific debate, and provides straightforward recommendations for optimizing secondary preventive strategies.

Although the earliest case of human CAD was identified in a 3,000-year-old female mummy earlier this century, the disease was of relatively low prevalence under our founding fathers. Industrialization brought dramatic lifestyle changes during the last 200 years, including increases in dietary fat, cholesterol, and salt and use of tobacco products and a marked decrease in physical activity. With increased prevalence, the devastating sequelae of CAD became recognized. The syndrome of angina pectoris was first described by Heberden in 1772 and acute MI diagnosed premortem by Herrick in 1912. Cardiovascular disease prevalence increased from approximately 125 to more than 400 deaths per 100,000 population in the first half of the 20th century (Fig. 1.1). The Framingham Heart Study launched in 1948 has systematically followed more than 5,000 men and women initially free of CAD. This and subsequent smaller studies firmly documented that CAD prevalence was associated with a number of modifiable and nonmodifiable patient parameters, termed "cardiac risk factors." Interpopulation studies, such as the Seven Countries Study, further supported the risk-factor concept (Table 1.1).

With recognition of the consequences of hypertension, tobacco abuse, and hypercholesterolemia, major public health campaigns were initiated in the United States and other countries during the 1960s. In 1964, the Surgeon General's Report on Smoking and Health summarized the mounting evidence on the health risks of tobacco abuse. Over the ensuing 30 years, cigarette smoking in men declined from 55 to less than 30%. Major programs were undertaken in hypertension management as well, including the Hypertension Detection and Followup Program, the National High Blood Pressure Education Program and the Reports of the National Committee on Detection, Evaluation and Treatment of High Blood Pressure. More recently, the importance of systolic hypertension has been emphasized, and reductions in CAD events resulting from blood pressure control have been documented,

Table 1.1   Major Coronary Risk Factors

Modifiable	Immutable
Smoking	Age
Hypertension	Male sex
High LDL-C	Family history
Low HDL-C	
Diabetes mellitus	
Sedentary lifestyle	
Obesity	

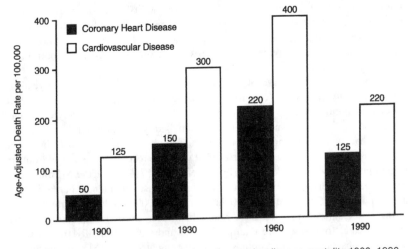

Figure 1.1.   Coronary heart disease and cardiovascular disease mortality 1900–1990.

in addition to beneficial effects on cerebrovascular and renal disease. Public recognition of the adverse effects of high fat and cholesterol diets increased during the past 30 years, resulting in a decrease in mean serum cholesterol from about 220 to 205 mg/dL. In 1988, the National Cholesterol Education Program reset the limits of a "desirable" cholesterol to less than 200 mg/dL, and also emphasized the importance of treating individuals with established heart disease. Weight reduction and regular exercise also became popular lifestyle modifications during the last 30 years. During this period, age-adjusted CAD mortality in the United States dropped by more than 40%, and cerebrovascular disease mortality declined by 50%. Although major changes also occurred in acute and chronic CAD management, it is estimated that more than half of this mortality decline is due to risk-factor changes in the general population (Table 1.2).

Table 1.2   Temporal Changes in Coronary Risk Factors

Cigarette Smoking	1960	Men: 55%
		Women: 33%
	1990	Men: 30%
		Women: 27%
Undiagnosed Hypertension	1960:	52%
	1980:	29%
Mean Serum Cholesterol	1960:	225 mg/dL
	1990:	208 mg/dL
Diabetes Mellitus	1970:	2.6%
	1990:	3.1%
Sedentary Lifestyle	1970:	41%
	1985:	27%
Obesity	1960:	25%
	1990:	33%

The 20th century has also been a period of remarkable progress in the under-standing of the pathogenesis of atherosclerosis. The lipid accumulation theory of Virchow and clot absorption theory of Rokitansky were followed by the induction of experimental atherosclerosis by Anitschkow and others. The response-to-injury hypothesis suggested by Ross and others synthesizes the earlier hypotheses and was complemented by the observations on low-density lipoprotein (LDL) oxidation by Steinberg and others. Finally, the theory of plaque rupture popularized by Davies and others has led to an understanding of the acute coronary disease syndromes.

The treatment of CAD also changed dramatically during the second half of the 20th century. An initial phase focused on diagnosis and a latter phase on aggressive management. Coronary arteriography was introduced by Sones in 1959. This allowed documentation of the presence and extent of coronary disease, leading to the important concept of risk stratification by the number of involved vessels. Scintigraphic and echocardiographic technology allowed noninvasive diagnosis of ventricular function and ischemic burden, both with important prognostic value. Treatment of CAD progressed rapidly after the introduction of saphenous vein coronary bypass surgery by Favalaro in 1967 and percutaneous transluminal coro-nary angioplasty (PTCA) by Grüntzig in 1977. Other key surgical interventions include cardiac transplantation (Barnard) and implanted defibrillators (Mirowsky). During the same period, pharmacologic management of CAD improved dramati-cally following the introduction of long-acting nitrates, β-adrenergic blocking agents, calcium channel blockers and angiotensin-converting enzyme (ACE) inhibitors. Treatment of acute MI was revolutionized by the introduction of the coronary care unit, electrical cardioversion and defibrillation, and pharmacologic and mechanical thrombolysis. The posthospitalization mortality of acute MI fell during this period from approximately 30% to less than 10%.

Therapeutic options for the treatment of hypercholesterolemia proliferated greatly during this period, as well. Early therapies such as bile acid sequestrants, thyroid hormone, nicotinic acid, and clofibrate had either modest effects on serum cholesterol or had a number of bothersome side effects. During the 1980s, the well-tolerated HMG CoA reductase inhibitors and other fibric acid derivatives were introduced.

Armed with improved therapeutic regimens, investigators undertook single and multifactorial coronary prevention studies to determine treatment efficacy (Fig. 1.2). In contrast to the disappointing results obtained in the early primary prevention trials (e.g., Multiple Risk Factor Intervention Trial (MRFIT) and VA Diet Study) the Lipid Research Clinics Coronary Primary Prevention Trial (cholestyramine) and Helsinki Heart Study (gemfibrozil) demonstrated significant reductions in cardiovascular events. Nevertheless, primary prevention studies were criticized because total mortality rates were unaltered. Because yearly CAD mortality rates are relatively low in otherwise healthy, hyperlipidemic middle-aged subjects, these results should not have been surprising. Therefore, emphasis began to shift from primary to secondary prevention trials. During the 1980s and early 1990s, 17 angiographic and echocardiographic studies of patients with established coronary and/or

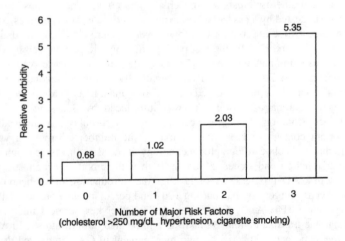

Figure 1.2. The Framingham Heart Study: Effect of multiple risk factors.

Table 1.3. Impact of Risk Factor Modification on Mortality

Factor	Modification	Decline in Mortality
Diastolic BP	1 mm Hg (1%)	2–4%
LDL-C	1.5 mg/dL (1%)	1–1.5%
HDL-C	0.5 mg/dL (1%)	1–1.5%
Smoking	1%	0.5%

carotid artery disease were undertaken using various forms of cholesterol lowering. The HMG-CoA reductase inhibitors, the most potent and well-tolerated of the lipid-lowering agents were employed in many of these trials. Sixteen of these 17 trials demonstrated significant evidence of reduction in atherosclerotic progression, and a few demonstrated angiographic evidence for disease regression. Recently, the Scandinavian Simvastatin Survival Study demonstrated a 29% reduction in *all-cause mortality* with HMG-CoA reductase inhibitor therapy. This study brought a sense of closure to the cholesterol hypothesis vis-à-vis atherosclerosis and firmed up the distinction between primary and secondary prevention.

Controlling risk factors other than the major three, hypertension, smoking, and hypercholesterolemia (Table 1.3), has also proven to be beneficial. The Diabetes Control and Complications Trial (DCCT) demonstrated reduced vascular complications with more rigid diabetes control. Meta-analysis of post-MI rehabilitation has demonstrated improved survival, although individual studies were not of sufficient size to demonstrate this outcome singly. Even a low level of physical exercise has been demonstrated to markedly reduce MI rates. There has been improvement in lay public awareness of "heart healthiness." Adults classified as sedentary decreased from 41% in 1971 to 27% in 1985. Unfortunately, today's children are undergoing the opposite trend. The lay public has become more interested in the fat, cholesterol, and salt content of packaged foods, resulting in better labeling owing to stricter guidelines imposed by the FDA. Unfortunately, obesity has increased in Americans and currently afflicts 33% of the population. This is especially prevalent in lower socioeconomic groups.

Physicians' interest in "heart healthiness" has clearly lagged behind the lay public. Despite the clear and well-justified recommendations of the national programs covering hypertension, smoking, and hypercholesterolemia, risk-factor modification is undertaken in the minority of patients with multiple risk factors and/or established CAD. Nationwide surveys suggest that only approximately one patient in four with CAD and a clear-cut lipid abnormality receives effective diet or drug management. This treatment gap extends to other proven cardioprotective treatment modalities, even simple and inexpensive ones. Less than 50% of patients with established heart disease are currently taking aspirin, and fewer still receive β-blocking agents following Q-wave MI. Whereas it can be argued that major lifestyle modification requires substantial physician and patient effort, there is little evidence that many physicians are routinely undertaking even the simplest of treatments proven to reduce cardiovascular morbidity and mortality. This handbook provides a simple guide for physicians interested in their patients' cardiovascular health.

Suggested Readings

AHA Committee Report. Risk factors and coronary disease. A statement for physicians. Circulation 1980;62:449A–455A.

Berlin JA, Colditz GA. A meta-analysis of physical activity in the prevention of coronary heart disease. Am J Epidemiol 1990;132:612–628.

Connor SL, Gustafson JR, Artaud-Wild SM, et al. The cholesterol-saturated fat index: An indication of the hypercholesterolemic and atherogenic potential of food. Lancet 1986;1:1229–1232.

Ekelund LG, Haskell WL, Johnson JL, et al. Physical fitness as a predictor of cardiovascular mortality in asymptomatic North American men. The Lipid Research Clinics Mortality Follow-up Study. N Engl J Med 1988;319:1379–1384.

Frick MH, Elo O, Happa K, et al. Helsinki Heart Study: Primary-prevention trial with gemfibrozil in middle-aged men with dyslipidemia: Safety of treatment, changes in risk factors, and incidence of coronary heart disease. N Engl J Med 1987;317:1237–1245.

Friedman LA, Kimball AW. Coronary heart disease mortality and alcohol consumption in Framingham. Am J Epidemiol 1986;124:481–489.

Gillum RF. Coronary heart disease in black populations. I. Mortality and morbidity. Am Heart J 1982;104:839–850.

Gordon T, Kannel WB. Premature mortality from coronary heart disease. The Framingham Study. JAMA 1971;215:1617–1625.

Haynes SG, Feinleib M, Kannel WB. The relationship of psychosocial factors to coronary heart disease in the Framingham Study. II. Eight-year incidence of coronary heart disease. Am J Epidemiol 1980; 111:37–58.

Herrick JB. Clinical features of sudden obstruction of the coronary arteries. JAMA 1912;59:2015–2020.

Hubert HB, Feinleib M, McNamara PM, Castelli WP. Obesity as an independent risk factor for cardiovascular disease: A 26-year follow-up of participants in the Framingham Heart Study. Circulation 1983;67:968–977.

Johansson S, Bergstrand R, Ulvenstam G, et al. Sex differences in pre-infarction characteristics and long-term survival among patients with myocardial infarction. Am J Epidemiol 1984;119:610–623.

Joseph A, Ackerman D, Talley JD, et al. Manifestations of coronary atherosclerosis in young trauma victims—An autopsy study. J Am Coll Cardiol 1993;22: 459–467.

Kannel WB, McGee DL. Diabetes and cardiovascular disease. The Framingham Study. JAMA 1979;241:2035–2038.

Keys A, Aravanis C, Blackburn H, et al. Epidemiological studies related to coronary heart disease. Characteristics of men aged 40-59 in seven countries. Acta Med Scand 1967;180:Suppl 460:1–392.

The Lipid Research Clinics Program. The Lipid Research Clinics Coronary Primary Prevention Trial Results. I. Reduction in incidence of coronary heart disease. JAMA 1984;251:351–364.

Pekkanen J, Linn S, Heiss G, et al. Ten-year mortality from cardiovascular disease in relation to cholesterol level among men with and without pre-existing cardiovascular disease. N Engl J Med 1990;322: 1700–1707.

Ross R. The pathogenesis of atherosclerosis— An update. N Engl J Med 1986;314: 488–500.

Scandinavian Simvastatin Survival Group. Randomised trial of cholesterol lowering in 4444 patients with coronary heart disease: The Scandinavian Simvastatin Survival Study (45). Lancet 1994;344: 1383–1389.

SHEP Cooperative Research Group. Prevention of stroke by antihypertensive drug treatment in older persons with isolated systolic hypertension; final results of the Systolic Hypertension in the Elderly Program (SHEP). JAMA 1991;265: 3255–3264.

Sparrow D, Dawber TR, Colton T. The influence of cigarette smoking on prognosis after a first myocardial infarction. J Chron Dis 1978;31:425–432.

Steinberg D, Witztum JL. Lipoproteins and atherogenesis. Current Concepts. JAMA 1990;264:3047–3052.

U.S. Department of Health and Human Services. The health consequences of smoking. Cardiovascular disease. A report of the Surgeon General, 1983. USDHHS publication (PHS) 84–50204.

Worth RM, Kato H, Rhoads GG, et al. Epidemiologic studies of coronary heart disease and stroke in Japanese men living in Japan, Hawaii and California: Mortality. Am J Epidemiol 1975;102:481–490.

2/ Pathobiology of Coronary Artery Disease

The seminal work by Virchow during the last century highlighted the importance of lipids in the pathophysiology of CAD. The evolutionary events accompanying atherosclerotic progression (i.e., fatty streak → fibrous plaque → complicated lesion → complete occlusion), however, do not take into account the pathobiology of the disease. More recent concepts have invoked the endothelium as a critical component in regulating plaque lesion growth and stabilization. Because an arteriographically "clean" coronary artery may generate a pathologic consequence if endothelial dysfunction exists, the definition of a disease-free coronary artery implies the absence of both anatomic and functional abnormalities. Intervention between the endothelium and the milieu to which it is exposed (e.g., risk factors) underlies the complex dynamic and intricate process involved in promoting atherosclerosis.

EARLY STUDIES

In 1915, Mönckeberg reported the presence of CAD in nearly 50% of soldiers (mean age 27.7 years) killed in action. These results were subsequently confirmed and extended during the Korean War. Autopsies of 300 U.S. servicemen (mean age 22.1 years) who died in the line of duty revealed that only a minority (23%) had "clean" coronary vessels. With anatomic CAD, 15% had significant occlusion defined by 50% or greater stenosis in at least one epicardial vessel. These landmark studies challenged the conventional wisdom that atherosclerosis was a "disease of aging." Rather, the data suggested that this process occurred early (atherogenic factors) and through the interplay of environmental stimuli was markedly accelerated (thrombogenic factors) (Fig. 2.1).

Beginning in the 1950s, studies demonstrated that atherosclerosis began in childhood. As a ubiquitous manifestation, aortic fatty streaks and fibrous plaques were observed by ages 3 and 15, respectively. Studies from Bogalusa, LA, disclosed that by age 20, more than 90% of adults (Caucasian and African-American) evidenced coronary fatty streaking, the progenitor of coronary atherosclerosis. Examination of early atherogenesis by the Pathobiological Determinants of Atherosclerosis in Youth (PDAY) Research Group disclosed a positive association between cigarette smoking, lipoprotein cholesterol concentration, and raised aortic and coronary lesions. The evidence from autopsied males aged 15–34 years suggested that modifiable risk factors influence the development of early atherosclerotic lesions. Important correlations were also drawn by the International Atherosclerosis Project (IAP). Following a systematic study of aortas and coronary and cerebral arteries from autopsied subjects in 14 countries, a strong association was demonstrated between extent of atherosclerotic lesions and cardiovascular

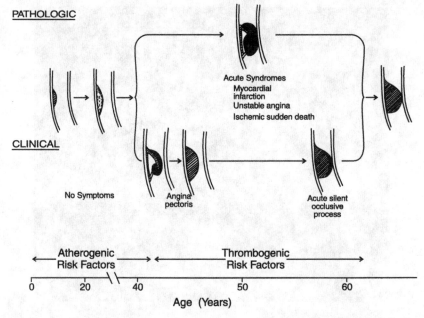

Figure 2.1. Schematic diagram of the natural history of the etiopathogenesis of athero-sclerotic coronary disease. When the progression of early atherosclerosis impairs the coronary blood flow, exertional angina may develop. Further progression will involve a) the existence of occlusive coronary thrombosis with significantly reduced myocardial perfusion expressed as unstable angina, myocardial infarction, or even sudden death or b) the thrombi may be mural and asymptomatic. In either case, plaque fissuring or ulceration triggers the thrombotic process. The subsequent fibrotic organization of the thrombi may account for the continuous growth of the plaque, which may become occlusive and associated with further chronic ischemic symptoms. From Badimon JJ, Fuster V, Chesebro JH, Badimon L. Coronary atherosclerosis: A multifactorial disease. Circulation 1993;87(suppl II):II–3–II–16. Reproduced with permission. Circulation. Copyright © 1993 American Heart Association.

death rate. These studies acknowledged that atherosclerosis commences at a young age, is progressive, and is influenced by risk factors. The scientific challenge in preventive cardiology is to unravel the fundamental mediators regulating and promoting this process.

ATHEROSCLEROTIC LESIONS

The earliest lesion is the fatty streak, which consists primarily of macrophage-derived foam cells (Fig. 2.2). The development of foam cells, whose composition

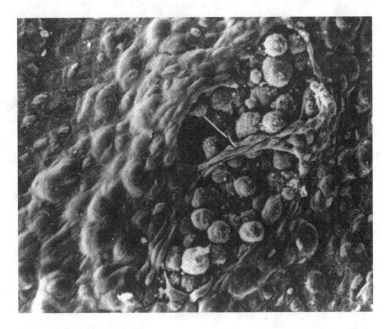

Figure 2.2. Scanning electron micrograph of the surface of a fatty streak in a pigtail monkey ($\times$600). The endothelium is retracted over a portion of the lesion, exposing underlying lipid-laden macrophages. A bridge of endothelial cells (*arrow*) can be seen over the center of the region of exposed macrophages. Reprinted by permission of The New England Journal of Medicine from Ross R. The pathogenesis of atherosclerosis—an update. N Engl J Med 1986;314(8):488–500, Copyright © 1986, Massachusetts Medical Society.

includes esterified cholesterol derived from modified LDL-C, may occur in the absence of endothelial damage or denudation. As noted above, the fatty streak begins in childhood and develops in the aorta, with a preference for the distal or abdominal segment. Because the aortic fatty streak occurs in both industrialized and poverty stricken societies, these lesions are not predictive of CAD. In contrast, fatty streaking in the coronary artery is associated with the subsequent development of coronary lesions.

The more advanced lesion is the fibrous plaque, consisting of a fibrous cap, rich in ground substance, collagen fibers, and reticulum fibrils that surround smooth muscle cells and T cells in the media. There are also macrophage-derived foam cells that surround a core of extracellular lipids (Fig. 2.3). The extracellular core is composed of intracytoplasmic material released from nonviable macrophages. In contrast to early atherosclerosis, advanced plaques are characterized by endothelial injury with associated platelet aggregation and mural thrombi. When luminal diameter is reduced by 70-80% the patient will often experience exertional angina. Rest angina occurs with more than 90% luminal diameter obstruction. Advanced lesions often develop calcification. There may be thinning and splitting of the fibrous cap resulting in plaque fissuring (Fig. 2.4). This event is more common when there is an associated large core of extracellular lipids. As fissuring occurs, contact is made

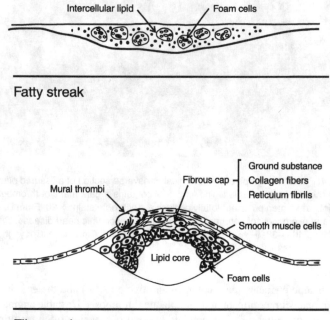

Figure 2.3. Microscopic pathology of atherosclerosis. **Top,** microscopic changes of the fatty streak. There is an accumulation of cells containing liquid droplets (foam cells) in the subintimal region. Finely dispersed extracellular lipids are present. **Bottom,** fibrous plaque has a fibrous cap containing ground substance, collagen fibers, and reticulum fibrils. Mural thrombi are sometimes present. Smooth muscle cells in the periphery show evidence of transformation into foam cells or connective tissue-secreting cells. Center of lesion is a core of necrotic material containing large quantities of extracellular cholesterol and other lipids. From Grundy SM. Atherosclerosis: Pathology, pathogenesis, and role of risk factors. Dis Mon 1983;29(9):6. Used with permission.

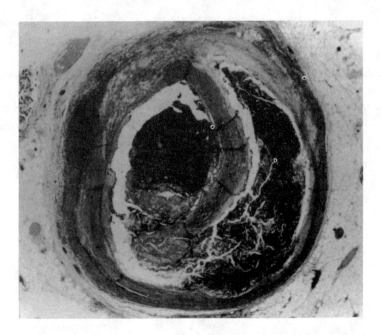

Figure 2.4. Photomicrograph of a histological transverse section of a fissured plaque. The fissure in the cap is at lower left. The lipid pool contains a dark mass of thrombus, which projects into the lumen but is not totally occlusive. Trichrome stain, ×20. From Davies MJ. A macro and micro view of coronary vascular insult in ischemic heart disease. Circulation 1990;82(suppl II):II–38–II–46. Reproduced with permission. Circulation. Copyright © 1990 American Heart Association.

between plaque elements (e.g., collagen and tissue factor) and the entering blood, leading to platelet recruitment and intraplaque thrombosis. Unstable angina implies the presence of stuttering or incomplete luminal obstruction often resulting from fissuring and instability of small plaques. Plaque instability is associated with an elevated extracellular lipid content and increase in macrophage-derived foam cells. The "soft plaques" comprising early atherosclerotic lesions are vulnerable to spontaneous rupture. Importantly, with aggressive risk-factor modification (e.g., lipid lowering), depletion of some of the excess lipid may stabilize the plaque and reduce the likelihood of subsequent fissuring (see Chapter 4).

With large plaque fissuring, the result is a large intraplaque thrombus that causes luminal compression, intraluminal thrombus with propagation, and complete occlusion (Fig. 2.5). Following endogenous or exogenous fibrinolysis (e.g., TPA), there

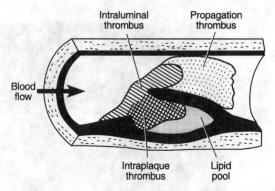

Figure 2.5. Diagrammatic representation of a longitudinal reconstruction from step histological sections of an occluding thrombus. Lipid is shown stippled, thrombus is shown cross-hatched. Much of the thrombus at the site of occlusion is contained within the plaque and compresses the lumen from outside. A plug of lipid has extruded into the lumen. From Davies MJ. A macro and micro view of coronary vascular insult in ischemic heart disease. Circulation 1990;82(suppl II):II–38–II–46. Reproduced with permission. Circulation. Copyright © 1990 American Heart Association.

is increased proliferation of smooth muscle cells and collagen, which aids in plaque stabilization.

Unfortunately, coronary arteriography is not a sensitive predictor for either early plaque detection or subsequent plaque rupture. For example, small intimal and eccentric plaques are often not visualized. The use of intravascular ultrasound is considerably more sensitive for early plaque detection (Fig. 2.6).

The presence of coronary calcification is a sensitive indicator of CAD, although the absence of calcification does not preclude the possibility of occlusive disease. From a therapeutic standpoint, aggressive risk-factor modification is more successful on noncalcified lesions. With calcification, the likelihood of plaque reversibility diminishes and surgical or mechanical revascularization becomes the primary reparative option.

ATHEROSCLEROSIS IN ANIMALS

Spontaneous atherosclerosis accelerated by an atherogenic diet occurs in pigeons, rabbits, and swine. The Watanabe rabbit has been extensively studied as a model for familial hypercholesterolemia because this rabbit lacks functional LDL-C receptors. In addition, there are strains of rabbits that overproduce VLDL-C, a characteristic feature of familial combined hyperlipidemia. Although dogs do not develop spontaneous atherosclerosis, cholesterol loading and suppression of thy-

Figure 2.6. Left coronary arteriogram (**A**) is entirely normal with no identifiable disease in the left main coronary artery; however, the intravascular ultrasound image of the left main coronary (**B**) reveals an eccentric noncalcified plaque (*arrow*). The central black circle and surrounding halo represent catheter artifact. For the detection and quantification of intramural atherosclerosis, intravascular ultrasound is superior to coronary arteriography, as demonstrated by this typical example. From Waters D, Lespérance J, Craven TE, Hudon G, Gillam LD. Advantages and limitations of serial coronary arteriography for the assessment of progression and regression of coronary atherosclerosis. Circulation 1993; 87(suppl II):II–38–II–47. Reproduced with permission. Circulation. Copyright © 1993 American Heart Association.

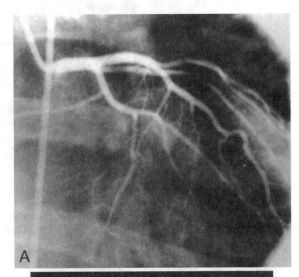

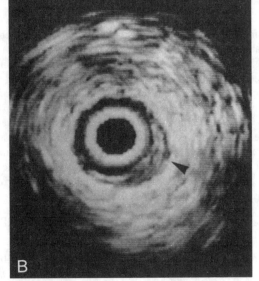

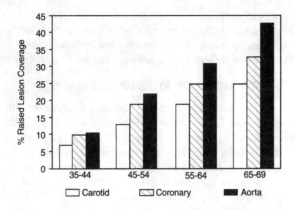

Figure 2.7. Relationship of raised atherosclerotic lesions in the aorta and in the carotid and coronary arteries in "basal" men, those who died of noncardiovascular causes. Adapted, by permission, from: Atherosclerosis of the aorta and coronary arteries in five towns. Bulletin of the World Health Organization, 53:509–518 (1976).

roid function will accelerate atherogenesis. Nonhuman primates develop atherosclerotic lesions that resemble human plaques and occur with chronic high-fat, high-cholesterol alterations. The inciting pathophysiologic cellular events are similar to those that occur in humans, with monocyte adherence, transendothelial migration, and development of foam cells.

LOCATION OF ATHEROSCLEROTIC LESIONS

There is a good correlation between the extent of atherosclerosis in the coronary and carotid arteries and the aorta. During aging, the percentage of raised lesions increases proportionately, with the degree of atherosclerosis greatest in the aorta and lowest in the carotids (Fig. 2.7). The presence of atherosclerosis in the carotid or large-vessel peripheral vascular beds is also associated with an elevated risk of CAD and cardiovascular death.

Branch points increase the development of atherosclerotic lesions as a result of shear stress and hemodynamic turbulence. These branch points include bifurcation of the carotids, aortic subdivisions (renal arteries), and the bifurcation of the left anterior descending (LAD) and circumflex artery off the left main coronary artery.

CONTENTS OF THE ATHEROSCLEROTIC PLAQUE

The two components of the atherosclerotic plaque, the fibrous cap and the lipid-rich core, have been extensively examined by immunohistochemistry. The fibrous cap consists primarily of smooth muscle cells as well as macrophages and T lymphocytes. The lipid-rich core is primarily derived from macrophages replete with cholesterol oleate. With advanced lesions, free cholesterol and cholesterol linoleate (normally present in plasma) are found and are primarily derived from circulating monocytes.

MEDIATORS OF ATHEROSCLEROSIS

There are several important mediators that initiate and accelerate atherosclerosis. Among the atherogenic factors are modified lipoproteins (e.g., oxidized LDL-C), inflammatory factors (e.g., monocytes/macrophages, T lymphocytes), smooth muscle cells, and growth factors. The thrombogenic factors include platelets and their activated contents, which promote aggregation and smooth muscle proliferation. The sequence of events involved in the initiation and propagation of atherosclerosis is summarized below and illustrated in Figure 2.8.

Atherogenic Factors

MODIFIED LDL-C

In the initial stages of atherosclerosis, LDL-C traverses the endothelial barrier by a process referred to as transcytosis. Direct endothelial injury as a result of mechanical (e.g., hypertension) or chemical (e.g., cigarette smoking) alterations accelerates this process. Upon entering the subendothelial space, LDL-C is anchored by glycosoaminoglycans, where chemical modification may take the form of oxidation via the generation of oxygen-reactive species by macrophages, smooth muscle cells, or endothelial cells. Other modifications include acetylation and glycosylation. In contrast to native (i.e., unmodified) LDL-C that binds to regulated, high-affinity receptors located on the surface of macrophages, modified LDL-C is bound and incorporated in an unregulated manner. Modified (i.e., oxidized, acetylated) LDL-C is relentlessly incorporated by macrophages and, to a lesser extent, smooth muscle cells, producing an engorged macrophage, or foam cell. Antibodies to the oxidatively modified LDL-C have been demonstrated in atherosclerotic plaques. Oxidized LDL-C has other properties, including a direct cytotoxic effect on macrophages and endothelial cells. It promotes the upregulation of gene expression for proteins that mediate adhesion and chemotaxis for monocytes: colony-stimulating factor (CSF) and monocyte chemotactic protein (MCP-1). Finally, oxidized LDL-C stimulates secretion of a putative atherogenic cytokine, interleukin-1 (IL-1). This cytokine upregulates endothelial expression of adhesion molecules by macrophages.

Inflammatory Factors

MONOCYTE-MACROPHAGES

Tissue macrophages are the predominant inflammatory factor in atherosclerosis. Prior to differentiation, blood monocytes are recruited by several chemotactic fac-

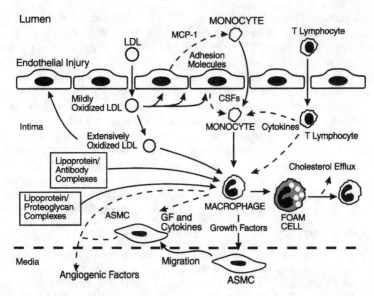

Figure 2.8. Overview of events involved in atherogenesis. Lipoprotein deposition in the intima may result from an excess of lipoproteins such as LDL in the circulation and occurs preferentially at sites of endothelial injury. The lipoproteins undergo mild oxidative modification in the subendothelial space to form mildly oxidized LDL, which can induce endothelial cell (EC) expression of chemotactic factors, which attract monocytes, and of mononuclear cell adhesion molecules. Monocytes and T lymphocytes enter the subendothelial space via these molecules. Colony-stimulating factors (CSFs) secreted by EC in response to stimulation by mildly oxidized LDL induce differentiation of monocytes into macrophages. Cytokines secreted by T lymphocytes activate macrophages, causing the release of several growth factors and cytokines, which act on both intimal and medial arterial smooth muscle (ASMC) to stimulate proliferation, migration, and synthesis of matrix proteins. Macrophages and ASMC secrete angiogenic factors that stimulate neovascular ingrowth from the vasa vasorum. This neovasculature provides routes for further lipoprotein deposition and mononuclear cell infiltration. Macrophages then differentiate into foam cells by ingestion of large amounts of lipid in the form of extensively oxidized LDL, lipoprotein-antibody complexes and/or complexes of proteoglycans secreted by ASMC and LDL. Efflux of excess cholesterol from foam cells may be mediated by HDL and by secretion of apo E-lipid vesicles. From O'Brien KD, Chait A. The biology of the artery wall in atherogenesis. Med Clin North Am 1994;78:41–67. Used with permission.

tors, including α-thrombin, MCP-1, and CSF. They are anchored at the endothelial surface by selectins, adhesion molecules that bind to carbohydrate groups. Monocytes are subsequently activated by adhesion molecules of the immunoglobulin superfamily, intercellular adhesion molecule-1 (ICAM-1) and vascular cell adhesion molecule-1 (VCAM-1). Both ICAM-1 and VCAM-1 facilitate transendothelial migration of monocytes to the subendothelial space (Fig. 2.8). Upon entering the subendothelial space, monocytes are transformed into macrophages. Macrophages generate free radicals leading to LDL-C oxidation and cytotoxicity. As actively phagocytic cells, they ingest LDL-C via the scavenger receptor and ultimately develop into lipid-laden foam cells. Macrophages also secrete cytokines such as IL-1, which stimulate smooth muscle cell proliferation. Acting like smooth muscle cells, foam cells retain the capacity to proliferate, thereby contributing to the growth of the atherosclerotic lesion. They may also egress to the circulation, where they may potentially cause further endothelial damage.

T LYMPHOCYTES

T cells accumulate during various stages of atherosclerosis. They comprise more than 20% of the early fatty streak and are present in considerable quantities in advanced fibrous plaque lesions. The T lymphocyte also secretes cytokines; interferon (IFN)-γ suppresses smooth muscle cell proliferation and has been shown to reduce restenosis following carotid angioplasty in the rat. T lymphocytes and macrophages also secrete tumor necrosis factor (TNF), which downregulates the scavenger receptor gene and limits formation of foam cells. Thus, cytokines are important mediators of atherosclerosis.

Smooth Muscle Cells

Although the macrophage is the primary cellular element in the fatty streak, the smooth muscle cell predominates with lesion progression to the fibrous plaque. Smooth muscle cells elaborate connective tissue matrix (e.g., collagen) and proteoglycans (e.g., chondroitin sulfate), substances that provide adhesive properties and enables plaque strength and durability.

Smooth muscle cells accumulate lipid and, like macrophages, may be transformed into foam cells. Moreover, they can oxidize LDL-C. However, unlike macrophages, scavenger receptors have not been identified in cultured human smooth muscle cells. The regulation of smooth muscle cell proliferation is mediated by growth factors and cytokines. One of the most potent mitogens is platelet-derived growth factor (PDGF). Released from the alpha granule of platelets, PDGF stimulates migration of smooth muscle cells from the media to the intimal region. PDGF also induces cellular proliferation, thereby converting the fatty streak to a more advanced atherosclerotic lesion. Other inducers of smooth muscle cell proliferation include fibroblast growth factor, insulin growth factor, transforming growth factor, IL-1, and TNF.

Thrombogenic Factors

PLATELETS

When vascular injury occurs, platelets are attracted to the region and adhere to form an initial hemostatic plug. The generation of thrombin stimulates platelets to release their granular contents. In addition to secondary hemostasis formed as a result of a platelet-fibrin plug, platelet-activated membrane phospholipases release arachidonic acid, which is subsequently converted to thromboxane A_2 (a potent inducer of platelet aggregation).

Vascular Factors

ENDOTHELIUM

The vascular endothelium secretes potent vasodilators and inhibitors of platelet aggregation. The two most notable agents are prostacyclin and endothelium-derived relaxing factor, or nitric oxide (EDRF-NO). Endothelial cells also secrete heparin sulfate, which maintains an anticoagulant environment by binding to antithrombin III.

The endothelium also produces factors that favor hemostasis, including plasminogen activator inhibitor and tissue factor. Interleukin-1 has also been shown to increase endothelial cell production of endothelin-1. Endothelin-1 is the most potent vasoconstrictor known (approximately 10-fold more potent than angiotensin II). It stimulates the release of renin and catecholamines, which contribute to its hypertensive effect. Plasma endothelin levels have been shown to be elevated in MI survivors.

PROSTACYCLIN

Prostacyclin (PGI_2) is the most powerful naturally occurring inhibitor of platelet aggregation. With endothelial damage or atherosclerosis, prostacyclin production is impaired. Prostacyclin also stimulates fibrinolytic activity and inhibits the release of platelet-mediated growth factors. Unfortunately, prostacyclin infusion has not been shown to be of clinical benefit in the treatment of acute MI, which may reflect its relatively short circulating half-life in plasma.

ENDOTHELIUM-DERIVED RELAXING FACTOR-NITRIC OXIDE

EDRF-NO is a potent mediator of endothelium-dependent relaxation of vascular smooth muscle. EDRF-NO also exerts direct effects on platelets, including inhibition of platelet adhesion and aggregation. Decreased production of EDRF-NO and reduced vasodilator response to acetylcholine have been reported with diabetes mellitus, hypertension, and hyperlipidemia.

Endothelial Vasoactivity

As a modulator of arterial tone, the endothelium plays a central role in the pathobiology of atherosclerosis and CAD. With an intact endothelium, the administration of acetylcholine stimulates EDRF-NO release, leading to smooth muscle cell relaxation and coronary vasodilation. Other agents that affect EDRF-NO release are thrombin, ADP, serotonin, and vasopressin (Fig. 2.9). With endothelial injury or ischemia, however, EDRF-NO release is inhibited, and unopposed endothelial contraction factors cause vasoconstriction. Recent studies have demonstrated a paradoxical vasoconstrictive response to acetylcholine in patients with angiographically normal coronary arteries, suggesting the presence of early endothelial dysfunction. This paradoxical response has also been produced in subjects with hypertension, diabetes mellitus, family history of premature CAD, and hyperlipidemia. Importantly, effective treatment of hyperlipidemia reversed the paradoxical response to intra-arterial acetylcholine, suggesting that endothelial restoration may coincide with lipid-lowering treatment.

As a surrogate for invasive arteriographic studies in assessing endothelial vasomotor function, noninvasive studies of the brachial arteries have been performed. Celermajer and colleagues noted impairment in flow-mediated vasodilation in patients with CAD or associated risk factors following blood pressure cuff occlusion. Results of studies examining the brachial artery response to risk-factor intervention are pending. However, estrogen replacement has recently been shown to restore the impaired flow-mediated vasodilatory response in postmenopausal women.

PATHOBIOLOGY OF RESTENOSIS

PTCA will be performed more than 500,000 times in 1995, and restenosis will occur in one-third of these cases. The process of restenosis is similar to native atherosclerosis in that there is endothelial injury denudation followed by platelet activation and release of mitogenic factors and cytokines, including PDGF, fibroblast growth factor, and IL-1. Proliferation of smooth muscle cells occurs within 3 days of the procedure, followed by smooth muscle migration, intimal invasion, and hyperplasia. Rheologic factors and the degree of smooth muscle cell proliferation are two important determinants that predict the extent of intimal hyperplasia and probability of restenosis.

Many pharmacologic trials have assessed the effect of platelet antagonists, anticoagulants, anti-inflammatory agents, and lipid-lowering medications. Unfortunately, none of these agents has consistently reduced restenosis rates. Although favorable responses were demonstrated in one study using an HMG-CoA reductase inhibitor, these results await validation in larger prospective studies. In a meta-analysis employing fish oil, clinical and arteriographic endpoints of restenosis were reduced by nearly 30%. More recently, gene therapy has been applied in animal models. In a recent report by Nabel and colleagues, PTCA was performed in the pig femoral artery.

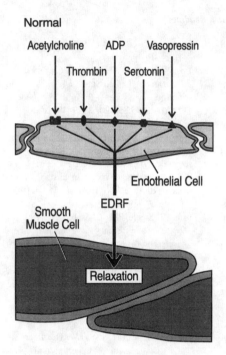

Normal

Figure 2.9. Acetylcholine, thrombin, ADP, serotonin, and vasopressin stimulate release of EDRF by vascular endothelium. Reproduced with permission. Vanhoutte PM. The endothelium and control of coronary arterial tone. HOSPITAL PRACTICE Volume 23, issue 5, page 87. Illustration by Ilil Arbel.

Following injection of an adenovirus containing a thymidine kinase gene and an antiviral drug (ganciclovir), there was a 90% reduction in intimal hyperplasia (see Ohno et al.). Similar results were also obtained by Finkel and associates who used a thymidine kinase adenovirus in the rat carotid artery (see Guzman et al.). Although a major limitation of adenoviral vector use is the requirement for repeated injections (because of rapid falls in viral expression levels), this does not appear to be a primary concern with restenosis, because initiation of smooth muscle proliferation and intimal hyperplasia occur within 72 hours following angioplasty. Therefore, pending the outcome of human trials, gene therapy may indeed hold considerable promise for the treatment of coronary restenosis (see also review by Nabel).

Suggested Readings

A preliminary report from the Pathobiological Determinants of Atherosclerosis in Youth (PDAY) Research Group. Relationship of atherosclerosis in young men to serum lipoprotein cholesterol concentrations and smoking. JAMA 1990;264:3018–3024.

Badimon JJ, Fuster V, Chesebro JH, Badimon L. Coronary atherosclerosis—A multifactorial disease. Circulation 1993;87(suppl II):II-3-II-16.

Bairati I, Roy L, Meyer F. Double-blind, randomized, controlled trial of fish oil supplements in prevention of recurrence of stenosis after coronary angioplasty. Circulation 1992;85:950–956.

Blankenhorn DH. Regression of atherosclerosis. In: Braunwald E, ed. Heart Disease Update. Philadelphia, Pa: W.B. Saunders Company, 1992:73–83.

Bulletin of the World Health Organization, 1976;53:509–518.

Bush DE, Bruza JM, Bass KM, Walters GK, Jones CE, Ouyang P. Estrogen replacement increases flow mediated vasodilation in post-menopausal women. Circulation 1994; 90(suppl 4):I–86.

Casino PR, Kilcoyne CM, Quyyumi AA, Hoeg JM, Panza JA. The role of nitric oxide in endothelium-dependent vasodilation of hypercholesterolemic patients. Circulation 1993;88:2541–2547.

Celermajer DS, Sorensen KE, Bull C, Robinson J, Deanfield JE. Endothelium-dependent dilation in the systemic arteries of asymptomatic subjects relates to coronary risk factors and their interaction. J Am Coll Cardiol 1994;24:1468–1474.

Chester AH, O'Neil GS, Moncada S, Tadjkarimi S, Yacoub MH. Low basal and stimulated release of nitric oxide in atherosclerotic epicardial coronary arteries. Lancet 1990;336:897–900.

Davies MJ. A macro and micro view of coronary vascular insult in ischemic heart disease. Circulation 1990;82(suppl II): II–38–II–46.

Enos WF, Holmes RH, Beyer J. Coronary disease among United States soldiers killed in action in Korea—Preliminary report. JAMA 1986;256(20):2859–2862.

Faruqi RM, DiCorleto PE. Mechanisms of monocyte recruitment and accumulation. Br Heart J 1993;69(suppl):S19–S29.

Fitzgerald DJ, Roy L, Catella F, FitzGerald GA. Platelet activation in unstable coronary disease. N Engl J Med 1986; 315:983–989.

Fuster V, Steele PM, Chesebro JH. Role of platelets and thrombosis in coronary atherosclerotic disease and sudden death. J Am Coll Cardiol 1985;5:175B–184B.

Fuster V, Stein B, Ambrose JA, Badimon L, Badimon JJ, Chesebro JH. Atherosclerotic plaque rupture and thrombosis—evolving concepts. Circulation 1990;82(suppl II): I–47–II–59.

Gotto AM, Jones PH, Scott LW. The diagnosis and management of hyperlipidemia. Dis Mon 1986;32:252–311.

Grundy SM. Atherosclerosis: Pathology, pathogenesis, and role of risk factors. Dis Mon 1983;29:3–58.

Guzman RJ, Hirschowitz EA, Brody SL, Crystal RG, Epstein SE, Finkel T. In vivo suppression of injury-induced vascular smooth muscle cell accumulation using adenovirus-mediated transfer of the herpes simplex virus thymidine kinase gene. Proc Natl Acad Sci USA 1994;91:10732–10736.

Hansson GK. Immune and inflammatory mechanisms in the development of atherosclerosis. Br Heart J 1993;69 (suppl): S38–S41.

Holman RL, McGill HC Jr, Strong JP, et al. The natural history of atherosclerosis: The early aortic lesions as seen in New Orleans in the middle of the 20th century. Am J Pathol 1958;34:209–235.

Ip JH, Fuster V, Badimon L, Badimon J, Taubman MB, Chesebro JH. Syndromes of accelerated atherosclerosis: Role of vascular injury and smooth muscle cell proliferation. J Am Coll Cardiol 1990;15: 1667–1687.

McGill HC Jr, ed. The Geographic Pathology of Atherosclerosis. Baltimore: Williams & Wilkins, 1968.

Mönckeberg JG. Über die Atherosklerose der Kombattanten (nach Obduktionsbefunden). Zentralbl Herz Gefässkrankheiten 1915; 7:7–10.

Mönckeberg JG. Anatomische Veränderungen am Kreislaufsystem bei Kriegsteilnehmern. Zentralbl Herz Gefässkrankheiten 1915; 7:336–343.

Nabel EG. Gene therapy for cardiovascular disease. Circulation 1995;9:541–548.

O'Brien KD, Chait A. The biology of the artery wall in atherogenesis. Med Clin North Am 1994;78:41–69.

Ohno T, Gordon D, San H, Pompili VJ, Imperiale MJ, Nabel GJ, Nabel EG. Gene therapy for vascular smooth muscle cell proliferation after arterial injury. Science 1994;265:781–784.

Raines EW, Ross R. Smooth muscle cells and the pathogenesis of the lesions of atherosclerosis. Br Heart J 1993;69(suppl): S30–S37.

Riessen R, Isner JM. Prospects for site-specific delivery of pharmacologic and molecular therapies. J Am Coll Cardiol 1994;23: 1234–1244.

Ross R. The pathogenesis of atherosclerosis—an update. N Engl J Med 1986;314:488–500.

Sahni R, Maniet AR, Voci G, Banka VS. Prevention of restenosis by lovastatin after successful coronary angioplasty. Am Heart J 1991;121:1600.

Steinberg D. Lipoproteins and the pathogenesis of atherosclerosis. Circulation 1987;3: 508–514.

Steinberg D, Parthasarathy S, Carew TE, et al. Modifications of low-density lipoprotein that increase its atherogenicity. N Engl J Med 1989;320:915–924.

Vane JR, Änggard EE, Botting RM. Regulatory functions of the vascular endothelium. N Engl J Med 1990;323: 27–36.

Vanhoutte PM. The endothelium and control of coronary arterial tone. Hosp Pract May 15, 1988;67–84.

Waters D, Lespérance J, Craven TE, Hudon G, Gillam LD. Advantages and limitations of serial coronary arteriography for the assessment of progression and regression of coronary atherosclerosis—implications for clinical trials. Circulation 1993;87 [suppl II]:II–38–II–47.

Werns SW, Walton JA, Hsia HH, Nabel EG, Sanz ML, Pitt B. Evidence of endothelial dysfunction in angiographically normal coronary arteries of patients with coronary artery disease. Circulation 1989;79:287–291.

Witztum JL. Role of oxidised low density lipoprotein in atherogenesis. Br Heart J 1993;69(suppl):S12–S18.

3/ Clinical Signs and Syndromes Associated with Premature Coronary Artery Disease

BALDNESS

The issue of whether male-pattern baldness is associated with premature CAD has been hampered by a lack of prospective data. Many of the case-control studies indicate a small increased risk of CAD. While data compiled from one recent large study did not demonstrate such an association with frontal baldness, baldness involving the vertex scalp (Fig. 3.1) was correlated with a 1.5–3.5 fold increased risk of MI in men below the age of 55. The active metabolite of testosterone, dihydrotestosterone, is believed to be the primary androgen responsible for male-pattern baldness. Men who have been castrated during adolescence or possess low levels of this androgen (e.g., 5α-reductase deficiency) do not develop baldness, although CAD rates in these individuals have yet to be uncovered.

CORNEAL ARCUS

Corneal arcus is a whitish-gray opacification located at the periphery of the cornea (Fig. 3.2). In contrast to the diffuse corneal opacification characteristic of low HDL-C, e.g., LCAT deficiency (see Chapter 5), the cholesteryl-ester enriched opacities do not extend into the limbus or corneoscleral junction. Corneal arcus is a particularly useful sign when present in young Caucasians (arcus juvenilis) because of its association with type II hyperlipidemia. In the elderly (arcus senilis) and in African-Americans, however, corneal arcus is a common and nonspecific finding.

EAR LOBE CREASE

The ear crease is defined by a 45° diagonal fold extending down the lower pole of the external auditory canal (Fig. 3.3). The incidence of ear lobe creases in hospitalized adults is approximately 15% and is more prevalent beyond age 60. Although the sensitivity of the test is not high (approximately 50%), the crease appears to be a specific marker for CAD. It remains unclear whether the crease represents an independent marker for CAD or is a primary effect to the aging process and elastin degeneration.

HAIRY EARS

Characterized by as many as 180 terminal hairs in the pinnae, hairy ears are prevalent in South Indian males (15–20%) (Fig. 3.4). The trait has also been reported in Europe, Africa, and Australia. It is believed to be inherited by autosomal dominant transmission and is under the influence of androgenic hormones. The inci-

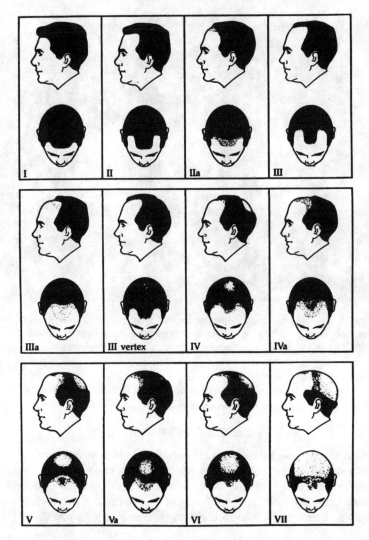

Figure 3.1. The Hamilton Baldness Scale as modified by Norwood. From Norwood OT. Hair Transplant Surgery, 1973. Courtesy of Charles C. Thomas, Publisher, Springfield, Illinois.

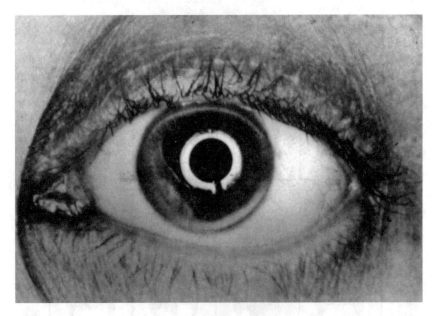

Figure 3.2. Corneal arcus in the heterozygote with hypercholesterolemia. From Gotto AM, Jones PH, Scott LW. The diagnosis and management of hyperlipidemia. Dis Mon 1986;32:252–311. Used with permission of Baylor College of Medicine.

dence of diabetes mellitus is increased in association with hairy ears raising the possibility of genetic linkage between these entities.

HOLLENHORST PLAQUES

Hollenhorst plaques are cholesterol emboli located within the retinal artery. Arising from the carotid circulation, these atherosclerotic plaques may invade and obstruct the central retinal artery. They may be visualized on fundoscopic examination in an asymptomatic individual (Fig. 3.5). The presence of Hollenhorst plaques is indicative of significant cerebral atherosclerosis and may also suggest underlying CAD.

RHEUMATIC DISORDERS

Various rheumatic manifestations have been described in association with hyperlipidemia. In type II familial hypercholesterolemia (FH), Achilles tendinitis or tenosynovitis may be accompanied by xanthomata and in some cases have preceded their emergence. Migratory polyarthritis has also been described with FH and

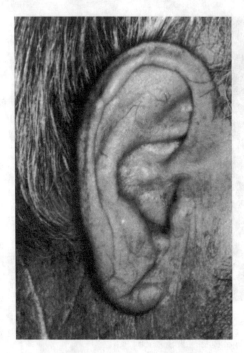

Figure 3.3. Ear lobe crease. From Moraes D, McCormack P, Tyrrell J, Feely J. Ear lobe crease and coronary heart disease. Ir Med J 1992;85 (4):131–132. Used with permission.

type IV hyperlipidemia. Other sites of rheumatic involvement, including the knees and great toes, may masquerade as pseudogout or gout. Because rheumatic manifestations may be the initial presenting feature of hyperlipidemia, a thorough musculoskeletal evaluation is warranted.

SHORT STATURE

Several studies have demonstrated an association between short stature and CAD. In the Physicians' Health Study, the risk of MI was increased 2–3% for each 1 inch decrement in height. Overall, there was an approximate one-third increase in MI rate among the shortest men (less than 67 inches) compared with the tallest (greater than 73 inches). Similar findings have also been demonstrated in women. Coronary vessel size and diameter, both of which are characteristically reduced with short stature, have been proposed to account for these findings.

XANTHOMAS

Xanthomas (or xanthomata) are cutaneous deposits of macrophage-derived foam cells that are present in association with marked hyperlipidemia (TC usually greater

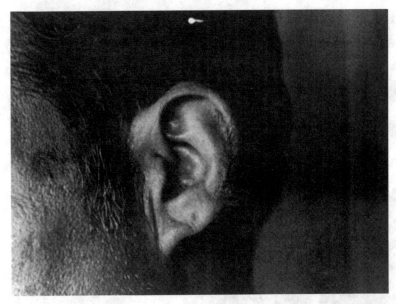

Figure 3.4. Terminal hairs over the middle of the helix of a man. From Kamalam A, Thambiah AS. Genetics of hairy ears in South Indians. Clin Exp Dermatol 1990;15:192–194. Used with permission of Blackwell Science Ltd.

than 400 mg/dL). Xanthomas most often deposit in tendons and ligaments but may occasionally be present in fascia and periosteum. The most common sites of tendinous xanthomas include the Achilles tendon and extensor surfaces of the hand, elbow, and knee (Figs. 3.6 and 3.7). Tendinous xanthomas are found in patients with Type II FH, cerebrotendinous xanthomatosis (CTX), and sitosterolemia (see below). Tuberous and tuberoeruptive xanthomas are characterized by soft cutaneous and subcutaneous nodules that occur on extensive surfaces and areas of previous trauma. In contrast to the colorless epidermis overlying tendinous xanthomas, tuberous xanthomas are circular, raised lesions that display a yellowish-orange hue (Fig. 3.8). These xanthomata are found with type II FH, CTX, sitosterolemia and type III familial dysbeta lipoproteinemia. Planar xanthomas are elevated cutaneous yellow-orange deposits located on the skin, palm (xanthoma striata palmaris), or eyelid (xanthelasma palpebrum) (Fig. 3.9). Planar skin xanthomas occur with type II FH, while planar palmar xanthomas are characteristic of type III familial dysbetalipoproteinemia. Xanthelasma palpebrum is associated with hyperlipidemia, as well as diabetes mellitus, hypothyroidism, and

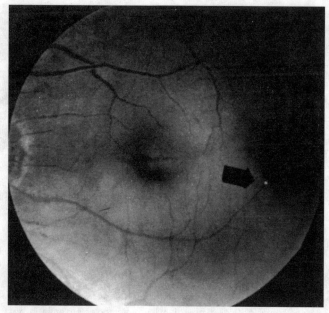

Figure 3.5. Cholesterol embolus (*arrow*) in the fundus of an asymptomatic woman. The embolus occurs at a bifurcation because it is trapped as the lumen of the artery narrows. From Brown GC. Retinal vascular disease. In Ryan SJ, ed. Retina. 2nd ed. St. Louis, Mo: CV Mosby, 1994:1362. Used with permission.

biliary cirrhosis. Approximately 50% of subjects with xanthelasma have no accompanying lipid abnormality.

SYNDROMES ASSOCIATED WITH CAD

Cerebrotendinous Xanthomatosis

This rare disease has been diagnosed in approximately 150 patients since its original description in 1937. It is characterized by early atherosclerosis, tendon and tuberous xanthomas, cataracts, and signs of CNS disease (e.g., ataxia, dementia) owing to a defect in bile acid synthesis. Accumulation of cholestanol in serum and CNS results from inhibition of 26-hydroxylase and a corresponding increase in 7α-hydroxylated intermediates. The treatment of choice is chenodeoxycholic acid, which inhibits 7α-hydroxylation of cholesterol and reduces cholestanol formation. Patients afflicted with this disorder have normal levels of serum cholesterol.

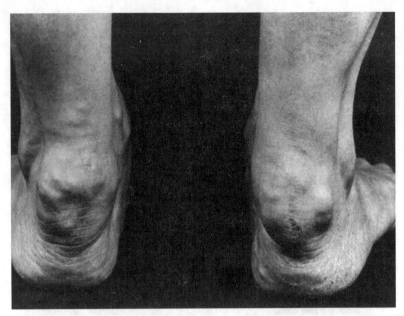

Figure 3.6. Xanthoma in heterozygous familial hypercholesterolemia in a 41-year-old woman. From Haber C, Kwiterovich PO. Dyslipoproteinemia and xanthomatosis. Pediatr Dermatol 1984;1(4):261–280. Reprinted by permission of Blackwell Scientific Publications, Inc.

Autopsies performed in patients who died following an MI have disclosed atheromatous plaque with an elevated content of cholestanol.

Homocystinuria (see Chapter 11)

Progeria (Hutchinson-Gilford Syndrome)

The classic manifestations of progeria (e.g., loss of eyebrows/eyelashes, baldness) begin in childhood. The facial appearance, as illustrated in Figure 3.10, demonstrates an enlarged skull and micrognathia. The preponderance of deaths are cardiovascular, resulting from either CAD or congestive heart failure (CHF); the median age at death is 12 years. Chromosomal aberration (inversion of chromosome 1) has been reported in one patient. Progeria patients excrete large amounts of hyaluronic acid in urine and endogenous growth hormone resistance was demonstrated in two affected subjects.

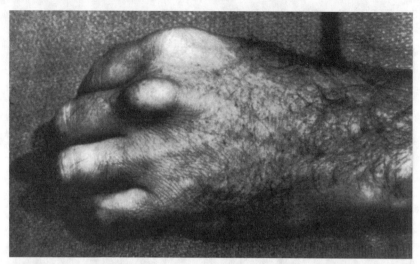

Figure 3.7. Tendinous xanthoma in the heterozygote with familial hypercholesterolemia. From Gotto AM, Jones PH, Scott LW. The diagnosis and management of hyperlipidemia. Dis Mon 1986;32:252–311. Used with permission.

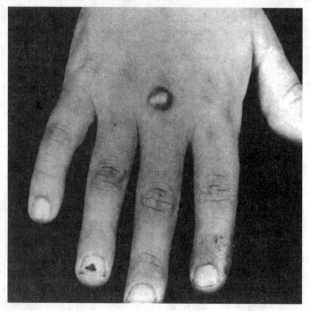

Figure 3.8. Tuberous xanthoma over the right hand in homozygous familial hypercholesterolemia in a 12-year-old girl. From Haber C, Kwiterovich PO. Dyslipoproteinemia and xanthomatosis. Pediatr Dermatol 1984;1(4):261–280. Reprinted by permission of Blackwell Scientific Publications, Inc.

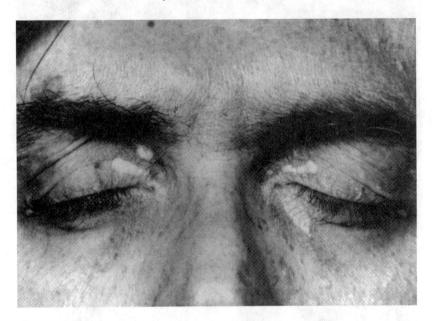

Figure 3.9. Bilateral xanthelasma in heterozygous familial hypercholesterolemia in a 44-year-old man. From Haber C, Kwiterovich PO. Dyslipoproteinemia and xanthomatosis. Pediatr Dermatol 1984;1(4):261–280. Reprinted by permission of Blackwell Scientific Publications, Inc.

Pseudoxanthoma Elasticum

This disorder is characterized by pseudoxanthoma or yellow-orange raised lesions located predominantly in flexure regions (e.g., neck) (Fig. 3.11). Atherosclerosis is accelerated by an excess of calcium deposits within the internal elastic laminae of arteries. Patients requiring coronary artery bypass surgery should have vein conduits rather than the internal mammary or gastroepiploic artery.

Sitosterolemia

This recently described (1973) autosomal recessive disorder is characterized by marked intestinal absorption of plant sterols. The major plant sterols, sitosterol, campesterol, and stigmasterol are found in fat-enriched vegetables, among other sources (see below); approximately 250 mg of these sterols are consumed daily. In normal individuals, less than 5% of plant-derived sterols are absorbed and 20% are subsequently converted to bile acids. The remaining sterols are metabolized in the

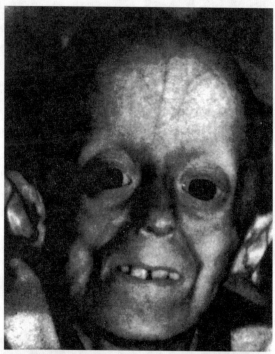

Figure 3.10. A 10-year-old girl with progeria who suffered a stroke and had bilateral hip dislocations. She died of cardiac arrest at age 13. From Brown WT. Progeria: A human-disease model of accelerated aging. Am J Clin Nutr 1992; 55(suppl): 1222S–1224S. Used with permission. Copyright © Am J Clin Nutr American Society for Clinical Nutrition.

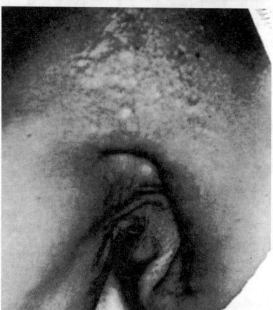

Figure 3.11. Pseudoxanthoma elasticum, an inherited disorder of connective tissue. Characteristic skin lesions can be seen in the axilla and anterior to the axilla. Typically, patients with this disease also have angioid streaks on retinal examination and are at risk for premature cardiovascular disease. Reprinted by permission of The New England Journal of Medicine from Lebwohl M. Pseudoxanthoma elasticum. N Engl J Med 1993;329:1240. Copyright © 1993, Massachusetts Medical Society.

intestine and excreted. In patients with sitosterolemia, however, up to 25–30% of sterols are absorbed. The metabolic basis underlying this disorder is not known.

As with cerebrotendinous xanthomatosis, patients may develop tendinous xanthomas despite normal TC levels. Two affected males, age 13 and 18 years, died following an MI. Patients with this disorder are asked to eliminate foods containing plant sterols (vegetable fats) from the diet. These foods include avocados, margarine, nuts, olives, certain shellfish (e.g., clams, oysters, scallops), and vegetable oils.

Werner's Syndrome

Referred to as "adult progeria," this autosomal recessive disorder is associated with premature aging. The characteristic habitus includes short stature, premature greying/baldness, juvenile cataracts, beaked nose, diabetes mellitus, scleroderma-like patches on the face and lower extremities (scleropoikiloderma), and accelerated atherosclerosis. As in Hutchinson-Gilford syndrome, urinary levels of hyaluronic acid are increased.

Suggested Readings

Björkhem I, Skrede S. Familial diseases with storage of sterols other than cholesterol: Cerebrotendinous xanthomatosis and phytosterolemia. In: Scriver CR, Beaudet AL, Sly WS, Valle D. The metabolic basis of inherited disease. New York: McGraw-Hill Information Services Company, 1989.

Brown WT. Progeria: A human-disease model of accelerated aging. Am J Clin Nutr 1992;55(suppl):1222S–1224S.

Glueck CJ, Levy RI, Fredrickson DS. Acute tendinitis and arthritis: A presenting symptom of familial type II hyperlipoproteinemia. JAMA 1968;206:2895–2897.

Gotto AM, Jones PH, Scott LW. The diagnosis and management of hyperlipidemia. Dis Mon 1986;32:252–311

Haber C, Kwiterovich PO. Dyslipoproteinemia and xanthomatosis. Pediatric Dermatology 1984:1:261–280.

Hebert PR, Rich-Edwards JW, Manson JE, et al. Height and incidence of cardiovascular disease in male physicians. Circulation 1993;88(part 1):1437–1443.

Herrera CR, Lynch C. Is baldness a risk factor for coronary artery disease? A review of the literature. J Clin Epidemiol 1990; 43:1255–1260.

Kamalam A, Thambiah AS. Genetics of hairy ears in South Indians. Clin Exp Dermatol 1990;15:192–194.

Kannam JP, Levy D, Larson M, Wilson PWF. Short stature and risk for mortality and cardiovascular disease events—The Framingham Heart Study. Circulation 1994;90:2241–2247.

Khachadurian AK. Migratory polyarthritis in familial hypercholesterolemia: Type II hyperlipoproteinemia. Arthritis Rheum 1968;11:385–393.

Lebwohl M, Halperin J, Phelps RG. Brief report: Occult pseudoxanthoma elasticum in patients with premature cardiovascular disease. N Engl J Med 1993; 329: 1237–1240.

Lesko SM, Rosenberg L, Shapiro S. A case-control study of baldness in relation to myocardial infarction in men. JAMA 1993;269:998–1003.

Moraes D, McCormack P, Tyrrell J, Feely J. Ear lobe crease and coronary heart disease. Ir Med J 1992;85:131–132.

Mudd SH, Skovby F, Levy HL, et al. The natural history of homocystinuria due to cystathionine beta-synthase deficiency. Am J Hum Genet 1985;37:1.

Polano MK. Xanthomatoses and dyslipoproteinemias. In: Fitzpatrick, ed. Dermatology in General Practice. New York: McGraw-Hill, 1993:1901–1916.

Salk D. Werner's syndrome: A review of recent research with an analysis of connective tissue metabolism, growth control of cultured cells, and chromosomal aberrations. Hum Genet 1982; 62:1–15.

4/ Total and Low-Density Lipoprotein Cholesterol

LIPOPROTEIN CLASSES

Dyslipidemias are one of the major modifiable CAD risk factors. The major circulating lipids are free and esterified cholesterol, triglycerides (TG), free fatty acids, and phospholipids (PL). Due to lipid insolubility in plasma, free fatty acids circulate with albumin and cholesterol, and TG and PL combine with apolipoproteins, forming large molecules called lipoproteins. Most circulating cholesterol is synthesized endogenously by the liver and is utilized as a component of cell membranes as well as a precursor for steroids and bile acids. In contrast, TG is predominately used as a source of energy.

Lipoproteins are generally spherical particles with polar surface layers made up of apolipoproteins, phospholipids, and free cholesterol (Fig. 4.1). Internally they contain esterified cholesterol and TG. The simplest circulating lipid measurements are TC and TG. Although epidemiologically useful, this approach disregards the pathophysiology of the heterogenous lipoproteins, some of which are pathogenic and others protective. Lipoproteins are generally classified by three techniques: density, electrophoresis, or apolipoprotein content. The most widely used approach is classification by density, dividing lipoprotein particles into increasingly dense fractions: chylomicrons, VLDL-C, LDL-C, and HDL-C (Table 4.1). Chylomicrons are very large, predominantly TG-containing molecules secreted by the intestine from dietary fat. Lipoprotein lipase (LPL) hydrolyzes free fatty acids from chylomicrons, forming chylomicron remnants. A second enzyme, hepatic triglyceride

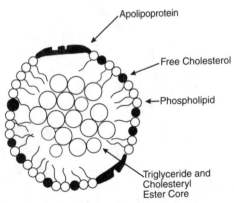

Figure 4.1. Lipoprotein cross-section.

Table 4.1. Composition of Lipoproteins

	CHYLO	VLDL	LDL	HDL
Triglyceride	90%	55%	5%	4%
Cholesterol	4%	21%	55%	21%
Phospholipid	4%	16%	20%	27%
Protein	2%	8%	20%	50%
Predominate Apoprotein	C-III C-II	C-III B-100	B-100	A-I A-II
	C-I B-48	E		

CHYLO = Chylomicron
VLDL = Very low density lipoprotein
LDL = Low density lipoprotein
HDL = High density lipoprotein

lipase, is also responsible for hydrolysis of TG. Acquisition of apolipoproteins and PL by TG hydrolysis facilitates maturation of HDL-C.

Lipoproteins of greater density than chylomicrons include VLDL-C, LDL-C, and HDL-C. VLDL-C is secreted predominately by the liver (Fig. 4.2). Hepatic VLDL-C contains apo B-100. VLDL-C, like chylomicrons, are TG-enriched lipoproteins. When hydrolyzed by LPL, VLDL-C is converted to a smaller particle or IDL-C (intermediate-density lipoprotein cholesterol). Some of the IDL-C is directly removed from the circulation by the liver through the B/E receptor, which recognizes both the apo E and apo B-100 configurations on the surface. The remainder is further hydrolyzed by hepatic triglyceride lipase producing the smaller, predominately cholesterol-enriched LDL-C. About 25% of LDL-C is cleared by the peripheral tissues, with the majority being returned to the liver, primarily via the B/E receptor.

Expression of the B/E receptor by hepatic cells is the primary mechanism in regulating cholesterol homeostasis. LDL-C binds to this receptor and is internalized and some of its contents degraded; LDL-C is hydrolyzed by lysosomes into unesterified cholesterol and amino acids. The B/E receptors become disassociated from the LDL-C and return to the cell surface. Expression of the B/E receptor is highly influenced by levels of dietary saturated fat and cholesterol intake, hormones, and increasing age. For example, dietary cholesterol and, to a greater extent, saturated

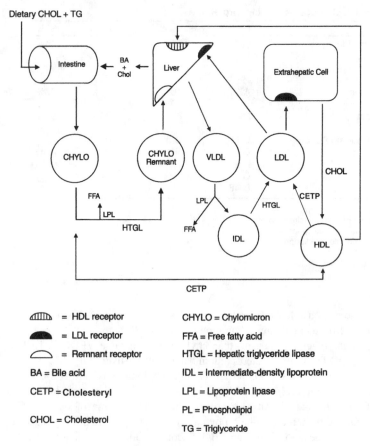

Figure 4.2. Lipoprotein transport.

fat intake decreases the production of hepatic LDL-C receptors, indirectly causing hypercholesterolemia. In contrast, a decreased level of cholesterol leads to an increase in B/E receptor density, causing additional plasma clearance of LDL-C. Bile acid sequestrants and HMG-CoA reductase inhibitors work independently by reducing the level of hepatic cholesterol via decrease in enterohepatic bile acid recirculation and direct synthesis, respectively.

Peripheral tissues are not able to degrade cholesterol directly. Reverse cholesterol transport is mediated by HDL_3 (see also Chapter 5). After removing excess free cholesterol from peripheral cells, HDL_3 is converted to a larger particle (HDL_2). Much of the esterified cholesterol is subsequently transferred to VLDL-C and LDL-C by cholesteryl ester transfer protein (CETP) for removal by the liver via the B/E receptor. Some is also taken up by the liver via nonreceptor mechanisms. Both components are converted into bile acids, which partly recirculate between the intestinal lumen and liver.

Thus, cholesterol circulates in three sizes of lipoprotein particles: VLDL-C, LDL-C, and HDL-C. TC is equal to the sum of these three fractions. TC and HDL-C are generally measured directly, and VLDL-C is estimated as TG divided by 5. Most laboratories calculate LDL-C as TC − HDL-C − TG/5. This relationship holds approximately true for fasting determinations with TG levels below 400 mg/dL. The measurement of TC, however, does not require a fasting state. In the setting of an acute MI, TC drops between 10–30% within 1 to 2 days and returns to normal by 12 wks. Moreover, hospitalization for either elective or emergent surgery may result in reduced TC levels. This has led to the misconception that many acute MI and bypass surgery patients have relatively low TC levels. TC and HDL-C measured (within 12 hours of an acute MI) provide better estimates of free-standing lipid values. However, it may still be useful to check lipoprotein levels beyond 12 hours of hospital admission because elevated levels of TC or LDL-C may enable the detection of a previously unrecognized dyslipidemia.

Using the second lipoprotein scheme based on electrophoresis, Fredrickson grouped the hyperlipidemias into six categories. The rare type I is familial hyperchylomicronemia and is due to LPL deficiency. Patients experience acute pancreatitis, hepatosplenomegaly, lipemia retinalis, and eruptive xanthomas. Type IIa, familial hypercholesterolemia (FH), is associated with either heterozygous (1 in 500 persons) or homozygous (1 in 1 million persons) deficiency or dysfunction of the B/E receptor. TC levels average 400 and 1000 mg/dL for the heterozygous and homozygous states, respectively. Patients experience premature CAD, corneal arcus, and tendinous xanthomas. Type IIb is associated with elevations of both LDL-C and VLDL-C, resulting from overproduction of apo B. This condition, also termed familial combined hyperlipidemia (1 in 200 persons), is associated with premature CAD and the most common lipoprotein phenotype in MI survivors (see Goldstein et al.). Type III or dysbetalipoproteinemia is associated with elevated chylomicron remnants resulting in a β-VLDL electrophoretic band. These patients (1 in 10,000 persons) have a high frequency of apo E_2E_2 phenotype, which has a lower receptor affinity. Manifestations include premature CAD, tuberous xanthomas, hyperuricemia, and glucose intolerance (see also Chapter 6). Type IV or familial hypertriglyceridemia results from an increased synthesis and decreased catabolism of VLDL-C. The condition is associated with premature CAD, glucose intolerance, and hyperuricemia. Type V patients (1 in 1000 persons) have elevations in TG resulting from both overproduction of VLDL-C and defective lipolysis of

TG-rich lipoproteins. This disorder is associated with diabetes, obesity, acute pancreatitis, eruptive xanthomas, glucose intolerance, hyperuricemia, and peripheral neuropathy.

Lipoprotein abnormalities can also be classified by apolipoprotein levels. Apolipoproteins more precisely categorize the number and nature of lipoprotein particles than does measurement of the cholesterol in the density subfractions. Apo B levels, especially the hepatic portion, apo B-100, indicate the amount of cholesterol synthesized and available for peripheral uptake. Reverse cholesterol transport is believed to be more precisely estimated by apo AI levels than by total HDL-C or HDL-C subfractions. Both the presence and severity of CAD is highly correlated with apo B and apo AI levels. From a clinical standpoint, however, it has not been determined whether patient management is improved by basing therapeutic decisions on apolipoprotein (vs lipoprotein) measurements and, therefore, lipoproteins are suitable for assessing CAD risk.

Lipoprotein(a) (Lp(a)) is an LDL subfraction containing a large side chain with homology to plasminogen (see also Chapter 11). As an inhibitor of intrinsic fibrinolytic activity, Lp(a) enhances thrombogenicity. Patients with Lp(a) levels above 30 mg/dL have an approximately threefold increase in CAD prevalence and may also exhibit a higher tendency for restenosis following angioplasty. LDL-C size also varies among individuals. A smaller, denser LDL-C form termed "phenotype B" is associated with an increased incidence of atherosclerosis, as reflected by low HDL-C, elevated TG, insulin resistance, HTN, and truncal obesity. This constellation of findings defines "Syndrome X."

EPIDEMIOLOGY AND CLINICAL TRIALS

Several lines of evidence suggest a pivotal role for cholesterol in the genesis of atherosclerosis. Following early identification of the presence of cholesterol in atheroma, Anitschkow demonstrated that atherosclerotic lesions could be induced in susceptible animals by high saturated fat and cholesterol diets and that these lesions regressed when low fat, low cholesterol diets were resumed. However, differences exist between human and experimental atherosclerosis. Experimental animal atherosclerosis tends to be more diffuse and concentric than human disease and less likely to result in vessel thrombosis. There is marked species variability in susceptibility to atherosclerosis by cholesterol feeding. Rabbits can be made grossly atherosclerotic in about 6 weeks, primates in about 2 years, but true carnivores such as dogs are extremely resistant to atherosclerosis. While regression occurs more readily in experimental animals than in humans, plaque reduction is variable, depending upon the experimental animal model, severity in composition of plaques, and the magnitude of cholesterol reduction. Armstrong demonstrated that plaque content of esterified cholesterol falls in response to dietary cholesterol reduction, followed by gradual changes in plaque collagen and elastin. However, the meager regression in stenosis severity (1–2%) in humans cannot account for the large reduction (75%) in clinical events observed. Brown and colleagues have therefore hypothesized that shrinkage of excess culprit intimal and core lipid results in plaque stabilization. Cholesterol reduction also leads to improvement of coronary flow reserve. Using positron emission tomography (PET), Gould observed enhanced myocardial perfusion in CAD subjects placed on a strict low-fat diet. This improvement in flow reserve appears to reflect reductions in plaque volume and restoration of endothelial function.

POPULATION STUDIES

The landmark Framingham Heart Study (see Castelli et al.) was initiated in 1948. It has followed more than 5,000 men and women who were initially without cardiovascular disease (ages 30–62). Twenty-one biennial examinations have been performed with 99% survival follow-up documentation. This study originated the coronary risk-factor concept, that is, development of CAD was enhanced by the following factors: male gender, increased age, family history of premature CAD, hypercholesterolemia, low HDL-C, cigarette smoking, HTN, DM, decreased physical activity, and obesity. Other studies have confirmed the validity of the risk-factor concept. Originating in the mid-1950s, the Seven Countries Study compared CAD morbidity and mortality in 12,500 middle-aged men living in countries with varying lifestyles: Finland, Greece, Italy, Japan, the Netherlands, the U.S., and Yugoslavia. Mean serum TC varied in these seven populations from approximately 150 to 250 mg/dL. CAD mortality varied approximately 10-fold and was shown to correlate closely with both TC and dietary fat and cholesterol consumption. The highest CAD prevalence rates were found in Finland and the U.S., with the lowest in Japan and Greece.

Epidemiological studies have also affirmed an important association between environment and CAD rates. In the NI-HON-SAN Migration Study of Japanese men inhabiting Honolulu and San Francisco, age-adjusted CAD mortality rose with migration to Honolulu and increased further in San Francisco. CAD rates correlated closely with lifestyle changes.

The 356,000 patients screened in the MRFIT constitutes the largest population followed for risk-factor evaluation. CAD risk was found to rise continuously; for each 50 mg/dL increment above 200 mg/dL, CAD rates doubled. In MRFIT, a "J" curve relationship between TC and total mortality was also observed and was most notable at TC levels below 160 mg/dL (Fig. 4.3). Some of the excess mortality (e.g., increased cancer, hepatic and pulmonary disease) was believed to reflect chronic debility process rather than result from its deficiency. A causal relationship may exist, however, between low TC and hemorrhagic stroke. The observation of the "J" relationship between TC and total mortality has resulted in controversy and caution regarding lipid-lowering therapy, especially as a tool in primary prevention. Several

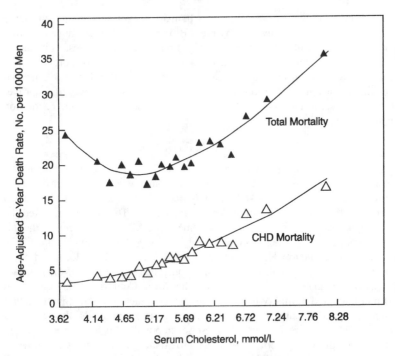

Figure 4.3. Age-adjusted total and coronary heart disease mortality in 361,662 men in the Multiple Risk Factor Intervention Trial. From Martin MJ, et al. Serum cholesterol, blood pressure, and mortality: Implications from a cohort of 361,662 men. To obtain mg/dL, multiply mmol/L by 38.6. Lancet 1986;2:933–936. Copyright by The Lancet Ltd. 1986. Used with permission.

lines of evidence suggest that this should not be a significant clinical problem. First, the MRFIT data observed maximum longevity at a TC of 122 mg/dL. Second, countries with mean TC < 150 mg/dL (e.g., China), have demonstrated lower CAD rates without increases in excess mortality. Perhaps more compelling, however, was the absence of enhanced mortality rates attributable to cancer, trauma, or suicide in the primary prevention West of Scotland Coronary Prevention Study (WOS) and the secondary prevention Scandinavian Simvastatin Survival Study (4S).

INTERVENTIONAL TRIALS

Numerous clinical trials have examined the effect of cholesterol reduction on CAD rates. The Lipid Research Clinic's Coronary Primary Prevention Trial (LRC-CPT) reported in 1984 studied 3,800 middle-aged men (35–59 years) with TC greater than 265 mg/dL and without symptomatic CAD. During the 7-year trial, patients were randomized to receive either placebo or up to 24 grams of cholestyramine daily. Approximately two-thirds of assigned drug therapy were consumed, resulting in a 13% decrease in total cholesterol and 20% decrease in LDL-C. Definite CAD death or MI occurred in 155 treated men and 187 control men (19% difference). Significant reductions were observed in angina (20%), positive exercise stress testing (25%), surgical revascularization (21%), and CHF (28%). The investigators in this important trial concluded that CAD and cholesterol have a continuous and graded relationship resulting in a reduction of approximately 2% in CAD occurrence for every 1% decrease in TC. As in other primary prevention trials, no difference in all-cause mortality was observed (see Chapter 1).

The 2nd major primary prevention trial, the Helsinki Heart Study, randomized 4,000 middle-aged men to either placebo or gemfibrozil. Use of gemfibrozil resulted in decreases in TC, LDL-C (8%), TG (35%) and increases in HDL-C (10%). In the drug-treated men there was a 34% decrease in CAD events, although no difference in all-cause mortality was observed. In the MRFIT trial, however, a 7.7% decline in all-cause mortality was found in the special intervention group. In the last 4 years of this 11-year, 13,000-patient study, all-cause mortality was reduced 16%.

The most touted of the primary prevention studies, the West of Scotland Study (WOS) (see Shepherd et al.), randomized nearly 6,600 men between the ages of 45 and 64 with elevated LDL-C (>155 mg/dL) to either pravastatin (40 mg) or placebo for 5 years. In addition to reductions in TC (20%) and LDL-C (26%), subjects treated with pravastatin evidenced significant reductions in nonfatal MI or death from CAD (31%), death from cardiovascular causes (32%), and revascularization procedures (37%). All-cause mortality, reduced by 22% (P = 0.051), became statistically significant (p = 0.039) after adjustment for baseline risk factors. Extrapolation of the data revealed that pravastatin use would prevent 20 MIs, 14 coronary arteriograms, 8 revascularization procedures, and 7 cardiovascular deaths for every 1,000 asymptomatic hypercholesterolemic middle-aged men treated. Interestingly, the time-to-event curves began to diverge nearly 6 months following initiation of treatment and was in contrast to the LRC-CPT and Helsinki trials where dichotomy was not apparent until the third year of the study.

Numerous secondary prevention studies have been undertaken acknowledging the 5–7 fold increase in CAD event rate in patients with established disease. Most of these trials have focused on arteriographic changes. The results of the first controlled angiographic progression study, the National Heart, Lung, and Blood Institute (NHLBI) Type II Trial, were published in 1984 (see Brensike et al.). TC levels were reduced by 25% in cholestyramine-treated patients, compared with a 6% reduction in diet-only treated subjects. Quantitative angiography revealed disease progression in 12% of significant lesions (≥ 50% stenoses) in the cholestyramine-treated group, compared with progression in 33% of significant lesions in the control group. No definitive evidence of disease regression was observed in this trial. Utilizing quantitative coronary arteriography, the Leiden Intervention Trial, published the following year, demonstrated improvement in vessel diameter related to the TC:HDL-C ratio among patients assigned to a high polyunsaturated fat diet. In a few patients CAD regression was observed.

The Cholesterol Lowering Atherosclerosis Study (CLAS) (see Blankenhorn, et al.), a randomized trial of colestipol and nicotinic acid vs placebo, demonstrated CAD progression in 39 and 62% of the patients in the drug treatment and control groups, respectively. Moreover, 16% of the treated patients demonstrated qualitative regression compared with 2% of the controls. One of the critical findings emerging from a retrospective analysis of CLAS was the benefit of drug treatment irrespective of the initial baseline TC or LDL-C level. This observation that cholesterol-lowering efficacy is angiographically independent of initial TC level has been confirmed in additional studies (see Table 5.3).

The Familial Atherosclerosis Treatment Study (FATS) (see Brown et al.) randomized patients into colestipol plus lovastatin, colestipol plus niacin, and placebo. This study found a correlation between LDL-C lowering and retarding CAD progression, HDL-C raising and regression. The Lifestyle Heart Trial, utilizing a strict low-fat diet (10% of calories), demonstrated overall angiographic disease regression, as well as improvement in coronary flow physiology. Six coronary arteriographic and two carotid ultrasound progression trials have utilized the highly effective HMG-CoA reductase inhibitors, introduced in the late 1980s (Tables 4.2 and 4.3). Taken together, these eight trials randomized treatment in 3,796 patients. All studies reported a lessening of coronary or carotid disease progression over the 2- to 4-year trial intervals. Individual studies varied in greater efficacy on more or less severe lesions. Importantly, a 36% reduction in cardiovascular events was observed

Table 4.2. Coronary Disease Progression (Minimum Lumen Diameter) in Selected Angiographic Progression Studies

Study	Agent	Duration (Years)	Placebo	Treatment
CCAIT[1]	Lovastatin	2	−0.09 mm	−0.05 mm*
PLAC I[2]	Pravastatin	3	−0.05 mm	−0.03 mm*
MAAS[3]	Simvastatin	4	−0.13 mm	−0.04 mm*

*p<0.05

1 Waters D, Higginson L, Gladsone P, et al for the CCAIT Study Group. Effects of monotherapy with an HMG-CoA reductase inhibitor on the progression of coronary atherosclerosis as assessed by serial quantitative arteriography. The Canadian Coronary Atherosclerosis Intervention Trial. Circulation 1994;89:9959–9968.
2 Pitt B, Mancini GBJ, Ellis SG, et al. for the PLAC I Investigators. Pravastatin Limitation of Atherosclerosis in the Coronary Arteries (PLAC I). Reduction in artherosclerosis progression and clinical events. J Am Coll Cardiol 1995;26(5):1133–1139.
3 MAAS Investigators. Effect of simvastatin on coronary atheroma: The Multicentre Anti-Atheroma Study. Lancet 1994;344:633–638.

Table 4.3. HMG-CoA Reductase Inhibitor Atherosclerosis Progression Trials

Study	N	Years	Drug	CVEs + Mort HMG	Placebo
ACAPS[1]	919	3	Lovastatin	5*	14
CCAIT[2]	331	2	Lovastatin	17	22
MARS[3]	270	2	Lovastatin	21	32
KAPS[4]	447	3	Pravastatin	11	14
PLAC I[5]	408	3	Pravastatin	8*	19
PLAC II[6]	151	3	Pravastatin	6*	16
REGRESS[7]	889	2	Pravastatin	59*	93
MAAS[8]	381	4	Simvastatin	40	51
	3796			167**	261

* $p < 0.05$
**$p < 0.01$

[1] Furberg CD, Adams, HP Jr, Applegate WB, et al. Effect of lovastatin on early carotid atherosclerosis and cardiovascular events. Circulation 1994;90:1679–1687.

[2] Waters D, Higginson L, Gladsone P, et al. for the CCAIT Study Group. Effects of monotherapy with an HMG-CoA reductase inhibitor on the progression of coronary atherosclerosis as assessed by serial quantitative arteriography. The Canadian Coronary Atherosclerosis Intervention Trial. Circulation 1994;89:9959–9968.

[3] Blankenhorn DH, Azen SP, Kramsch, et al. Coronary angiographic changes with lovastatin therapy: The Monitored Atherosclerosis Regression Study (MARS). Ann Intern Med 1993;119:969–976.

[4] Salonen R, Nyyssönen, K, Porkkala E, et al. for the Kuopio Atherosclerosis Prevention Study (KAPS). A population-based primary preventive trial of the effect of LDL lowering on atherosclerotic progression in carotid and femoral arteries. Circulation 1995;92:1758–1764.

[5] Pitt B, Mancini GBJ, Ellis SG, et al. for the PLAC I Investigators. Pravastatin Limitation of Atherosclerosis in the Coronary Arteries (PLAC I). J Am Coll Cardiol 1995;26:1133–1139.

[6] Crouse JR III, Byington RP, Bond MG, et al. Pravastatin, Lipids, and Atherosclerosis in the Carotid Arteries (PLAC-II). Am J Cardiol 1995;75:455–459.

[7] Jukema JW, Bruschke AVG, Jukema JW, van Boven AJ, et al. Effects of lipid lowering by pravastatin on progression and regression of coronary artery disease in symptomatic men with normal to moderately elevated serum cholesterol levels. The Regression Growth Evaluation Statin Study (REGRESS). Circulation 1995;91:2528–2540.

[8] MAAS Investigators. Effect of simvastatin on coronary atheroma: The Multicentre Anti-Atheroma Study. Lancet 1994;344:633–638.

in the treated patients in which a 50–75% reduction in disease progression was observed (Table 4.3). Although the number of women taking part in the progression trials was small, available data suggested equal efficacy between the sexes.

In 1994, the Scandinavian Simvastatin Survival Study group (4S) reported the results of a secondary prevention trial with all-cause mortality as the primary endpoint. The trial studied 4,444 men and women aged 35 to 70 with prior acute MI or angina with abnormal stress electrocardiography and TC between 212 and 300 mg/dL. A 30% decrease in all-cause mortality was observed over a mean 5.4-year followup, an effect which was independent of initial TC or age (Table 4.4). Significant reductions in coronary deaths (42%), acute MI (37%), revascularization procedures (37%), stroke (30%), incidence of CHF (20%), and hospital length of

Table 4.4. Scandinavian Simvastatin Survival Study Results

T Chol	Simvastatin 189	Placebo 260
Total Mortality	182	256
MI	380	553
PTCA/CABG	252	383
Stroke or TIA	66	103
Unstable Angina	295	331
Total Events	1175	1626

Data from Scandinavian Simvastatin Survival Study Group. Randomised trial of cholesterol lowering in 4444 patients with coronary heart disease: The Scandinavian Simvastatin Survival Study (4S). Lancet 1994;344:1383–1389.

stay were observed. Four hundred fifty-one fewer cardiovascular events were observed in the drug-treated group who, on average, had a 25% lower TC level. As noted above, rates of cancer, suicide, and trauma did not increase.

In addition to the traditional hygienic and pharmacologic routes, other modalities for lowering LDL-C and TC have been employed. The Program on the Surgical Control of the Hyperlipidemias (POSCH) was a long-term trial which randomized patients for ileal bypass. In addition to demonstrating a reduction in disease progression, this trial was the first to demonstrate an effect on cardiovascular events. CAD mortality and MI rates were reduced in the patients assigned to ileal bypass.

More recently, LDL apheresis and liver transplantation have been tried with familial hypercholesterolemia (FH). FH patients have also begun to undergo LDL receptor gene transfer therapy with successful, although transient, results. It is anticipated that these pioneering efforts in molecular biology will eventually play an important contributing role in retarding the process otherwise destined to lead to premature CAD and cardiovascular death.

TREATMENT

Goals

The National Cholesterol Education Program (NCEP) Adult Treatment Panel divides cholesterol management into three classes of decreasing priority: (1) patients with established CAD, (2) patients with multiple CAD risk factors, and (3) patients without CAD risk factors. Risk is acknowledged for men over 45 and women over 55 years of age. HDL-C greater than 60 mg/dL is considered a negative risk factor (see Chapter 5). All adults and high-risk children should have TC measured periodically as part of general medical care. Measurement of LDL-C, HDL-C, and TG in addition to TC should be performed in the fasting (12-hour) state in all patients with TC greater than 240 mg/dL (abnormal), multiple risk-factors and TC between 200 and 240 mg/dL (borderline), and in all CAD patients. As depicted in Figure 4.4, treatment is based on LDL-C rather than TC levels.

Diet therapy should be used for CAD patients with LDL-C levels between 100 and 130 mg/dL, and diet and drug therapy should be reserved for those with LDL-C above 130 mg/dL. In patients with multiple risk factors, LDL-C should be reduced below 130 mg/dL. Diet should be employed for multiple-risk-factor patients with LDL-C levels between 130 and 160 mg/dL, and diet followed by drug therapy if necessary with LDL-C above 160 mg/dL. Low-risk patients without multiple risk factors should maintain an LDL-C below 160 mg/dL. For LDL-C exceeding 160 mg/dL, drugs should be added to diet if levels remain above 190 mg/dL. Less evidence for modifying other lipoproteins is available, with more conservative treatment recommendations. Recommendations for HDL-C and TG management are provided in Chapters 5 and 6. In general, for high-risk and CAD patients, desirable apo B levels are less than 125 mg/dL and Lp(a) below 30 mg/dL.

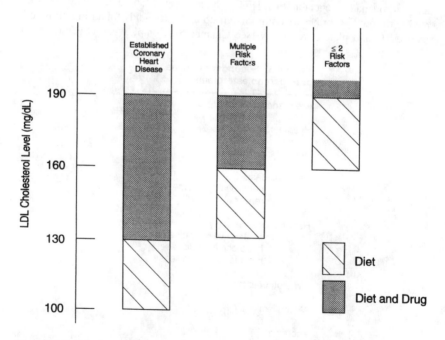

Figure 4.4. National Cholesterol Education Program LDL cholesterol treatment recommendations.

Before patient management is undertaken, secondary causes of hypercholesterolemia should be excluded. These are listed in Table 4.5. Of these, hypothyroidism and diabetes are the most common underlying problems.

Dietary Treatment

Monounsaturated and polyunsaturated fatty acids lower TC and the latter may lower HDL-C as well. In addition to the benefits on TC, appropriate diet can achieve weight loss and improve blood pressure and hyperglycemia. The physician plays a pivotal role in suggesting diet modification, but implementation is usually carried out by nurses and/or dietitians. As outlined above, the NCEP recommends two stages of diet modification to achieve target LDL-C levels. These are summarized in Table 4.6. In addition to reductions in total and saturated fat, total caloric intake should be adjusted to achieve and maintain desirable weight. For comparison, the average American diet consists of 37% of total calories derived from fat, 15% of which is saturated; cholesterol intake is 450 mg per day. Reduction in saturated fat can be achieved by decreasing meat, tropical oils (e.g., palm and coconut) and hydrogenated vegetable oils. High polyunsaturated fatty acid intake is associated with low CAD rates. Among this group ω-3 fatty acids found in marine oils reduce TG and platelet reactivity (see Chapter 6). Complex carbohydrate intake

**Table 4.5. Secondary Causes
of Hypercholesterolemia**

Pregnancy

Hypothyroidism

Diabetes mellitus

Renal disease
　　　　nephrotic syndrome
　　　　renal failure

Hepatic disease
　　　　obstructive liver disease
　　　　hepatocellular disease
　　　　hepatic storage disease

Dysproteinemias

Alcoholism

Anorexia

Porphyria

Table 4.6. National Cholesterol Education Program Diet Modification
Recommendations

	Average American Diet	NCEP* Step I Diet	NCEP* Step 2 Diet
Total Fat:	37%	<30%	<30%
Saturated Fat:	15%	<10%	< 7%
Cholesterol:	450 mg/day	<300 mg/day	<200 mg/day

% = % of total calories
*NCEP Adult Treatment Panel guidelines

(e.g., starches and soluble fiber) is strongly encouraged in a "heart healthy" diet. Modest intake (1 oz/day) of alcohol is associated with reduced CAD prevalence in comparison with abstinence or excess (see Chapter 12). Regular physical activity decreases weight, increases cardiovascular conditioning, improves a sense of well-being and lessens the risk of sudden death and acute MI.

In contrast to the generally prudent recommendations of the NCEP, stricter diets (e.g., Pritikin) containing approximately 10% of calories from fat have been undertaken by a minority of patients sufficiently motivated to undertake this major lifestyle modification. American vegetarians have an average cholesterol of 140 mg/dL, and angiographic data has documented comparable efficacy of such diets with drug therapy for reducing TC. Although scientifically sound, few patients and physicians are willing and/or able to implement these diets. It should be remembered that there is marked patient variability to diet adherence. Although up to a 25% reduction in TC may result from strict dietary fat restriction, there is an overall mean 5% reduction in TC with adherence to an NCEP Step diet.

Dietary behavior is a complex, slowly changing process involving multiple factors and adaptations. Culture, geography, and food availability are important factors. The American diet has substantially changed over the past several decades with some reduction in fat intake, although total calories and prevalence of obesity have increased. Successful diet modification requires both patient and physician motivation. If patient motivation can be achieved, the next step involves developing patient awareness of existing eating habits through use of detailed food diaries (3–7 days). This initiates a patient empowerment process. Following documentation, concrete, practical advice regarding necessary changes needs to be given both in verbal and written form. This is best provided by nurses and dietitians knowledgeable in nutrition and patient motivation. Several good, simple recipe books are available (see suggested reading). Finally, long- term reinforcement and followup with patient and food preparer are mandatory. Again, both adherence to and results of diet modification vary substantially among patients.

Treatment

Drug treatment of lipid disorders is generally more effective than dietary treatment but is associated with added cost and potential side effects. Cholesterol-modifying drugs can be divided into three general classes. HMG-CoA reductase inhibitors ("statins") and bile acid sequestrants predominately lower LDL-C. In addition, HMG-CoA reductase inhibitors may modestly raise HDL-C as a secondary effect. The second class, nicotinic acid and fibric acid derivatives (e.g., gemfibrozil), lower TG and have a secondary effect on lowering LDL-C and raising HDL-C. The third class, probucol, lowers both LDL-C and HDL-C and is a potent antioxidant. The comparative effects of these drugs are shown in Table 4.7. Treatment of HDL-C and TG is covered in Chapters 5 and 6.

A suggested clinical algorithm for lowering LDL-C is seen in Table 4.8. Introduced in the U.S. in 1987, HMG-CoA reductase inhibitors are the most potent drugs for lowering LDL-C. HMG-CoA reductase inhibitors reduce TC by inhibiting the rate-limiting enzyme involved in the hepatic synthesis of cholesterol. Four HMG-CoA reductase inhibitors are currently available in the U.S.: lovastatin, pravastatin, simvastatin, and fluvastatin. Approximately equivalent doses of HMG-CoA reductase inhibitors are simvastatin 10 mg, pravastatin 20 mg, lovastatin 20 mg, and fluvastatin 40 mg. These doses will lower LDL-C approximately 20–25%. Some patients who are able to adhere to cholesterol-lowering diets may achieve target LDL-C levels with lower doses. If further reduction is required, the recommended second step is to increase the dose, e.g., lovastatin 40 mg, pravastatin 40 mg, or simvastatin 20 mg. Dividing these doses into b.i.d. administration is slightly more efficacious than single-dose administration. For additional LDL-C lowering, supplementation with a bile acid sequestrant may be tried and is generally more

Table 4.7. Drug Effects on Lipoproteins

Drug	Dose	TC	LDL	HDL	TG
Pravastatin/Lovastatin	40 mg	–30%	–35%	5%–10%	–20%
Cholestyramine/Colestipol	24–30 g	–20%	–23%	3%–5%	+10%
Nicotinic Acid	3 g	–18%	–20%	10%–30%	–35%
Gemfibrozil	1.2 g	–10%	–12%	10%–20%	–35%
Probucol	1 g	–10%	–10%	–20%	–3%

HDL = high density lipoprotein
LDL = low density lipoprotein
TC = total cholesterol
TG = triglycerides

Table 4.8. Stepwise Low-Density Lipoprotein Cholesterol Drug Management

1. Low dose HMGRI
2. Moderate dose HMGRI
3. Moderate dose HMGRI + BAS
4. High dose HMGRI + BAS
5. Consider low-moderate dose HMGRI + nicotinic acid

<u>HMGRI-Intolerant Individuals</u>

1. BAS
   or
2. Nicotinic acid
3. BAS + nicotinic acid

HMGRI = HMG-CoA reductase inhibitor
BAS = Bile acid sequestrant

effective than using a high dose of an HMG-CoA reductase inhibitor. The combination of a moderate dose of an HMG-CoA reductase inhibitor and 8–12 grams of a bile acid sequestrant will generally lower LDL-C 40–45%. For management of concomitant elevated TG/low HDL-C, nicotinic acid or gemfibrozil may be added. Patients must be monitored closely and warned about the possibility of myositis or rhabdomyolysis (see below).

HMG-CoA reductase inhibitors are generally well tolerated, with a 95–98% patient acceptance. This class is associated with an infrequent occurrence of two recognized side effects, hepatocellular injury and myositis. Occurring from the time of drug initiation up to 2 years later, hepatocellular injury has been observed. The frequency ranges from approximately 0.1% at lower dose ranges to 1% at higher dose ranges. Elevation in liver enzymes (SGOT, SGPT) three times the upper limit of normal should lead to its discontinuance. Hepatic dysfunction is reversible on drug cessation and some patients are able to tolerate other reductase inhibitors or lower doses of the same agent. Monitoring of hepatic function every 2–4 months for 1 to 2 years is recommended.

A second recognized side effect of HMG-CoA reductase inhibitors is myositis and, potentially, rhabdomyolysis. This occurs infrequently (0.1%) in patients on monotherapy, but more frequently when HMG-CoA reductase inhibitors are given in conjunction with nicotinic acid, fibric acid derivatives, immunosuppressant therapy, or erythromycin. The clinical manifestations of myositis are diffuse muscle pain and weakness associated with marked elevations of creatine phosphokinase (CPK). In the extreme, rhabdomyolysis associated with renal failure has been reported. Practitioners should be aware that the Federal Drug Administration (FDA) cautions against use of an HMG-CoA reductase inhibitor with either gemfibrozil or nicotinic acid. Although such combinations are effective for lowering LDL-C and raising HDL-C, the 2–5% risk of myositis must be considered in clinical decision making. Patients receiving combination therapy outlined above should be monitored closely with LFTs every 2–3 months for the first 1–2 years and then 3–6 months thereafter.

Bile acid sequestrants (BAS), such as cholestyramine and colestipol, increase cholesterol excretion by binding bile acids during enterohepatic recirculation. These agents lower LDL-C approximately 20–25% when used in maximum doses. Gastrointestinal side effects are common with use of bile acid sequestrants, including constipation, bloating, and flatulence. These agents may also interfere with the absorption of other drugs, including coumadin and other cholesterol-lowering agents. Patients should be advised to take medication(s) 45 minutes to 1 hour prior to BAS or 4–5 hours afterwards. Low doses (4–12 g) are usually well tolerated and useful in conjunction with HMG-CoA reductase inhibitor administration (see above). Occasionally, bile acid sequestrants may raise TG and should not be used as single line agents in patients with fasting TG > 200 mg/dL.

Too Low Cholesterol?

Although the risk of CAD decreases in a continuous and graded manner with reduced TC levels, all-cause mortality increases at TC levels below 160 mg/dL. Cancer and hepatic and respiratory diseases account for most of the excess mortality. Considerable controversy has arisen regarding a cause/effect relationship between excess cholesterol lowering and enhanced non-CAD mortality rate. Most of the excess mortality is believed to be an associated rather than a causally related phenomenon. Although not totally resolved, this concern should not prevent aggressive lipid lowering, especially in patients with CAD, because of the 80% risk of cardiovascular death in this subgroup. Moreover, in the 4S Trial (see above), there were no excess cancer, hepatic, respiratory, or traumatic deaths associated with 5 years of HMG-CoA reductase inhibitor use among CAD participants. As illustrated in the MRFIT Registry (see above), the longest overall patient survival was found to be associated with a total cholesterol of 122 mg/dL. Furthermore, Klag and coworkers observed the lowest mortality rates among medical students followed for 25 years with the lowest TC levels at baseline. Concern has also arisen for a possible association between low TC and hemorrhagic stroke, as noted in the Pacific Rim populations. (This may reflect concomitant hypertension or excess consumption of ω-3 fatty acids (see Chapter 12)). Again, in the 4S Trial, overall stroke rate was reduced in the treated patients, along with all aspects of CAD risk.

Special Populations

Considerable debate has also focused on TC lowering in older individuals and in women (see also Chapters 13 and 14). While absolute risk of CAD increases continuously with advanced age, elevated TC levels appear to be less predictive of future CAD events in subjects older than 75 years of age. In this population, it is useful to differentiate between primary and secondary prevention. Older individuals without CAD are at low priority for aggressive cholesterol lowering. Generally, prudent diet constitutes adequate clinical management. It is our view, however, that older "youthful" individuals with CAD should be treated as aggressively as younger patients. The efficacy of cholesterol lowering for reducing subsequent cardiovascular events in patients with established heart disease is strongly supported by data from the 4S Trial.

Most epidemiological studies have demonstrated a poorer correlation between CAD events and TC in women than in men. Unfortunately, data is not available regarding all-cause mortality rates in women following lipid-lowering therapy. However, nonfatal cardiovascular events and angiographic progression of disease have been observed equally in women and men. As such, we recommend an aggressive approach to risk factor modification in women with CAD.

TREATMENT GAP

Despite the widespread lay and physician education programs stressing the importance of cholesterol management over the past decade, many patients potentially benefiting from lipid lowering therapy remain untreated. This is true in both primary and secondary prevention. In the U.S., adequate treatment is provided for only about 10% of patients with CAD with TC between 200 and 240 mg/dL, 40% of patients with TC between 240 and 300 mg/dL, and 75% of patients with TC higher than 300 mg/dL. Because most CAD patients fall within the first two categories, only about one-quarter of CAD patients are adequately treated at the present time.

Several explanations for this treatment gap have been put forth (Table 4.9). To some extent, failure to treat represents a lack of belief in the importance of risk-factor management. To this end, we explored the extent to which risk factors are assessed by medical and surgical house-officers prior to CABG. To our surprise, certain risk factors, notably hyperlipidemia, were markedly underassessed by both the medical and surgical housestaff (Table 4.10) (see Miller et al.). Deficits in the recognition and management of cardiovascular disorders are not limited to cholesterol. Only about one-half of patients with CHF receive ACE inhibitors, and the majority are dosed inadequately. Less than one-half of patients with known CAD receive daily aspirin, and a 1994 Health Care Financing Administration (HCFA) survey demonstrated that only one American in three receives aspirin within 24 hours of the diagnosis of acute MI. Therefore, it appears that cost, side effects, and demonstrated clinical utility are not the major underlying reasons for medical treatment gaps. Interestingly, nurses and other health care workers tend to follow treatment guidelines more frequently than do physicians. The solutions to these problems are neither simple nor necessarily fostered by current trends in health care

Table 4.9. Reasons for Lack of Cardiologist Interest in Cholesterol Management

- Lack of belief in cholesterol hypothesis

- Routine nature of cholesterol management

- Lack of knowledge of lifestyle and drug management

- Confusion regarding guidelines

- Lipid experts aren't cardiologists

- Expense of drug treatment

- Adverse effects of drug treatment

- Poor reimbursement for cholesterol management

Data from Roberts WC. Getting cardiologists interested in lipids. Am J Cardiol 1993;72:744–745.

Table 4.10. Prevalence of Risk Factor Identification by Medical and Surgical Admitting Interns in Patients with Coronary Artery Disease Before Coronary Artery Bypass Grafting

Variable	House Staff		p Value
	Surgery No. (%)	Medicine No. (%)	
Systemic hypertension	166 (79)	92 (73)	NS
Cigarette smoker	166 (92)	92 (84)	NS
Diabetes mellitus	166 (76)	92 (57)	0.001
Premature menopause	46 (54)	32 (44)	NS
Family history of CAD in patient aged <55 years	166 (22)	92 (36)	NS
Hyperlipidemia	165 (23)	92 (53)	0.0001

reform. Independent of primary or tertiary patient treatment responsibilities, however, it is imperative that physicians develop more uniform risk-factor management practices (Table 4.11).

Table 4.11. Comparative Clinical Consequences of Treatment

	Lipid Management*	PTCA	CABG
Stenosis (2 yr)	–2%	–50%	**
CFR (1 yr)	6%	60%	90%
Exercise Tolerance (2 yr)	10%	40%	50%
Nonfatal CVEs (5 yr)	–35%	?	10%
Mortality (5 yr)	–30%	?	–35%***

PTCA = Percutaneous transluminal coronary angioplasty
CABG = Coronary artery bypass graft
CFR   = Coronary flow reserve
CVE   = Cardiovascular event
*   0-30% Cholesterol reduction
**   Increases proximal vessel stenosis, provides collateral revascularization
*** Depends on high-risk features

Adapted from Vogel RA et al. Comparative clinical consequences of aggressive lipid management, coronary angioplasty and bypass surgery in coronary heart disease. Am J Cardiol 1992;69:1229–1233.

Suggested Readings

American Heart Association. American Heart Association Cookbook. New York, NY: David McKay Co, 1984.

Anitschkow N. Experimental atherosclerosis in animals. In: Cowdry EV, ed. Arteriosclerosis: A study of the problem. New York: Macmillan, 1933;271–322.

Arnntzenius AC, Kromhout D, Barth JD, et al. Diet, lipoproteins, and the progression of coronary atherosclerosis: The Leiden Intervention Trial. N Engl J Med 1985; 312:805–811.

Blankenhorn DH, Azen SP, Kramsch et al. Coronary angiographic changes with lovastatin therapy: The Monitored Atherosclerosis Regression Study (MARS). Ann Intern Med 1993; 119:969–976.

Blankenhorn DH, Nessim SA, Johnson RL, et al. Beneficial effects of combined colestipol-niacin therapy on coronary atherosclerosis and coronary venous bypass grafts. JAMA 1987;257:3233–3240.

Brensike JF, Levy RI, Kelsey SF, et al. Effects of therapy with cholestyramine on progression of coronary arteriosclerosis: Results of the NHLBI Type II Coronary Intervention Study. Circulation 1984; 289:220–223.

Brown BG, Zhao X-Q, Sacco DE, Albers JJ. Lipid lowering and plaque regression. New insights into prevention of plaque disruption and clinical events in coronary disease. Circulation 1993;87:1781–1791.

Brown G, Albers JJ, Fisher LD, et al. Regression of coronary artery disease as a result of intensive lipid-lowering therapy in men with high levels of apolipoprotein B. N Engl J Med 1990;323:1289–1298.

Buchwald H, Varco RL, Matts JP, et al. Effect of partial ileal bypass surgery on mortality from coronary heart disease in patients with hypercholesterolemia: Report of the Program on the Surgical Control of the Hyperlipidemias (POSCH). N Engl J Med 1990;323:946–955.

Cashin-Hemphill L, Mack WJ, Pogoda JM, et al. Beneficial effects of colestipol-niacin on coronary atherosclerosis: A 4 year follow-up. JAMA 1990;264:3013–3017.

Castelli WP, Garrison RJ, Wilson PFW, et al. Incidence of coronary heart disease and lipoprotein cholesterol levels: The Framingham Study. JAMA 1986;256: 2835–2838.

Clarkson TB, Bond MG, Bullock BC, et al. A study of atherosclerosis regression in Macaca mulatta: IV. Changes in coronary arteries from animals with atherosclerosis induced for 19 months and then regressed for 24 or 48 months at plasma cholesterol concentrations of 300 and 200 mg/dl. Exp Molec Pathol 1981;34:345–368.

Cohen MV, Byrne M-J, Levine B, et al. Low rate of treatment of hypercholesterolemia by cardiologists in patients with suspected and proven coronary artery disease. Circulation 1991;83:1294–1304.

Conner PL, Berge KG, Wenger NK, et al. Fifteen year mortality in Coronary Drug Project patients: Long-term benefit with niacin. J Am Coll Cardiol 1986; 8:1245–1255.

Connor SL, Gustafson JR, Artaud-Wild, et al. The cholesterol/saturated-fat index: An indication of the hypercholesterolemic and atherogenic potential of food. Lancet 1986;327:1229–1232.

Connor W, Connor S. The New American Diet. New York, NY: Simon & Schuster, 1986.

Crouse JR III, Byington RP, Bond MG, et al. Pravastatin, Lipids, and Atherosclerosis in the Carotid Arteries (PLAC-II). Am J Cardiol 1995;75:455–459.

Davies MJ, Thomas AC. Plaque fissuring—the cause of acute myocardial infarction, sudden ischemic death, and crescendo angina. Br Heart J 1985;53:363–373.

Egashira K, Hirooka Y, Kai H, et al. Reduction in serum cholesterol with pravastatin improves endothelium-dependent coronary vasomotion in patients with hypercholesterolemia. Circulation 1994;89: 2519–2524.

Frederickson DS, Levy RI, Lees RS. Fat transport in lipoproteins. An integrated approach to mechanisms and disorders. N Engl J Med 1967;276:32–44, 94–103, 148–156, 215–224, 273–281.

Frick MH, Elo O, Haapa K, et al. Helsinki Heart Study: Primary-prevention trial with gemfibrozil in middle-aged men with dyslipidemia: Safety of treatment, changes in risk-factors, and incidence of coronary heart disease. N Engl J Med 1987;317: 1237–1245.

Furberg CD, Adams HP, Jr, Applegate WB, et al. Effect of lovastatin on early carotid atherosclerosis and cardiovascular events. Circulation 1994;90:1679–1687.

Furberg CD, Byington RP, Crouse JR, et al. Pravastatin, lipids, and major coronary events. Am J Cardiol 1994;73:1133–1134.

Fuster V, Badimon L, Badimon JJ, et al. Mechanism of disease: The pathogenesis of coronary artery disease and the acute coronary syndromes. N Engl J Med 1992;326(5):310–318.

Goldman L, Cook EF. The decline in ischemic heart disease mortality rates: An analysis of the comparative effects of medical interventions and changes in lifestyle. Ann Intern Med 1984;101:825–836.

Goldstein JL, Schrott HG, Hazzard WR, Bierman EL, et al. Hyperlipidemia in coronary heart disease. II. Generic analysis of lipid levels in 176 families and delineation of a new inherited disorder, combined hyperlipidemia. J Clin Invest 1973;52:1544.

Goor R, Goor N. Eater's choice: A food lover's guide to lower cholesterol. Rev ed. New York, NY: Houghton Mifflin Co, 1989.

Gordon T, Kannel WB. Premature mortality from coronary heart disease. The Framingham Study. JAMA 1971;215: 1617–1625.

Gould KL, Martucci JP, Goldberg DI, et al. Short-term cholesterol lowing decreases size and severity of perfusion abnormalities by positron emission tomography after dipyridamole in patients with coronary artery disease. A potential noninvasive marker of healing coronary endothelium. Circulation 1994;89:1530–1538.

Holme I. An analysis of randomized trials evaluating the effect of cholesterol reduction on total mortality and coronary heart disease incidence. Circulation 1990;82: 1916–1924.

Hunninghake DB, Stein EA, Dujovne CA, et al. The efficacy of intensive dietary therapy alone or combined with lovastatin in outpatients with hypercholesterolemia. N Engl J Med 1993;328:1213–1219.

Jacobs D, Blackburn H, Higgins M, et al. Report of the conference on low blood cholesterol: Mortality associations. Circulation 1992;86:1046–1060.

Jukema JW, Bruschke AUG, van Boven AJ, et al. Effects of lipid lowering by pravastatin on progression and regression of coronary artery disease in symptomatic men with normal to moderately elevated serum cholesterol levels. The Regression Growth Evaluation Statin Study (REGRESS). Circulation 1995;91:2528–2540.

Kane JP, Malloy MJ, Ports TA, et al. Regression of coronary atherosclerosis during treatment of familial hypercholesterolemia with combined drug regimens. JAMA 1990;264:3007–3012.

Keys A. Coronary heart disease in seven countries. Circulation 1970;41(suppl 1): I–1–I–211.

Klag MJ, Ford DE, Mead LA, He J, et al. Serum cholesterol in young men and subsequent cardiovascular disease. N Engl J Med 1993;328:313–318.

LaRosa JC. Cholesterol lowering, low cholesterol and mortality. Am J Cardiol 1993;72:776–786.

Leaf A, Weber PC. Cardiovascular effects of N-3 fatty acids. N Engl J Med 1988;318:549–557.

Lipid Research Clinics Program. The Lipid Research Clinics Coronary Primary Prevention Trial results: I. Reduction in incidence of coronary heart disease. JAMA 1984;251:351–364.

Loscalzo J. Regression of coronary atherosclerosis. N Engl J Med 1990;323:1337–1339.

MAAS Investigators. Effect of simvastatin on coronary atheroma: The Multicentre Anti-Atheroma Study (MAAS). Lancet 1994; 344:633–638.

Miller M, Konkel K, Fitzpatrick D, Burgan R, Vogel RA. Divergent reporting of coronary risk factors before coronary artery bypass surgery. Am J Cardiol 1995;75:736–737.

The Multiple Risk Factor Intervention Trial Research Group. Mortality rates after 10.5 years for participants in the Multiple Risk Factor Intervention Trial: Findings related to a priori hypotheses of the trial. JAMA 1990;263:1795–1801.

Ornish D, Brown SE, Scherwitz LW, et al. Can lifestyle changes reverse coronary heart disease? The Lifestyle Heart Trial. Lancet 1990;336:129–133.

Pitt B, Mancini GBJ, Ellis SG, et al. for the PLAC I Investigators. Pravastatin Limitation of Atherosclerosis in the Coronary Arteries (PLAC I). Reduction in atherosclerosis progression and clinical events. J Am Coll Cardiol 1995;26:1133–1139.

The Pravastatin Multinational Study Group for Cardiac Risk Factors. Effects of pravastatin in patients with serum total cholesterol levels from 5.2 to 7.8 mmol/liter (200 to 300mg/dl) plus two additional risk factors. Am J Cardiol 1993;72:1031–1037.

Report from the Committee of Principal Investigators: A co-operative trial in the primary prevention of ischemic heart disease using clofibrate. Br Heart J 1978;40:1069–1118.

Roberts WC. Lipid-lowering therapy after an atherosclerotic event. Am J Cardiol 1990;65:16–18F.

Roberts WC. Getting cardiologists interested in lipids. Am J Cardiol 1993;72:744–745.

Rossouw JE, Lewis B, Rifkind BM. The value of lowering cholesterol after myocardial infarction. N Engl J Med 1990;323: 1112–1119.

Salonen R, Nyyssönen K, Porkkala E, et al for the Kuopio Atherosclerosis Prevention Study (KAPS). A population-based primary preventive trial of the effect of LDL lowering on atherosclerotic progression in carotid and femoral arteries. Circulation 1995; 92:1758–1764.

Scandinavian Simvastatin Survival Study Group. Randomised trial of cholesterol lowering in 4444 patients with coronary heart disease: The Scandinavian Simvastatin Survival Study (4S). Lancet 1994;344: 1383–1389.

Schectman G, Hiatt J, Hartz A. Evaluation of the effectiveness of lipid-lowering therapy (bile acid sequestrants, niacin, psyllium and lovastatin) for treating hypercholesterolemia in veterans. Am J Card 1993;71:759–765.

Shear CL, Franklin FA, Stinnett S, et al. Expanded clinical evaluation of lovastatin (EXCEL) study results: Effect of patient characteristics on lovastatin-induced changes in plasma concentration of lipids and lipoproteins. Circulation 1992;85: 1293–1303.

Shepherd J, Cobbe SM, Ford I, Isles CG, et al. Prevention of coronary heart disease with pravastatin in men with hypercholesterolemia. N Engl J Med 1995;333: 1301–1307.

Stamler J, Wentworth D, Neaton JD. Is relationship between serum cholesterol and risk of premature death from coronary heart disease continuous and graded? Findings in 356,222 primary screenees of the Multiple Risk Factor Intervention Trial (MRFIT). JAMA 1986;256:2823–2828.

Steinberg D, Pearson TA, Juller LH. Alcohol and atherosclerosis. Ann Intern Med 1991;114:967–976.

Summary of the second report of the National Cholesterol Education Program (NCEP) Expert Panel on Detection, Evaluation and Treatment of High Blood Cholesterol in Adults (Adult Treatment Panel II). JAMA 1993;269:3015–3023.

Superko HR, Krauss RM. Coronary artery disease regression. Convincing evidence for the benefit of aggressive lipoprotein management. Circulation 1994;90:1056–1069.

Vogel RA, et al. Comparative clinical consequences of aggressive lipid management, coronary angioplasty and bypass surgery in coronary heart disease. Am J Cardiol 1992;69:1229–1233.

Waters D, Higginson L, Gladsone P, et al. for the CCAIT Study Group. Effects of monotherapy with an HMG-CoA reductase inhibitor on the progression of coronary atherosclerosis as assessed by serial quantitative arteriography. The Canadian Coronary Atherosclerosis Intervention Trial. Circulation 1994;89:9959–9968.

Wood PD, Stefanick ML, Dreon DM, et al. Changes in plasma lipids and lipoproteins in overweight men during weight loss through dieting as compared with exercise. N Engl J Med 1988;319:1173–1179.

Worth RM, Kato H, Rhoads GG, et al. Epidemiologic studies of coronary heart disease and stroke in Japanese men living in Japan, Hawaii and California: Mortality. Am J Epidemiol 1975;102:481–490.

5/ High-Density Lipoprotein

High-density lipoprotein cholesterol (HDL-C), a protein-enriched particle (approximately 50% by mass), plays a pivotal role in reverse cholesterol transport. Viewed within the context of hyperlipidemia, HDL-C poses the greatest risk for CAD when accompanied by high TC and LDL-C. More recent studies have demonstrated that even in the presence of "desirable" total cholesterol (levels less than 200 mg/dL), low HDL-C appears to be an important CAD risk factor (see below). Nevertheless, many unsettled issues remain. Perhaps chief among them is that not all HDL-C syndromes are associated with premature CAD. Moreover, the pharmacological armamentarium to treat low HDL-C is limited; raising low HDL-C is considerably more difficult than lowering LDL-C. Although raising low HDL-C reduces CAD event rate in hyperlipidemic subjects, there are presently no data showing whether raising an isolated low HDL-C reduces (primary or secondary) CAD event rate. An ongoing VA secondary prevention study examining this question should be completed by the end of the decade. With respect to arteriographic endpoints, the CLAS Study (see Blankenhorn, et al.) reported reduced progression of CAD in patients with desirable TC. Moreover, subgroup analysis from the 4S trial (see Scandinavian Simvastatin Survival Study Group) found reduction in CAD event rate even at the lowest baseline TC levels, suggesting that aggressive lipid-lowering therapy may be useful even without marked hyperlipidemia. This chapter will elaborate on the advances in HDL-C metabolism, and provide recommendations for the management of low HDL-C.

BIOCHEMISTRY

As noted in Chapter 4, HDL-C mediates cellular cholesterol removal. HDL-C originates as an intestinal or hepatically derived disk-like particle enriched with PL and apolipoprotein(s) (apo) (Fig. 5.1). Free cholesterol is acquired from extrahepatic cells and esterified by the enzyme LCAT. Apo AI, the primary apolipoprotein of HDL-C, serves as an important cofactor for LCAT activation. Hydrolysis of TG-rich lipoproteins, chylomicrons and VLDL-C, contributes surface components (PL, apos) with which continued acquisition of extrahepatic free cholesterol converts HDL_3 into a larger cholesteryl-ester-enriched HDL_2 particle. The mature HDL-C particle exchanges cholesteryl esters for TG by CETP; the cholesteryl ester is transferred to apo B-containing lipoproteins (VLDL-C remnants and LDL-C) for hepatic uptake and biliary excretion. Reverse cholesterol transport, the certified antiatherogenic property conferred by HDL-C, may be impeded with significant coronary luminal narrowing because cholesterol is trapped and immobilized within the atherosclerotic plaque. Therefore, low HDL-C with established CAD is a poor prognosticator vis-à-vis future CAD events (see below).

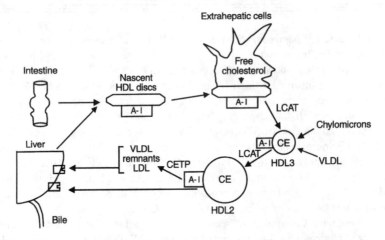

Figure 5.1. Schematic representation of HDL-C formation and transport. A-I = apolipoprotein A-I, CE = cholesteryl esters. From Leighton RF. Management of the patient with a low HDL-C-cholesterol. Clin Cardiol 1990;13:521–532. Copyrighted © and reprinted with the permission of Clinical Cardiology Publishing Company, Inc., and/or the Foundation for Advances in Medicine and Science, Inc.

HIGH-DENSITY LIPOPROTEIN SUBFRACTIONS

As noted above, HDL-C consists of two main subfractions, HDL_2 and HDL_3. HDL_3 mediates cholesterol removal from extrahepatic tissues; HDL_2 exchanges cholesteryl esters for TG via CETP. Some epidemiologic studies have shown an inverse correlation between elevated levels of HDL_2 and CAD. Levels of HDL_2 are elevated with lipoprotein lipase activation (e.g., conditioned athletes) or hepatic lipase inhibition (e.g., estrogen mediated). They are also increased with nicotinic acid, hepatic microsomal inducing agents, and heavy alcohol use. Levels of HDL_2 are low in subjects with CAD and those at increased risk (e.g., with familial hypoalphalipoproteinemia). A low HDL_2 is also associated with abnormal clearance of postprandial fat, commonly observed with CAD-prone syndromes (e.g., endogenous hypertriglyceridemia/Syndrome X). It has been postulated that the cardioprotection afforded by HDL_2 represents an epiphenomenon, reflecting enhanced efficiency of TG-rich lipoprotein catabolism and heightened clearance of atherogenic chylomicron remnants (see Chapter 6).

In the Physicians' Health Study (PHS), (see Stampfer et al.) among others, HDL_3 was the more important subfraction in predicting an initial MI. Moderate alcohol consumption and cardioprotective agents such as gemfibrozil raise HDL_3.

Thus, while either HDL-C subfraction has been shown to inversely predict CAD event rate, the clinician is advised to focus on total HDL-C in assessing CAD risk until more definitive data becomes available.

High-Density Lipoprotein and Endothelial Regulation

When Yui et al. reported that apo AI was structurally homologous to prostacyclin stabilizing factor (PSF) in 1988 an additional cardioprotective mechanism was ascribed for HDL-C. As PGI_2 (see Chapter 2) is very unstable in the circulation, its duration of action is accentuated by binding to PSF. Previous studies had demonstrated that the activity of PSF was reduced during an acute MI and unstable angina. Aoyama and colleagues subsequently showed that the addition of Apo AI to cell culture media stabilized the activity of prostacyclin (PGI_2) suggesting a role for HDL-C in endothelial vasodilation. Other reported actions of HDL-C include facilitating release of PGI_2 from cultured endothelial cells, antagonizing the EDRF-NO inhibition mediated by oxidized LDL-C, and stimulation of fibrinolysis by urokinase-induced plasminogen activation. Recently, Kuhn and coworkers at Georgetown demonstrated enhancement acetylcholine-induced coronary vasoconstriction in normal and diseased vessels in patients with low HDL-C. Whether raising HDL-C restores endothelial vasomotor function, however, awaits further study.

GENETIC STUDIES

Familial Hypoalphalipoproteinemia

Familial hypoalphalipoproteinemia, the most common disorder associated with low HDL-C, is characterized by CAD that is often manifest before age 55. Levels of HDL-C in these subjects generally range from 20 to 35 mg/dL. While an autosomal dominant mode of transmission has been postulated, complex segregation analysis has revealed significant genetic variation and a probable polygenic influence. To date, there have been no mutations in the apo AI gene associated with this disorder. Moreover, there are no specific clinical signs associated with this disorder.

High-Density Lipoprotein Mutations Associated With Premature Coronary Artery Disease

The primary apolipoprotein of HDL-C, apo AI, is complexed to two other apolipoprotein genes, apo CIII and AIV on chromosome 11. Complete absence of apo AI has been reported in several unrelated families. These subjects had severe premature CAD resulting from either inversion within the apo AI-CIII-AIV gene complex, complete deletion of the apo AI-CIII-AIV gene complex, or specific mutations in the apo AI gene resulting in apo AI deficiency. In these affected young (< 40 yrs) subjects, CAD developed in the absence of other risk factors. Planar xanthomas have been reported with HDL-C deficiency.

High-Density Lipoprotein Mutations Not Associated With Premature Coronary Artery Disease

Isolated low HDL-C is not always associated with premature CAD. Included in this group are LCAT deficiency, fish eye disease, Tangier disease, apo AI variants, and associated low total cholesterol (less than 150 mg/dL; see Rader et al.). Although apo AI catabolism is increased, apo AI production is normal and reverse cholesterol transport appears to be operative.

LECITHIN-CHOLESTEROL ACYLTRANSFERASE DEFICIENCY

As noted above, cholesterol is esterified and sequestered into the polar core of HDL-C by the LCAT. This enzyme transfers an acyl group from the second carbon of lecithin to esterify cholesterol (Fig. 5.2). LCAT stabilizes apo AI in plasma, and when deficient, apo AI is rapidly catabolized. The consequence is a very low HDL-C (less than 10 mg/dL in homozygotes). The clinical findings are based on the accumulation of free cholesterol (and lecithin) in selected tissues. They include anemia, corneal opacities, and renal failure due to enhanced mesangial deposition of free cholesterol. Although premature atherosclerosis has developed in some patients, CAD is uncommon below age 60. To date, approximately 30 families have been reported worldwide, and at least 15 different mutations within the LCAT gene have been identified. Most cases have been reported from Scandinavia, although the disease has been observed in Europe, Japan, and the United States. Heterozygotes for the disorder (estimated frequency, 1 in 500) have low HDL-C (approximately 30 mg/dL) but do not develop clinical manifestations of the disease. The homozygous state is estimated to be present in approximately 1 in 1 million people. That so few mutations have been reported to date may in part be attributable to the relative lack of screening for low HDL-C. This will likely be obviated in the near future because of the increased emphasis on complete lipid and lipoprotein analysis. Unfortunately, there is no effective therapy for this disorder at present. Renal transplantation remains only palliative owing to the systemic nature of the disease. Gene therapy may be an option in the future.

FISH EYE DISEASE

Fish eye disease is recognized as a mild form of LCAT deficiency as cholesterol esterification is reduced in HDL-C. Subjects afflicted with this disorder have severe corneal opacities resembling fish eyes (Fig. 5.3) but do not develop renal insufficiency. As in LCAT deficiency, the prevalence of premature CAD is not increased. Two different genetic mutations, both located in the LCAT gene, have been reported in this disorder (see Klein et al.).

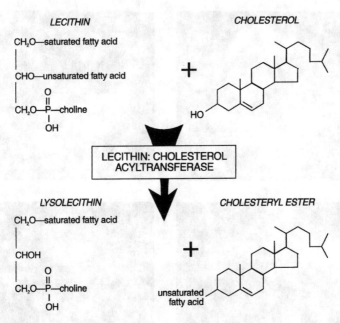

Figure 5.2. Principal lipid reactants in the plasma lecithin:cholesterol acyltransferase (EC 2.3.1.43) reaction. From Stanbury JB, Wyngaarden JB, Fredrickson DS, Goldstein JL, Brown MS. The Metabolic Basis of Inherited Disease. 5th ed. New York, NY: McGraw-Hill Book Co, 1983. Reproduced with permission of McGraw-Hill, Inc.

TANGIER DISEASE

The clinical description of this disorder, identified on Tangier Island off the Chesapeake Bay, was initially reported by Fredrickson in 1961. Affected subjects develop an abnormal accumulation of cholesteryl ester in reticuloendothelial tissues manifesting as orange tonsils, corneal opacities, hepatosplenomegaly, and peripheral neuropathy. Affected subjects have rapid catabolism of HDL-C owing to abnormal posttranslational processing of apo AI precursors (prepro apo AI).

APO AI VARIANTS

In recent years, apo AI variants identified by screening "healthy" subjects have often failed to disclose an association with either low HDL-C or CAD. One of these variants, apo AI Milano, may in fact be cardioprotective.

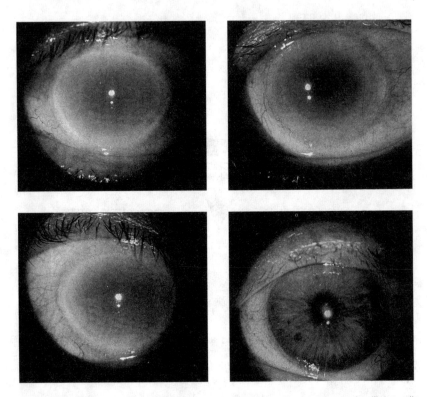

Figure 5.3. Fish eye disease. From Carlson LA. Fish eye disease: A new familial condition with massive corneal opacities and dyslipoproteinaemia. Eur J Clin Invest 1982;12:41–53. Used with permission of Blackwell Science Ltd.

APO AI MILANO

An apo AI variant was reported in the northern Italian village of Lucerne. A family with nearly 50 affected members displayed very low HDL-C but no evidence of CAD. The apo AI variant (known as apo AI Milano) is a point mutation resulting in substitution of cysteine for arginine (at amino acid position 173), causing AI dimerization and enhanced stabilization in plasma. The apo AI Milano dimer is more efficient than normal apo AI in promoting cholesterol efflux. In addition, this variant has been shown to provide greater fibrinolytic activity than normal apo AI. Recently, Ameli et al. administered human recombinant apo AI Milano to rabbits fed a high cholesterol diet and subjected the iliofemoral tree to numerous angioplasty lesions. In contrast to normal apo AI, rabbits receiving apo AI Milano evidenced significant reduction in intimal thickening following PTCA injury.

High High-Density Lipoprotein Disorders

FAMILIAL HYPERALPHALIPOPROTEINEMIA

An elevated HDL-C syndrome associated with longevity was initially reported by Glueck and coworkers. A study of 62 living members from 18 unrelated families in Cincinnati disclosed no history of CAD. Among subjects with familial hyperalphalipoproteinemia, the mean HDL-C and LDL-C were 81 and 105 mg/dL, respectively. The near 1:1 ratio of LDL-C:HDL-C was also reported in familial hypobetalipoproteinemia (a cardioprotective disorder characterized by very low levels of LDL-C).

CHOLESTERYL ESTER TRANSFER PROTEIN DEFICIENCY

As discussed above, CETP transfers cholesterol from HDL-C to lower-density lipoproteins (LDL-C, VLDL-C) in exchange for TG. Reduction in CETP activity is associated with very high HDL-C. A gene-splicing defect causing CETP deficiency occurs commonly in Japan with HDL-C levels exceeding 100 mg/dL. Longevity has been reported with this disorder.

HEPATIC LIPASE DEFICIENCY

This uncommon disorder is associated with elevation in HDL-C and premature CAD. The molecular defect was recently reported in one family due to a mutation in the hepatic lipase gene. The mechanism for accelerated atherosclerosis is presently unknown.

EPIDEMIOLOGY

Observational Studies Without Preexisting Coronary Artery Disease

The relationship of HDL-C and CAD has been the topic of numerous epidemiologic and arteriographic studies. Gordon and coworkers reviewed four major U.S. prospective studies. They included more than 10,000 participants in the Framingham Heart Study (FHS), the Coronary Primary Prevention Trial (CPPT), the Lipid Research Clinics Follow-Up Study (LRCF), and MRFIT. Illustrated in Figure 5.4 are initial CAD events in men and women (FHS and LRCF only) stratified by HDL-C. Meta-analysis of these studies revealed that for each 1 mg/dL rise in HDL-C, the risk of CAD was reduced by 2–3%. Alternatively, a 1% increase in HDL-C was associated with a 1.5–2% decrement in CAD risk. Many other cross-sectional and longitudinal cohort studies in the U.S. and Europe confirmed these

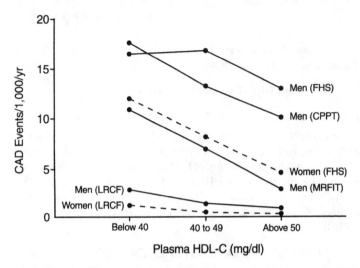

Figure 5.4. Plasma HDL-C cholesterol (HDL-C) levels and incidence of CAD in four American studies. (MRFIT usual-care group only.) From Rifkind BM. High-density lipoprotein cholesterol and coronary artery disease: Survey of the evidence. Am J Cardiol 1990;66:3A–6A. Used with permission.

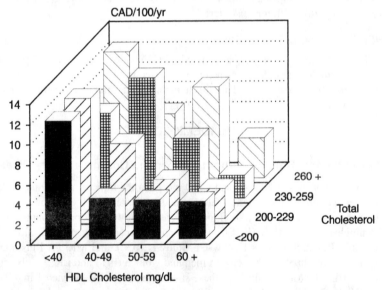

Figure 5.5. Incidence of CAD by total and HDL-C cholesterol levels in subjects aged 50 to 79 years. From Castelli WP, Garrison RJ, Wilson PWF, Abbott RD, Kalousdian S, Kannel WB. Incidence of coronary heart disease and lipoprotein cholesterol levels. The Framingham Study. JAMA 1986;256:2835–2838.

findings. One of the largest studies in Europe, the Prospective Cardiovascular Münster (PROCAM) Trial, an ongoing study launched in 1979 of nearly 20,000 men and women, found that HDL-C was the single best predictor of initial MI in middle-aged (40–65 years) men. The Israeli Ischemic Heart Disease Study demonstrated an inverse association between HDL-C and both CAD and total mortality. In the U.S., similar results have been reported (Fig. 5.5). HDL-C is a particularly important predictor of CAD events over age 50. In general, for each 5 mg/dL reduction in HDL-C, the risk of CAD increases 25%. Importantly, a high HDL-C appears to confer protection even when LDL-C levels are relatively high (Fig. 5.6). Conversely, a low HDL-C may be associated with CAD even when the LDL-C level is desirable (100 to 130 mg/dL). As LDL-C levels fall below 100 mg/dL and enter the physiologic range (approximately 60 to 80 mg/dL), CAD is exceedingly uncommon. Under these circumstances, as commonly observed in Third World countries, HDL-C assumes a Lilliputian role.

Percentiles of HDL-C levels in adults are depicted in Table 5.1. Mean HDL-C levels are 45 to 50 mg/dL in men and 50 to 60 mg/dL in women. A low HDL-C is defined as less than 35 mg/dL in men and less than 45 mg/dL in women. Another important parameter in assessing CAD risk is the TC:HDL-C ratio (Fig. 5.7). The

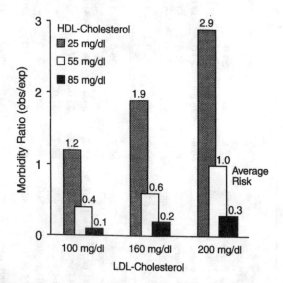

Figure 5.6. Risk of developing CHD in 4 years by HDL-C and LDL-C cholesterol (Framingham men, aged 50 to 70 years). From Kannel WB. Clin Chem 1988:34(suppl B):53B–59B. Used with permission.

Table 5.1. High-Density Lipoprotein Cholesterol in Milligrams per Deciliter for Persons 20 Years of Age and Older by Sex and Age: United States, 1988–1991

Sex and age	Number of examined persons	Mean	Selected percentile									
			5th	10th	15th	25th	50th	75th	85th	90th	95th
Men												
20 years and older	3,920	46.5	28.0	31.0	34.0	37.0	44.1	53.1	59.1	64.0	73.0
20–34 years	1,178	47.1	30.0	34.0	35.1	38.0	46.0	54.0	60.1	64.0	71.0
35–44 years	642	46.3	28.0	30.0	33.0	37.0	44.0	53.0	58.1	63.0	73.0
45–54 years	502	46.6	28.0	30.0	33.0	36.0	43.1	53.0	61.0	66.1	77.1
55–64 years	533	45.6	29.0	31.0	33.0	36.1	43.0	53.0	59.0	62.0	72.0
65–74 years	553	45.3	28.0	31.0	32.0	36.0	43.0	53.0	58.0	62.1	71.0
75 and older	512	47.2	28.0	32.0	34.0	38.0	45.0	54.0	62.0	67.0	75.1
Women												
20 years and older	3,855	55.7	34.0	38.0	41.0	44.1	54.0	65.0	71.0	76.1	83.0
20–34 years	1,167	55.7	34.0	38.0	41.0	44.1	54.0	64.1	70.1	75.1	83.1
35–44 years	701	54.3	33.0	37.0	40.0	44.0	53.0	64.1	69.1	72.1	79.0
45–54 years	459	56.7	37.0	38.1	41.0	46.0	56.0	65.0	72.1	77.1	84.1
55–64 years	500	56.1	33.0	37.0	40.0	44.0	53.0	66.0	73.0	79.0	87.1
65–74 years	492	55.7	34.0	37.0	40.0	44.1	54.0	65.1	73.0	78.0	83.1
75 and older	536	57.1	33.0	39.0	41.0	44.1	56.0	66.1	73.1	78.1	87.0

From National Cholesterol Education Program. Second Report of the Expert Panel on Detection, Evaluation, and Treatment of High Blood Cholesterol in Adults (Adult Treatment Panel II). National Heart, Lung, and Blood Institute; September 1993. Publication NIH 93–3095.

mean TC:HDL-C in CAD and non-CAD subjects is approximately 5.5 and 5.0 respectively. A desirable ratio is below 4.5 and the optimal TC:HDL-C ratio is less than 3.5.

Observational Studies With Pre-existing CAD

Coronary arteriographic studies have demonstrated a dose-response relationship between HDL-C levels and number and severity of diseased vessels (see reviews by Moore and Pearson). Undoubtedly, the most important variable associated with an increased coronary death rate is the presence of CAD at study baseline. Pekkanen and colleagues reviewed the mortality rates from the Lipid Research Clinics Program Prevalence Study and found that while death rates were always highest in men at the lowest HDL-C tertile, the overall rate was magnified with preexisting CAD (Fig. 5.8).

One interesting observation has been the association between low HDL-C and increased rate of coronary restenosis following angioplasty. In one study from Cedars-Sinai, an HDL-C less than 40 mg/dL was associated with a restenosis rate

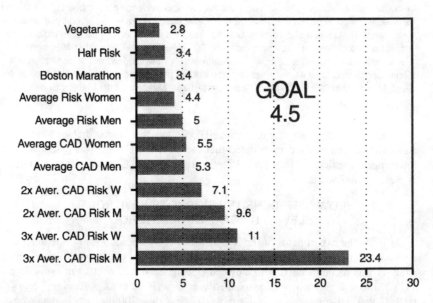

Figure 5.7. Total cholesterol:HDL-C ratio from the Framingham Heart Study. Reproduced with permission from Castelli WP. Cholesterol and lipids in the risk of coronary artery disease—The Framingham Heart Study. Can J Cardiol 1988;4(suppl A):5A–10A.

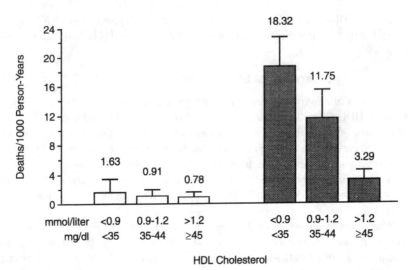

Figure 5.8. Age-adjusted rates of death from CHD per 1000 person-years of followup, according to HDL-C level, for men with and men without evidence of cardiovascular disease at baseline. Men without cardiovascular disease at baseline are represented by open bars, and men with evidence of cardiovascular disease by shaded bars. The T bars indicate the standard errors. Reprinted by permission of The New England Journal of Medicine from Pekkanen J, Linn S, Heiss G, et al. Ten-year mortality from cardiovascular disease in relation to cholesterol level among men with and without preexisting cardiovascular disease. N Engl J Med. 1990;322:1700–1707. Copyright © 1990, Massachusetts Medical Society.

of 64%, a fourfold greater rate than with HDL-C more than 40 mg/dL (see Shah and Amin). A second study demonstrated that the TC:HDL-C ratio was a significant independent predictor of restenosis. Whether raising HDL-C affects restenosis rates is presently unknown.

LOW HIGH-DENSITY LIPOPROTEIN WITHOUT ELEVATED TOTAL CHOLESTEROL

In 1988, the expert panel of the NCEP issued recommendations for the diagnosis and treatment of hyperlipidemia in adults. Whereas a complete lipoprotein analysis was recommended with elevated (greater than 240 mg/dL) or borderline TC (200 to 240 mg/dL), with associated coronary risk factors, screening for low HDL-C was not suggested with desirable TC (less than 200 mg/dL). In data from FHS, however, approximately 20% of MI survivors evidenced desirable TC (Fig. 5.9). Abbott and coworkers from Framingham had shown that the incidence of an

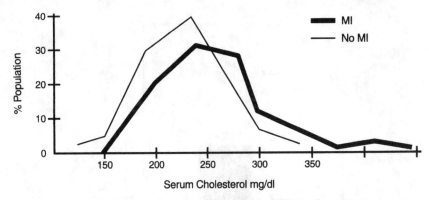

Figure 5.9. The distribution of baseline serum total cholesterol levels among Framingham men according to whether the men did (bold line) or did not (fine line) have a myocardial infarction within the first 16 years of the study. Entry ages were 30 to 40 years. The great deal of overlap between the plotted distributions underscores the uncertainty of using total cholesterol as the sole lipid screen for CHD risk. Further discrimination of risk is particularly important in the total cholesterol range of 200 to 250 mg/dL, where MI occurrence peaks yet there is full overlap between the distributions. Reprinted from Castelli WP, et al. A population at risk. Prevalence of high cholesterol levels in hypertensive patients in the Framingham study. American Journal of Medicine Supplement: 80:2A; February 14, 1986; 23 to 32.

initial MI was significantly elevated in normocholesterolemic subjects with low HDL-C. Subsequently, in PHS, a threefold increased risk of initial MI was observed in low HDL-C subjects with TC < 212 mg/dL (Fig. 5.10).

To examine the prevalence of low HDL-C in patients with documented CAD, data were reviewed from 1,000 patients who had diagnostic coronary arteriography performed at the Johns Hopkins Hospital. Approximately 35% of patients had desirable TC levels. Among individuals with a desirable TC and CAD, two-thirds of the men and four-fifths of the women also had a low HDL-C (less than 35 mg/dL and less than 45 mg/dL, respectively) (Fig. 5.11). Similar results were obtained by Ginsberg and associates at the Beth Israel Hospital in Boston. The high prevalence of low HDL-C in CAD patients (see also Aronow & Ahn, BIP Study Group, French et al., Genest et al., and Romm et al.) verified that a low HDL-C was the most common lipoprotein abnormality in CAD patients, irrespective of TC.

To evaluate the long-term implications of low HDL-C in the setting of desirable TC and CAD, 107 men and women were followed for 13 years. There was a markedly reduced survival rate from subsequent cardiovascular events with HDL-C less than 0.9 mmol/L (35 mg/dL) (Fig. 5.12) and a twofold increase in events compared with a baseline HDL-C exceeding 35 mg/dL. As a result of accumulating

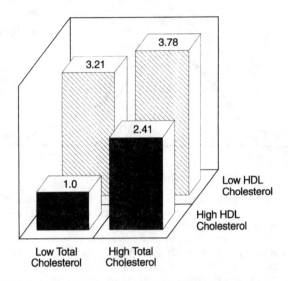

Figure 5.10. Relative risks of MI for subjects with values above and below the median for total and HDL-C cholesterol levels. The median for total cholesterol was 5.49 mmol per liter. The interaction of total cholesterol and HDL-C cholesterol was statistically significant in a model that also included total cholesterol and HDL-C cholesterol as separate terms. P = 0.01. Reprinted by permission of The New England Journal of Medicine from Stampfer MJ, Sacks FM, Salvini S, Willett WC, Hennekens CH. A prospective study of cholesterol, apolipoproteins, and the risk of myocardial infarction. N Engl J Med 1991;325:373–381. Copyright © 1991, Massachusetts Medical Society.

data and validated accuracy of HDL-C measurements, the expert panel of the NCEP reconvened and recommended that HDL-C be tested in all subjects at risk for CAD. In addition, the revised guidelines published in 1993 added an elevated HDL-C (greater than 60 mg/dL) as a negative cardiac risk factor (Fig. 5.13).

DETERMINANTS OF HIGH-DENSITY LIPOPROTEIN LEVELS

Table 5.2 summarizes the primary determinants influencing HDL-C levels. They include genetic, metabolic, dietary/environmental factors, and pharmaceuticals. Dietary/environmental factors and pharmaceuticals will be discussed in the treatment section below. An important caveat is that physiologic stress brought on by an acute illness (e.g., MI) may significantly reduce HDL-C levels (15–30%). A patient presenting with acute chest pain and suspected MI may have HDL-C levels mea-

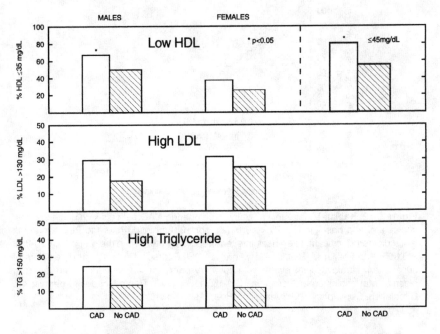

Figure 5.11. Prevalence of lipid and lipoprotein abnormalities with or without CAD and total cholesterol ≤200 mg/dL. From Miller M, Mead LA, Kwiterovich PO, Pearson TA. Dyslipidemias with desirable plasma total cholesterol levels and angiographically demonstrated coronary artery disease. Am J Cardiol 1990;65:1–5. Used with permission.

sured with reasonable accuracy provided they are drawn within 12 hours of initial presentation. A dietary fat load can also reduce HDL-C transiently (see Chapter 6).

RANDOMIZED TRIALS

Numerous trials have evaluated the efficacy of LDL-C lowering on CAD event rate, but much less information has been available on HDL-C raising in assessing clinical outcome. In the Helsinki Heart Study (see Frick et al.) there was a 34% reduction in primary CAD events among subjects assigned to gemfibrozil. Overall, HDL-C rose approximately 10% with the greatest increases (25%) observed at the lowest baseline HDL-C (less than 35 mg/dL). Importantly, raising HDL-C was independently associated with CAD event reduction; each 1% rise in HDL-C with gemfibrozil was associated with a 3% reduction in CAD event rate.

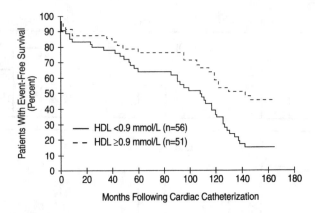

Figure 5.12. Kaplan-Meier survival analysis comparing CAD patients with desirable total cholesterol and baseline HDL-C <0.9 mmol/L or ≥0.9 mmol/L. Peto and Peto's log-rank test indicates significant differences in event-free survival between the groups. Z=-2.80; P = 0.005. From Miller M, Seidler A, Kwiterovich PO, Pearson TA. Long-term predictors of subsequent cardiovascular events with coronary artery disease and 'desirable' levels of plasma total cholesterol. Circulation. 1992;86:1165–1170. Reproduced with permission. Circulation. Copyright © 1992 American Heart Association.

While a number of arteriographic studies such as CLAS & FATS (see Brown et al.) evidenced reduced progression or CAD regression, these effects coincided with both significant LDL-C lowering and HDL-C raising; thus, it is difficult to dissect out the individual contribution of HDL-C. Interestingly, beneficial arteriographic changes may extend to subjects without marked baseline hyperlipidemia. In FATS, more regression was observed with lower (152 mg/dL) LDL-C levels (see Table 5.3). More recently, subgroup analysis from 4S revealed reductions in CAD rate for patients with the lowest entering LDL-C levels.

RAISING AN ISOLATED LOW HIGH-DENSITY LIPOPROTEIN

There have now been five randomized studies examining the effect of raising low HDL-C (less than 35 mg/dL) in "normolipidemic" (TC less than 240 mg/dL) subjects (Table 5.4). Gemfibrozil raised HDL-C modestly (9%) in the two studies using this medication. In the 1993 study, the entry criteria were stringent and included fasting TC of less than 200 mg/dL and TG less than 150 mg/dL. In subjects with TG greater than 95 mg/dL, a 15% increase in HDL-C was observed. The 30% increase in HDL-C reported with niacin use is noteworthy, although a paradoxical 10% rise in TG was also observed. Moreover, in the study by King et al.,

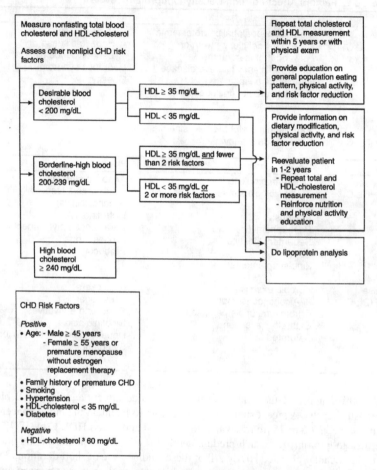

Figure 5.13. Primary prevention in adults without evidence of CHD: Initial classification based on total cholesterol and HDL-C cholesterol. From the National Cholesterol Education Program. Second Report of the Expert Panel on Detection, Evaluation, and Treatment of High Blood Cholesterol in Adults (Adult Treatment Panel II): Executive Summary. National Heart, Lung, and Blood Institute; September 1993. Publication NIH 93–3096.

Table 5.2. Factors Affecting High-Density Lipoprotein Levels

	Genetic	Metabolic
Low HDL-C	Familial hypoalphalipoproteinemia Apo A-I deficiency (with or without planar xanthomas) LCAT deficiency/fish eye disease Tangier disease Apo A-I variants (includes Apo A-I Milano)	Diabetes mellitus Hepatic disease Hypertriglyceridemia Nephrotic syndrome Obesity
High HDL-C	Familial hyperalphalipoproteinemia CETP deficiency	

	Dietary/Environmental	Pharmaceuticals
Reduce HDL-C	Cigarette smoking Physiologic stress Polyunsaturated fat Postprandial lipemia Sedentary lifestyle Sepsis Zinc supplementation	Anabolic steroids β-Blockers (especially nonselective) Isotretinoin A Parasympatholytic agents Progesterone Probucol
Raise HDL-C	Aerobic exercise Alcohol consumption Chromium supplementation Cigarette cessation Saturated fat	α-Blockers Estrogen Fibric acid derivatives Nicotinic acid Hepatic microsomal inducers Sympathomimetics

only 60% completed the study due to adverse side effects and abnormal blood chemistry results. A recent study using phenytoin to maintain the blood concentrations between 7.5 to 15 μg/mL was well tolerated and raised HDL-C by 12.4%. In contrast to gemfibrozil, which predominantly raised HDL_3, the niacin and phenytoin significantly elevated HDL_2. All of these studies were of short duration (3 to 4 months). A Veterans Administration multicenter trial is currently examining whether the use of gemfibrozil will reduce CAD event rates in normolipidemic subjects with low HDL-C.

Listed below are some of the more important exogenous factors affecting HDL-C levels.

Aerobic Exercise

Elite athletes maintain HDL-C levels approximately 20 mg/dL higher than sedentary individuals. However, the effect of aerobic conditioning on HDL-C lev-

Table 5.3. Stenosis Regression Dependence on Initial Lipid Levels

	Control	Treatment
CLAS[1] (TC <240)	0.7	0.3
CLAS (TC >240)	0.9	0.3
MARS[2] (TC <240)	0.7	0.4
MARS (TC >240)	1.1	0.5
FATS[3] (LDL-C = 152)	2.4%	−1.4%
FATS (LDL-C = 220)	1.8%	−0.2%

[1] Cashin-Hemphill L, Mack WJ, Pogoda JM, Sanmarco ME, et al. Beneficial effects of colestipol-niacin on coronary atherosclerosis: A 4-year followup. JAMA 1990;264:3013–3017.
[2] Blankenhorn DH, Azen SP, Kramsch et al. Coronary angiographic changes with lovastatin therapy: the Monitored Atherosclerosis Regression Study (MARS). Ann Intern Med 1993;119:969–976.
[3] Brown G, Albers JJ, Fisher LD, Schaefer SM, et al. Regression of coronary artery disease as a result of intensive lipid-lowering therapy in men with high levels of apolipoprotein B. N Engl J Med 1990;323:1289–1298.

Table 5.4. Randomized, Placebo-Controlled Trials Examining the Effect of High-Density Lipoprotein-Raising Medications in Normolipidemic Subjects With Low High-Density Lipoprotein

	Year	N	Pharmaceutical	% HDL-C Increase
Vega and Grundy[1]	1989	22	Gemfibrozil	9%
Lavie et al[2]	1992	19	Niacin	27%
Miller et al[3]	1993	14	Gemfibrozil	9%
King et al[4]	1994	15	Niacin	30%
Miller et al[5]	1995	39	Phenytoin	12%

[1] Vega GL, Grundy SM. Comparison of lovastatin and gemfibrozil in normolipidemic patients with hypoalphalipoproteinemia. JAMA 1989;262:3148–3153.
[2] Lavie CJ, Mailander L, Milani RV. Marked benefit with sustained-release niacin therapy in patients with "isolated" very low levels of high-density lipoprotein cholesterol and coronary artery disease. Am J Cardiol 1992;69:1083–1085.
[3] Miller M, Bachorik PS, McCrindle BW, Kwiterovich PO Jr. Effect of gemfibrozil in men with primary isolated low high-density lipoprotein cholesterol: a randomized, double-blind, placebo-controlled, crossover study. Am J Med 1993;94:7–12.
[4] King JM, Crouse JR, Terry JG, Morgan TM, Spray BJ, Miller NE. Evaluation of effects of unmodified niacin on fasting and postprandial plasma lipids in normolipidemic men with hypoalphalipoproteinemia. Am J Med 1994;97:323–331.
[5] Miller M, Burgan R, Osterlund L, Segrest JP, Garber DW. A prospective, randomized trial of phenytoin in non-epileptic subjects with reduced HDL cholesterol. Arteriosclerosis, Thrombosis, and Vascular Biology 1995;15:2151–2156.

els is dependent on the intensity and duration of training. Williams and coworkers observed that sedentary men (median HDL-C = 48.0 mg/dL) had to jog 10 to 12 miles weekly for 1 year to derive the biggest increase (10 mg/dL) in HDL-C. Thompson et al., however, reported more modest increases in HDL-C (5 mg/dL or 13%) in sedentary men (mean HDL-C = 37 mg/dL) who instituted stationary bicycling (more than 4 hours of intense exercise weekly). The increase in HDL-C, evident in the 3rd month, occurred in the absence of weight loss. Among trained athletes, significant increases (10 mg/dL) in HDL-C were reported in women (mean HDL-C = 60 mg/dL) who quadrupled their training distance (1.5 to 6 miles/day) over a 15-month period. The results of short-term studies (less than 6 months) and less vigorous training (e.g., walking) have been variable and inconsistent. Aerobic exercise stimulates LPL activity, leading to increases in HDL_2, enhanced hydrolysis of TG-rich lipoproteins, and reduction of postprandial lipemia. As Krauss noted, the benefit of aerobic conditioning on HDL-C appears to be greatest in subjects with the highest baseline HDL-C levels. In view of the cardiovascular and psychological benefits attributable to exercise, aerobic conditioning should be recommended, even if the HDL-C raising response is meager.

Alcohol

There is a dose-response relationship between alcohol consumption and HDL-C. Compared to a teetotaler, the consumer of two drinks or 1 ounce of alcohol daily (e.g., 24 oz of beer, 8 oz of table wine, 2 shots of 80 proof spirits) will experience, on average, a 6 to 7 mg/dL increase in HDL-C. Increases in HDL-C induced by alcohol (up to 2 drinks daily) account for approximately 50% of its purported cardioprotective effect. Above 2 drinks daily, however, the risk of adverse cardiovascular (i.e., arrhythmias) and other health consequences begin to accelerate. Moreover, alcohol raises TG levels and should be used sparingly when fasting TG exceeds 200 mg/dL. Consumption of alcohol is associated with increases in both HDL-C subfractions. At moderate doses, the HDL-C raising effect appears to predominate in the HDL_3 subfraction (elevation in hepatic lipase activity), but in higher quantities and in chronic alcoholics, disproportionate elevations in HDL_2 occur, due to LPL stimulation.

Cigarette Cessation

Cigarette smoking is associated with reduced HDL-C. Criqui and coworkers reported that 1 pack/day male smokers showed an approximately 5 mg/dL, or 11% lowering of HDL-C. Results of the Framingham Offspring Study demonstrated similar decrements. HDL-C levels were also lower in pubescent children inhaling the passive smoke of their parents. Importantly, smoking cessation produces increases in HDL-C of 10–30%, an effect that may be observed within several weeks of quitting.

Steroid Hormones

ANABOLIC STEROIDS

The potency of HDL-C reduction by anabolic steroids is highly dependent on the route of administration. Orally administered anabolic steroids stimulate hepatic lipase activity; Thompson and associates reported HDL-C reductions of 33% with stanozolol. In contrast, increased hepatic metabolism following intramuscular administration limits HDL-C reduction; modest (9%) lowering was observed following testosterone injection.

HORMONE REPLACEMENT THERAPY

Estrogenic compounds raise HDL-C (particularly HDL_2) by inhibiting hepatic lipase activity. The use of 0.625 mg of conjugated estrogens daily has been associated with up to a 16% increase in HDL-C. Ethinyl estradiol has been shown to raise HDL-C by 21%. Similarly, transdermal estrogens also have a favorable impact on HDL-C. Stanczyk et al. reported a 23% increase in HDL-C following 6 months of estradiol-17β use. Thus, in contrast to the relative impotency of nonoral anabolic steroids on HDL-C, the avid binding of certain estrogenic compounds to hepatic receptors provides similar effects on HDL-C whether administered by oral or transdermal route.

The effect of progestational agents on HDL-C is related to dosage and potency. Medroxyprogesterone acetate (Provera), the most widely prescribed progestogen in the U.S., has been observed with an approximate 5–10% reduction in HDL-C. The use of other progestational agents (e.g., 19-nortestosterone), as shown by Hirvonen et al., has been associated with up to a 20% reduction in HDL-C.

ORAL CONTRACEPTIVES

The effect of oral contraceptives on lipids and lipoproteins was evaluated in more than 1,000 women by Godsland et al. The percent difference in HDL-C with oral contraceptive use based on the various combinations employed is illustrated in Figure 5.14. Decrements in HDL-C were observed with 250LG/30EE (not available in the U.S.), 150LG/30EE (Nordette, Levlen), and 1000NE/35EE (Ortho-Novum 1/35, Norinyl 1 + 35), although the latter was not significant. Small but nonsignificant increments in HDL-C were found with 50–125LG/30–40EE (Triphasil, Tri-levlen) and 500–1000NE/35EE (Ortho-Novum 7/7/7). Significant increases in HDL-C (10–15%) were reported with 500NE/35EE (Modicon, Brevicon) and 150DG/30EE (not available in the U.S.).

Obesity

There is a negative correlation between body mass index and HDL-C. In the Framingham Offspring Study, a 5-lb weight gain was associated with a 5% reduc-

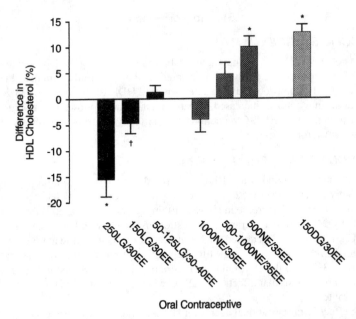

Figure 5.14. Percent differences in HDL-C cholesterol levels in response to oral glucose-tolerance tests between women taking one of seven combination oral contraceptives and those not taking oral contraceptives. The T bars indicate 1 SD. The asterisk (P<0.001) and dagger (P<0.01) indicate significant differences between users and nonusers in the mean values for the principal metabolic variables. Reprinted by permission of The New England Journal of Medicine from Godsland IF, Crook D, Simpson R, et al. The effects of different formulations of oral contraceptive agents on lipid and carbohydrate metabolism. N Engl J Med 1990;323:1375–1381. Copyright © 1990, Massachusetts Medical Society.

tion in HDL-C. Low HDL-C is also a common feature in Syndrome X, a disorder characterized by regional adiposity, insulin resistance, hyperglycemia, hypertension, and hypertriglyceridemia. HDL-C is positively correlated with adipose tissue levels of LPL. With weight loss, LPL activity is stimulated and HDL-C is increased; subjects with elevated TG exhibit the most pronounced increases in HDL-C. Importantly, a weight loss maintenance period of several months may elapse before HDL-C increases (up to 20%) are observed. Weight loss also improves insulin sensitivity, yielding favorable reductions in plasma glucose, blood pressure, and TG-rich lipoproteins. Unfortunately, not all individuals will experience increases in HDL-C with weight loss. Included in this group are relatively lean subjects with normal TG.

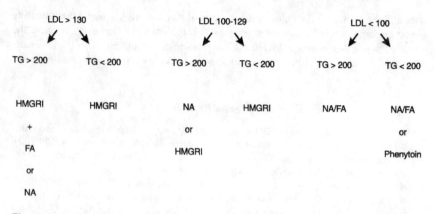

Figure 5.15. Algorithm for treatment of low HDL-C/CAD. TG = TR; HMGRI = HMG-CoA reductase inhibitor; FA = fibric acid; NA = nicotinic acid.

RECOMMENDATIONS

Pharmacologic therapy for dyslipidemia is focused on reducing elevated LDL-C. Although no formal recommendations for raising HDL-C exist, the authors believe that with CAD, a low HDL-C (defined as less than 35 mg/dL in men and less than 40 mg/dL in women) should be intensively addressed. Stratified by LDL-C and TG, the algorithm in Figure 5.15 addresses the pharmacologic management of low HDL-C. All patients should receive instruction regarding hygienic measures, including cigarette cessation, dietary reduction of total and saturated fat intake (less than 30% and 10% respectively, as outlined by the NCEP), and exercise/rehabilitation. Barring contraindications, hormone replacement therapy should be considered in all postmenopausal women.

Subjects with CAD are aggressively treated to reduce LDL-C to less than 100 mg/dL and TG to less than 200 mg/dL. This may necessitate combination or triple-drug therapy. When a second agent is added to an HMG-CoA reductase inhibitor, low doses of each medication should be initiated. The administration of more than one lipid-lowering agent necessitates regular monitoring of liver function tests (q 2–3 months), and patients must be informed of the potential undesirable effects such as myositis and rhabdomyolysis. These effects are most likely to occur with concomitant immunosuppressive therapy. Subjects receiving immunosuppressive agents must be closely monitored when systemic lipid-lowering drugs are used. Patients with low HDL-C and isolated TG or LDL-C elevation may effectively be managed with single-agent therapy as outlined. One CAD subgroup not addressed by the NCEP is isolated low HDL-C (e.g., LDL-C less than 100 mg/dL and TG less than 200 mg/dL). Unfortunately, there are no data currently available documenting whether aggressive management reduces CAD event rate. However, because the risk of new CAD events is increased, we recommend treatment with HDL-C raising agents, such as nicotinic acid, fibric acid derivatives, or microsomal inducers (e.g., phenytoin).

Suggested Readings

Abbott RD, Wilson PWF, Kannel WB, Castelli WP. High density lipoprotein cholesterol, total cholesterol screening, and myocardial infarction—The Framingham Study. Arteriosclerosis 1988;8:207–211.

Ameli S, Hultgardh-Nilsson A, Cercek B, Shah PK, et al. Recombinant apolipoprotein A-I Milano reduces intimal thickening after balloon injury in hypercholesterolemic rabbits. Circulation 1994;90:1935–1941.

Aoyama T, Yui Y, Morishita H, Kawai C. Prostaglandin I_2 half-life regulated by high density lipoprotein is decreased in acute myocardial infarction and unstable angina pectoris. Circulation 1990;81:1784–1791.

Aronow WS, Ahn C. Correlation of serum lipid with the presence or absence of coronary artery disease in 1,793 men and women aged ≥62 years. Am J Cardiol 1994; 73:702–703.

Assmann G, Schulte H, Funke H, von Eckardstein A, Seedorf U. The Prospective Cardiovascular Münster (PROCAM) Study: Identification of high-risk individuals for myocardial infarction and the role of HDL-C. In: Miller NE, ed. High density lipoproteins and atherosclerosis II. New York: Elsevier Science Publishers BV, 1989: 51–65.

Assmann G, von Eckardstein A, Funke H. High density lipoproteins, reverse transport of cholesterol, and coronary artery disease—insights from mutations. Circulation 1993;87(suppl III):III–28–III–34.

Benzafibrate Infarction Prevention (BIP) Study Group, Israel. Lipids and lipoproteins in symptomatic coronary heart disease.

Distribution, intercorrelations, and significance for risk classification in 6,700 men and 1,500 women. Circulation 1992;86: 839–848.

Black MR, Medeiros DM, Brunett E, Welke R. Zinc supplements and serum lipids in young adult white males. Am J Clin Nutr 1988;47:970–975.

Blankenhorn DH, Azen SP, Kramsch, et al. Coronary angiographic changes with lovastatin therapy: The Monitored Atherosclerosis Regression Study (MARS). Ann Intern Med 1993;119:969–976.

Brown G, Albers JJ, Fisher LD, Schaefer SM, et al. Regression of coronary artery disease as a result of intensive lipid-lowering therapy in men with high levels of apolipoprotein B. N Engl J Med 1990;323:1289–1298.

Carlson LA, Holmquist L. Fish eye disease. A lesson on plasma cholesterol esterification. In: Miller NE, ed. High density lipoproteins and atherosclerosis II. New York: Elsevier Science Publishers BV, 1989:95–102.

Cashin-Hemphill L, Mack WJ, Pogoda JM, Sanmarco ME, et al. Beneficial effects of colestipol-niacin on coronary atherosclerosis: A 4-year followup. JAMA 1990; 264:3013–3017.

Castelli WP, Anderson K. A population at risk. Prevalence of high cholesterol levels in hypertensive patients in the Framingham Study. Am J Med 1986;80(suppl 2A):23–32.

Castelli WP, Garrison RJ, Wilson PWF, Abbott RD, Kalousdian S, Kannel WB. Incidence of coronary heart disease and lipoprotein cholesterol levels—The Framingham Study. JAMA 1986;256:2835–2838.

Castelli WP, Wilson PWF, Levy D, Anderson K. Serum lipids and risk of coronary artery disease. Atherosclerosis Reviews 1990;21: 7–19.

Criqui MH, Wallace RB, Heiss G, Mishkiel M, Schonfeld G, Jones GTL. Cigarette smoking and plasma high-density lipoprotein cholesterol. The Lipid Research Clinics' Program Prevalence Study. Circulation 1980;62 (suppl IV):70–76.

Dammerman M, Breslow JL. Genetic basis of lipoprotein disorders. Circulation 1995; 91:505–512.

Frederickson DS, Altrocchi PH, Avioli LV, Goodman DS, et al. Tangier Disease. Ann Int Med 1961;55:1016–1031.

French JK, Elliott JM, Williams BF, Nixon DJ, et al. Association of angiographically detected coronary artery disease with low levels of high-density lipoprotein cholesterol and systemic hypertension. Am J Cardiol 1993;71:505–510.

Frick MH, Elo O, Haapa K, et al. Helsinki Heart Study: Primary-prevention trial with gemfibrozil in middle-aged men with dyslipidemia: Safety of treatment, changes in risk-factors, and incidence of coronary heart disease. N Engl J Med 1987;317: 1237–1245.

Garrison RJ, Kannel WB, Feinleib M, Castelli WP, McNamara PM, Padgett SJ. Cigarette smoking and HDL-C cholesterol: The Framingham Offspring Study. Atherosclerosis 1978;30:17.

Gaziano JM, Buring JE, Breslow JL, et al. Moderate alcohol intake, increased levels of high-density lipoprotein and its subfractions, and decreased risk of myocardial infarction. N Engl J Med 1993;329: 1829–1834.

Genest JJ, McNamara JR, Salem DN, Schaefer EJ. Prevalence of risk factors in men with premature coronary artery disease. Am J Cardiol 1991;67:1185–1189.

Genest JJ, Corbett HM, McNamara JR, Schaefer MM, Salem DN, Schaefer EJ. Effect of hospitalization on high-density lipoprotein cholesterol in patients undergoing elective coronary angiography. Am J Cardiol 1988;61:998–1000.

Ginsburg GS, Safran C, Pasternak RC. Frequency of low serum high-density lipoprotein cholesterol levels in hospitalized patients with "desirable" total cholesterol levels. Am J Cardiol 1991;68:187–192.

Glueck CJ, Gartside P, Fallat RW, Sielski J, Steiner PM. Longevity syndromes: Familial hypobeta and familial hyperalpha lipoproteinemia. J Lab Clin Med 1976;88:941–957.

Godsland IF, Crook D, Simpson R, et al. The effects of different formulations of oral contraceptive agents on lipid and carbohydrate metabolism. N Engl J Med 1990;323: 1375–1381.

Goldbourt U, Medalie JH. High density lipoprotein cholesterol and incidence of coronary heart disease—the Israeli Ischemic Heart Disease Study. Am J Epidemiol 1979;109:296–308.

Gordon DJ, Probstfield JL, Garrison RJ, et al. High-density lipoprotein cholesterol and cardiovascular disease—Four prospective American studies. Circulation 1989; 79:8–15.

Hirvonen E, Malkonen M, Manninen V. Effects of different progestogens on lipoproteins during postmenopausal replacement therapy. N Engl J Med 1981; 304:560–563.

Inazu A, Brown ML, Hesler CB, et al. Increased high-density lipoprotein levels caused by a common cholesteryl-ester transfer protein gene mutation. N Engl J Med 1990;323:1234–1238.

Kannel WB. Contribution of the Framingham Study to preventive cardiology. J Am Coll Cardiol 1990;15:206–211.

King JM, Crouse JR, Terry JG, Morgan TM, Spray BJ, Miller NE. Evaluation of effects of unmodified niacin on fasting and post-prandial plasma lipids in normolipidemic men with hypoalphalipoproteinemia. Am J Med 1994;97:323–331.

Klein H, Lohse P, Pritchard PH, Bojanovski D, Schmidt H, Brewer HB Jr. Two different allelic mutations in the lecithin-cholesterol acyltransferase gene associated with the fish eye syndrome. J Clin Invest 1992; 89:499–506.

Krauss RM. Exercise, lipoproteins, and coronary artery disease. Circulation 1989; 79:1143–1145.

Kuhn FE, Mohler ER, Satier LF, Reagan K, Lu DY, Rackley CE. Effects of high-density lipoprotein on acetylcholine-induced coronary vasoreactivity. Am J Cardiol 1991;68:1425–1430.

Lavie CJ, Mailander L, Milani RV. Marked benefit with sustained-release niacin therapy in patients with "isolated" very low levels of high-density lipoprotein cholesterol and coronary artery disease. Am J Cardiol 1992;69:1083–1085.

Livshits G, Weisbort J, Meshulam N, Brunner D. Multivariate analysis of the twenty-year follow-up of the Donolo-Tel Aviv prospective coronary artery disease study and the usefulness of high density lipoprotein cholesterol percentage. Am J Cardiol 1989;63:676–681.

Matsuda Y, Hirata K, Inoue N, et al. High density lipoprotein reverses inhibitory effect of oxidized low density lipoprotein on endothelium-dependent arterial relaxation. Circ Res 1993;72:1103–1109.

Miller M, Bachorik PS, McCrindle BW, Kwiterovich PO Jr. Effect of gemfibrozil in men with primary isolated low high-density lipoprotein cholesterol: A randomized, double-blind, placebo-controlled, crossover study. Am J Med 1993;94:7–12.

Miller M, Burgan R, Osterlund L, Segrest JP, Garber DW. A prospective, randomized trial of phenytoin in non-epileptic subjects with reduced HDL cholesterol. Arteriosclerosis, Thrombosis, and Vascular Biology 1995;15:2151–2156.

Miller M, Mead LA, Kwiterovich PO Jr, Pearson TA. Dyslipidemias with desirable plasma total cholesterol levels and angiographically demonstrated coronary artery disease. Am J Cardiol 1990;65:1–5.

Miller M, Seidler A, Kwiterovich PO, Pearson TA. Long-term predictors of subsequent cardiovascular events with coronary artery disease and 'desirable' levels of plasma total cholesterol. Circulation 1992;86:1165–1170.

Miller M, Zeller K, Kwiterovich PO, Albers JJ, Feulner G. Lecithin:cholesterol acyltransferase deficiency:identification of two defective alleles in fibroblast cDNA. J Lipid Res 1995;36:931–938.

Miller NE. Associations of high-density lipoprotein subclasses and apolipoproteins with ischemic heart disease and coronary atherosclerosis. Am Heart J 1987; 113:589–597.

Miller NE, Thelle DS, Førde OH, Mjøs OD. The Tromsø Heart-Study—High-density lipoprotein and coronary heart-disease: A prospective case-control study. Lancet 1977;1:965–970.

Moore RD, Pearson TA. Moderate alcohol consumption and coronary artery disease—a review. Medicine 1986;65(4):242–267.

Morishita H, Yui Y, Hattori R, Aoyama T, Kawai C. Increased hydrolysis of cholesteryl ester with prostacyclin is potentiated by high density lipoprotein through the prostacyclin stabilization. J Clin Invest 1990;86:1885–1891.

Moskowitz WB, Mosteller M, Schieken RM, et al. Lipoprotein and oxygen transport alterations in passive smoking preadolescent children: The MCV Twin Study. Circulation 1990;81:586–592.

Norum KR, Gjone E, Glomset JA. Familial lecithin:cholesterol acyltransferase deficiency, including fish eye disease. In Metabolic Basis of Inherited Disease. Ed. Scriver 1989, chapter 46:1181–1194.

Pearson TA. Coronary arteriography in the study of the epidemiology of coronary artery disease. Epidemiol Rev 1984; 6:140–166.

Pekkanen J, Linn S, Heiss G, et al. Ten-year mortality from cardiovascular disease in relation to cholesterol level among men with and without preexisting cardiovascular disease. N Engl J Med 1990;322: 1700–1707.

Rader DJ, Ikewaki K, Duverger N, et al. Very low high-density lipoproteins without coronary atherosclerosis. Lancet 342;1993: 1455–1458.

Reis GJ, Kuntz RE, Silverman DI, Pasternak RC. Effects of serum lipid levels on restenosis after coronary angioplasty. Am J Cardiol 1991;68:1431–1435.

Roeback JR Jr, Hla KM, Chambless LE, Fletcher RH. Effects of chromium supplementation on serum high-density lipoprotein cholesterol levels in men taking beta-blockers. Ann Intern Med 1991; 115:917–924.

Romm PA, Green CE, Reagan K, Rackley CE. Relation of serum lipoprotein cholesterol levels to presence and severity of angiographic coronary artery disease. Am J Cardiol 1991;67:479–483.

Rönnemaa T, Viikari J, Irjala K, Peltola O. Marked decrease in serum HDL-C cholesterol level during acute myocardial infarction. Acta Med Scand 1980;207:161–166.

Sacks FM, Pasternak RC, Gibson CM, Rosner B, Stone PH. Effect on coronary atherosclerosis of decrease in plasma cholesterol concentrations in normocholesterolaemic patients. Lancet 1994;344:1182–1186.

Saku K, Ahmad M, Glas-Greenwalt P, Kashyap ML. Activation of fibrinolysis by apolipoproteins of high density lipoproteins in man. Thromb Res 1985;39:1–8.

Scandinavian Simvastatin Survival Study Group. Randomised trial of cholesterol lowering in 4444 patients with coronary heart disease: The Scandinavian Simvastatin Survival Study (4S). Lancet 1994;344: 1383–1389.

Shah PK, Amin J. Low high density lipoprotein level is associated with increased restenosis rate after coronary angioplasty. Circulation 1992;85:1279–1285.

Stampfer MJ, Sacks FM, Salvini S, Willett WC, Hennekens CH. A prospective study of cholesterol, apolipoproteins, and the risk of myocardial infarction. N Engl J Med 1991;325:373–381.

Stanczyk FZ, Shoupe D, Nunez V, et al. A randomized comparison of nonoral estradiol delivery in postmenopausal women. Am J Obstet Gynecol 1988;159:1540.

Takahashi K, Jiang X, Sakai N, et al. A missense mutation in the cholesteryl ester transfer protein gene with possible dominant effects on plasma high density lipoproteins. J Clin Invest 1993;92:2060–2064.

Taylor PA, Ward A. Women, high-density lipoprotein cholesterol, and exercise. Arch Intern Med 1993;153:1178–1184.

Thompson PD, Cullinane EM, Sady ST, et al. Contrasting effects of testosterone and stanozolol on serum lipoprotein levels. JAMA 1989;261:1165–1168.

Thompson PD, Cullinane EM, Sady SP, et al. Modest changes in high-density lipoprotein concentration and metabolism with prolonged exercise training. Circulation 1988;78:25–34.

Vega GL, Grundy SM. Comparison of lovastatin and gemfibrozil in normolipidemic patients with hypoalphalipoproteinemia. JAMA 1989;262:3148–3153.

Williams PT, Wood PD, Haskell WL, Vranizan K. The effects of running mileage and duration on plasma lipoprotein levels. JAMA 1982;247:2674–2679.

Yui Y, Aoyama T, Morishita H, Takahashi M, Takatsu Y, Kawai C. Serum prostacyclin stabilizing factor is identical to apolipoprotein A-I (Apo A-I)—a novel function of Apo A-I. J Clin Invest 1988;82:803–807.

6/ Triglycerides

While the evidence linking elevated LDL-C and low HDL-C to CAD is incontrovertible, the importance of triglycerides (TG) as a CAD risk factor remains speculative. Notwithstanding, there are several conditions where elevated TG is associated with CAD. They include diabetes mellitus (DM) and endogenous hypertriglyceridemia (Type IV). This chapter will summarize the evidence and the controversies relating CAD risk to hypertriglyceridemia.

BIOCHEMISTRY

Metabolism of TG-rich lipoproteins results from lipase induced hydrolysis followed by biliary solubilization and emulsification. After absorption within the intestinal villi, free fatty acids (FFAs) and partially hydrolyzed di- and monoglycerides are re-esterified and presented to the lymphatic circulation for packaging as chylomicrons. These particles enter the venous circulation via the thoracic duct and are rapidly cleared from the circulation by lipoprotein lipase (LPL) (see Chapter 4). The products of hydrolysis are smaller, cholesteryl-ester enriched chylomicron-remnant particles. A small percentage of hydrolyzed fatty acids, including small- and medium-chain glycerides, may instead be transported directly to the portal vein. Commercially available medium-chain TG products are available to subjects with impaired fat absorption or LPL deficiency.

In contrast to the smaller chylomicron remnant particles, which, like LDL-C, penetrate the endothelial barrier (see Chapter 2), the larger chylomicron particles are unable to traverse the endothelium. This may, in part, explain the paradox relating hypertriglyceridemia and CAD. For example, with very high TG (>1,000 mg/dL), chylomicrons predominate, and pancreatitis, rather than CAD, is the primary concern. On the other hand, moderate elevations in TG (200 to 500 mg/dL), enhance CAD risk owing to the predominance of smaller, atherogenic chylomicron remnants.

In the endogenous cascade of TG metabolism, hepatically synthesized VLDL-C is hydrolyzed by LPL, producing smaller cholesteryl-ester enriched particles, i.e., VLDL-C remnants, IDL-C, and LDL-C.

When TG is hydrolyzed by LPL, the following occurs:

1. FFAs are stored (e.g., in adipose tissue) or used as an energy source (e.g., muscle).
2. Transfer of surface components from chylomicrons or VLDL-C, including apos, PL, and FC, aid in the formation of HDL-C. Thus, efficient catabolism of TG-rich particles, as commonly observed in conditioned athletes, may be associated with low TG and high HDL-C levels. Conversely, when LPL activity is inhibited or reduced, both fasting and postprandial TG are elevated and HDL-C is low.

FASTING VS POSTPRANDIAL LIPEMIA

Although we routinely measure lipids and lipoproteins in the fasting state, the majority of each 24-hour period is, in fact, expended in the postabsorptive (post-

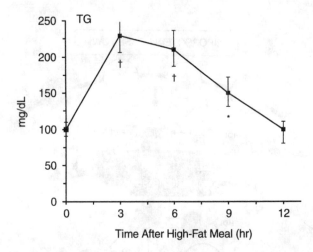

Figure 6.1. Postprandial changes in triglycerides are shown for 22 healthy subjects given a high-fat meal. TG = triglycerides. *p <0.01, †p <0.001 vs zero time. Adapted from Cohn JS, McNamara JR, Schaefer EJ. Lipoprotein cholesterol concentrations in the plasma of human subjects as measured in the fed and fasted states. Clin Chem 1988; 34:2456–2459. Used by permission.

prandial) state. Zilversmit hypothesized that atherogenesis is a postprandial phenomenon and postprandial rather than fasting TG measurements might provide a more accurate reflection of CAD risk. In subjects ingesting a high-fat meal, for example, the postprandial TG peak occurs between 2 and 4 hours and returns to baseline by 12 hrs (Fig. 6.1). Delayed clearance of postprandial fat has been reported with elevated fasting TG (>200 mg/dL), CAD, DM and with hyperapobetalipoproteinemia (hyperapoB). Recently, Uiterwaal and colleagues demonstrated that healthy adult men (mean age 25 years) with a familial predisposition to CAD displayed a prolonged postprandial TG response compared to control subjects, suggesting a link between postprandial lipid metabolism and familial risk of CAD. The delayed clearance of chylomicron remnants results in their avid non-regulated uptake by scavenger cells, thereby contributing to accelerated atherogenicity.

The metabolic relationship between postprandial TG and HDL-C is complex. As proposed by Patsch and colleagues (Fig. 6.2), elevated LPL is associated with effective transfer of surface components between TG-rich particles and HDL-C. However, with reduced LPL activity, the CETP mediated exchange of TG for CE is enhanced, producing a TG-rich HDL. The HDL_2 particle is further hydrolyzed by hepatic lipase to HDL_3. The associated LDL-C particles are small, dense and pro-

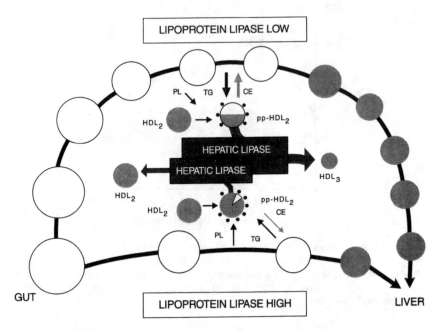

Figure 6.2. Metabolic relationship of HDL and triglyceride metabolism in postprandial state. Hepatic lipase removes phospholipids from triglyceride-rich lipoprotein surface and hydrolyzes core triglycerides. PL = phospholipids; TG = triglycerides; CE = cholesteryl ester; pp = postprandial. From Patsch W. Plasma triglycerides and coronary artery disease. Newspaper of Cardiology. March 1991:26. Used with permission.

tein-enriched. These particles appear to have an inherent greater tendency to be more avidly oxidized and taken up by macrophages. Thus, in addition to elevated TG and low HDL-C, hypertriglyceridemic subjects may also possess elevations in small, dense LDL-C particles thereby enhancing CAD risk (see Austin).

In addition to the fasting TG level, it has been proposed that HDL-C is an important inverse predictor of the postprandial response to fat. However, when subjects with isolated low HDL-C were administered a fat load, a reduced rather than increased postprandial response was observed (Fig. 6.3).

In general, postprandial studies provide an additional index for CAD risk assessment. Unfortunately, they are also very time consuming and less feasible to routinely perform by clinicians through fasting TG measurements.

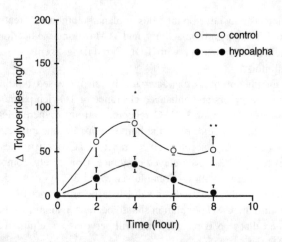

Figure 6.3. Line plot of change in postprandial plasma triglyceride levels. Increases over baseline (0 time) in control and hypoalphalipoproteinemia (hypoalpha) subjects are shown. Significantly different from baseline at *P=0.02, **P=0.03. From Miller M, Kwiterovich PO, Bachorik PS, Georgopoulos A. Decreased postprandial response to a fat meal in normotriglyceridemic men with hypoalphalipoproteinemia. Arterioscler Thromb 1993;13:385–392. Used with permission. Arteriosclerosis and Thrombosis. Copyright © 1993 American Heart Association.

MECHANISMS OF TRIGLYCERIDE ELEVATION AND CORONARY ARTERY DISEASE

Apolipoprotein E Phenotypes

Apo E, located on the surface of TG-rich remnant particles (e.g. IDL-C, chylomicron, VLDL-C) mediates their uptake by specific hepatic receptors. There are three different alleles in the apo E gene with a following population frequency: Σ2 (10%), Σ3 (75%), and Σ4 (15%). The frequency of each phenotype is 4/4 (2%), 4/3 (23%), 4/2 (3%), 3/3 (56%), 3/2 (15%), and 2/2 (1%). Patients with type III (familial dysbetalipoproteinemia) are homozygous for the E2 allele (E2/E2). As apo E2 is defective in binding to hepatic remnant receptors, affected subjects have impaired removal of cholesterol-enriched TG-rich remnants, or β-VLDL, from the circulation. Elevation in TG and TC contribute to the higher rate of premature CAD and peripheral vascular disease. Interestingly, only 2% of subjects with apo E2 homozygosity develop the typical clinical manifestations. Familial dysbetalipoproteinemia may be unmasked by hypothyroidism, DM, or renal insufficiency. As noted in

Chapter 3, subjects may develop tuberous or planar xanthomas. Treatment includes a low-saturated-fat diet, aerobic activity, and TG-lowering medications (e.g., gemfibrozil), often in combination with LDL-C reducing agents (e.g., HMG-CoA reductase inhibitors).

The apo E4 phenotype is characterized by an increased binding affinity to hepatic remnant receptors and enhanced clearance of TG-rich particles. However, owing to downregulation of LDL-C receptor activity, hypercholesterolemia is often manifest. Thus, in contrast to the homozygous E3 phenotype, E4 heterozygosity (e.g., E4/3) displays accelerated clearance of TG-rich particles, whereas E2 heterozygotes (e.g., E3/2) have delayed clearance. Conversely, compared to E3/3, LDL-C levels are higher with E4/3 and lower with E3/2. As methodology for apo E phenotyping has only recently been validated, the prevalence of the various apo E isoforms within the CAD population should become available in the near future. It is anticipated that apo E phenotyping will serve as an adjunctive measure in assessing CAD risk.

THROMBOGENIC EFFECTS

The association between hypertriglyceridemia and enhanced thrombogenicity stems from associated elevations in fibrinogen and clotting factors VII, VIII, and X. Reduced levels of endogenous tissue plasminogen activator (TPA) owing to increased plasminogen activator inhibitor (PAI) have also been observed with high TG. Hamsten and coworkers correlated elevated TG and low endogenous TPA activity in survivors (less than 45 years) of initial MI. In a subsequent study, they demonstrated that PAI was a risk factor for recurrent MI in this subgroup.

TG MEASUREMENTS

In contrast to other lipoproteins, TG measurements yield greater biologic (10–20%) and analytic (5–10%) variability. The following factors acutely raise TG: alcohol, certain medications (see below), illness or physiologic stress, postprandial state (see below), and posture (Fig. 6.4). Several fasting (more than 12 hours) samples obtained in the same postural position and measured by the same laboratory would minimize this variability.

Triglyceride Levels

As outlined by the Adult Treatment Panel of the NCEP, the definition and stratification of TG as adopted from the 1992 NIH Consensus Development Conference are listed in Table 6.1.

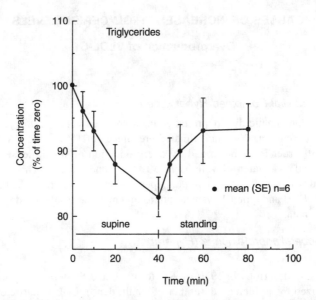

Figure 6.4. Changes in triglyceride concentrations in six subjects assuming the supine or standing position. Values (mean, SE) are expressed as percent of baseline. From Miller M, Bachorik PS, Cloey TA. Normal variation of plasma lipoproteins: Postural effects on plasma concentrations of lipids, lipoproteins, and apolipoproteins. Clin Chem 1992;38:569–574. Used with permission.

Table 6.1. Definition and Stratification of Triglyceride Levels

Category	Triglyceride Level
Normal	<200 mg/dL
Borderline	200–400 mg/dL
High	400–1,000 mg/dL
Very High	>1,000 mg/dL

CAUSES OF INCREASED TRIGLYCERIDE LEVELS

Overproduction of VLDL-C

GENETIC

Type IIb Familial Combined Hyperlipidemia

Among the genetic dyslipoproteinemias associated with CAD, type IIb FCH is the most common. With an estimated prevalence of 15% in the CAD population, the disorder is characterized by overproduction of small, dense VLDL-C particles and associated elevations in VLDL-C and LDL-C. This disorder is associated with familial dyslipidemic hypertension and Syndrome X. In contrast to type IIa FCH and type III dysbetalipoproteinemia, these subjects do not develop xanthomata.

Hyperapobetalipoproteinemia (HyperapoB)

Originally described in 1980 by Kwiterovich and Sniderman, hyperapoB is characterized by an increased number of small, dense, LDL-C particles. In this disorder, apo B levels are elevated (>120 mg/dL) in the presence of normal or mildly elevated LDL-C (<160 mg/dL). The ratio of apo B:LDL-C is > 1.2:1. In addition to mild elevations in TG, HDL-C is low. The prevalence of premature CAD is increased (see Kwiterovich et al.). As with familial combined hyperlipidemia, patients with hyperapoB do not develop specific physical stigmata. Postprandial lipemia commonly accompanies these syndromes.

Type IV Familial Hypertriglyceridemia

Overproduction of VLDL-C is also associated with type IV familial hypertriglyceridemia. In this disorder, TG exceeds 200 mg/dL, in the absence of hypercholesterolemia. The disorder is autosomal dominant and associated with premature CAD.

ENVIRONMENTAL

Causes for enhanced VLDL-C production include alcohol, bile acid sequestrants, carbohydrate diet (more than 65% of total caloric intake), diuretics, estrogen, glucocorticoids, hepatic microsomal inducers (e.g., phenytoin), obesity, and retinoids. In contrast to the small/dense VLDL-C particles overproduced in type IIb familial combined hyperlipidemia (see below) and the hyperapo B syndrome, VLDL-C particles are larger and are not believed to be atherogenic. The mechanism of β-blocker induced TG elevation is discussed in Chapter 10.

Reduced Catabolism of VLDL-C

GENETIC

Type III Familial Dysbetalipoproteinemia

Delayed clearance of TG-rich particles has also been reported with paraproteinemias (systemic lupus erythematosus (SLE), multiple myeloma) and renal failure (including hemodialysis and peritoneal dialysis). (See page 89.)

Systemic Diseases Associated With Elevated Triglycerides

DIABETES

Insulin-Dependent

Diabetic ketoacidosis may be associated with hypertriglyceridemia owing to attenuated LPL activity. Insulin serves to enhance adipocyte-derived FFA supply, which drives hepatic VLDL-C production. Conversely, complete insulin deficiency leads to FFA mobilization. The degree of TG elevation, however, is predicated on both FFA mobilization and hepatic VLDL-C synthesis which may be impaired with insulin deficiency. Therefore, it is not uncommon to observe TG levels ranging from normal to elevated among insulin-dependent subjects.

Non-Insulin-Dependent

Elevated insulin levels are characteristic of the non-insulin-dependent state. Hyperinsulinemia stimulates VLDL-C and may lead to very high TG. It is associated with Syndrome X.

HYPOTHYROIDISM

The elevated TG reported in hypothyroidism occurs by either enhanced production of remnant particles (e.g., IDL-C) or reduced clearance of VLDL-C remnants due to reduction in hepatic lipase activity (see Abrams et al.). The addition of thyroxine normalizes TG.

NEPHROTIC SYNDROME

Overproduction of hepatic VLDL-C is the primary mechanism causing elevated TG and LDL-C (see Appel et al.). Abnormalities in remnant catabolism have also been proposed.

GENETIC STUDIES

As noted above, a primary regulator of TG metabolism is LPL. The LPL gene consists of 10 exons on the short arm of chromosome 8. Genetic deficiencies of

LPL (type I hyperlipidemia) results in TG > 1,000 mg/dL and are associated with pancreatitis. Partial defects in the LPL gene produce moderate TG elevations and/or low HDL-C. One recently reported mutation in the LPL gene may be associated with premature CAD (see Reymer et al.).

The molecular basis of other familial disorders associated with elevated TG remains elusive. While mutations in the apo B gene have been associated with FCH and hyperapoB, most studies have not uncovered genetic defects attributed to these disorders. Similarly, little information is presently available regarding genetic defects associated with type IV familial hypertriglyceridemia.

EPIDEMIOLOGY

The correlation between plasma TG and CAD observed in univariate analysis tends to weaken or disappear with adjustment for HDL-C. In the Prospective Cardiovascular Münster (PROCAM) study (see Assmann and Schulte), CAD event rates increased with elevation in TG (Fig. 6.5). The high CAD rates were observed with elevated TG and low HDL-C (Fig. 6.6). While hypertriglyceridemia was an additional risk factor in the presence of low HDL-C, it was not an independent pre-

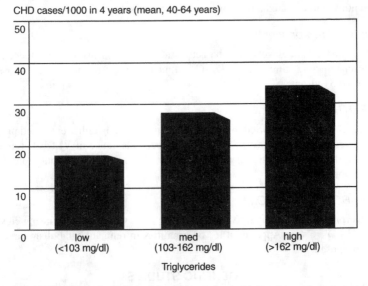

CHD cases/1000 in 4 years (mean, 40-64 years)

Triglycerides

Figure 6.5. PROCAM study: CHD incidence according to triglycerides. From Assmann G, Schulte H. Triglycerides and atherosclerosis: Results from the Prospective Cardiovascular Münster study. Atherosclerosis Reviews 1991;22:51–57. Used with permission.

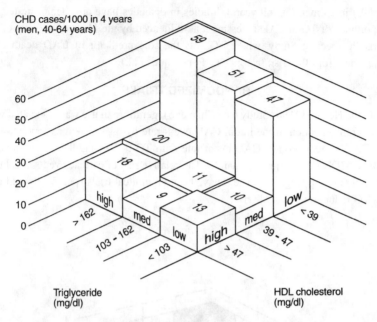

Figure 6.6. PROCAM study: CHD incidence according to triglycerides and HDL cholesterol. From Assmann G, Schulte H. Triglycerides and atherosclerosis: Results from the Prospective Cardiovascular Münster study. Atherosclerosis Reviews 1991;22:51–57. Used with permission.

dictor of CAD events in multiple regression analysis. Similarly, Criqui and coworkers analyzed the relationship between TG and CAD mortality from the Lipid Research Clinics (LRC) Follow-up Study. Although CAD death rate was positively correlated to TG levels, there was no overall independent association between TG and CAD mortality.

Some studies, however, have provided compelling evidence for TG as an independent predictor of CAD. They include studies performed in Scandinavia (see Carlson and Böttinger; Tverdal et al.) and the United Kingdom (see Bainton et al.). Indeed, TG appears to confer increased risk in certain subgroups. In the Paris Prospective Study, an independent effect of TG on CAD death was found only with TC ≤ 220 mg/dL (see Cambien et al.). Moreover, the Framingham Heart Study found TG to independently predict CAD in older women (>50 years). Similarly, the LRC follow-up study reported a near twofold increased mortality with moderate TG elevations (200–399 mg/dL) and a 3.5-fold excess death rate with higher TG (> 400 mg/dL) in women (50–69 years). Studies in diabetics have also demonstrated the importance of TG in CAD assessment as evidenced by the 11-year followup of the Paris Prospective Study, where TG was the sole predictor of CAD death after adjustment for other risk factors (see Fontbonne et al.).

RANDOMIZED TRIALS

In the Helsinki Heart Study (see Chapter 5), gemfibrozil use was associated with an overall reduction in the initial CAD event rate by 34%. Upon extrapolation of data, a 71% reduction in CAD event rate with TG > 200 mg/dL and an elevated LDL-C:HDL-C ratio (greater than 5). The relative risk of cardiac events was highest in this group (Fig. 6.7). There have been no clinical trials specifically addressing TG reduction and CAD risk.

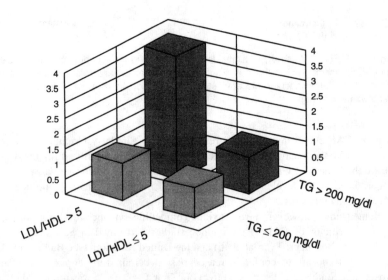

Figure 6.7. Helsinki Heart Study analysis: Relative risk of cardiac events. TG = triglycerides. From Manninen V, Tenkanen L, Koskinen P, et al. Joint effects of serum triglyceride and LDL cholesterol and HDL cholesterol concentrations on coronary heart disease risk in the Helsinki Heart Study. Circulation. 1992;85:37–45. Reproduced with permission. Circulation. Copyright © 1992 American Heart Association.

MANAGEMENT OF ELEVATED TRIGLYCERIDES

Nonpharmacologic

DIET

While reduction in total and saturated fat intake result in modest TC lowering (5–10%), the impact on TG may be considerable (~20%). Substitution of polyunsaturates (up to 10% of total calories) and monounsaturates (up to 15% of total calories) for saturated fat (less than 7% of calories) is outlined in the NCEP Step II Diet and is recommended with TG > 200 mg/dL. Examples of Step II menus for men and women aged 25 to 49 years are shown in Tables 6.2 and 6.3.

ω-3 FATTY ACIDS

Certain cold-water fish contain ω-3 fatty acids; the three primary ω-3 fatty acids are α-linolenic acid, docosahexaenoic acid (DHA), and eicosapentaenoic acid (EPA). Reduction in TG (30–50%) has been observed with ω-3 fatty acids due to reduction in hepatic VLDL-C and apo B synthesis. There is also attenuation in the postprandial TG response. Table 6.4 lists the ω-3 fat content of selected fish. Alternatively, fish-oil capsules may be used. Six fish-oil capsules contain the equivalent in ω-3 fatty acids to a 3.5-oz portion of Norwegian sardines. Unfortunately, the dose required to normalize TG in patients with FCH, 20 to 30 g/day, may also increase body weight, because the estimated 40 to 60 capsules required adds nearly 500 calories. The American Heart Association advocates consumption of fish three times weekly. In view of the lack of proven efficacy (compared with fish consumption) and potential side effects (e.g., GI distress, weight gain) fish-oil capsules are usually reserved for exceedingly high TG levels (greater than 1,000 mg/dL).

EXERCISE

Physical activity reduces TG by activating LPL. These effects occur after both acute and endurance training. The weight loss that often coincides with exercise is associated with reduction in VLDL-C synthesis.

SMOKING CESSATION

Cigarette smoking is associated with an elevation in TG (approximately 10%) because of catecholamine-mediated lipolysis of adipocytes. Smoking cessation is also associated with weight gain (mean = 10 lbs).

Pharmacologic

The primary TG-lowering medications are nicotinic acid and fibric acid derivatives (e.g., gemfibrozil and clofibrate). Nicotinic acid is a potent TG-lowering agent. It inhibits hepatic VLDL-C secretion by reducing FFA mobilization from

Table 6.2. Step II Sample Menus: Traditional American Cuisine, Males 25–49 Years

Breakfast

        Bagel, plain (1 medium)
                Margarine (2 tsp)
                Jelly (2 tsp)
        Cereal, shredded wheat (1 1/2 cups)
        Banana (1 small)
        Milk, skim (1 cup)
        Orange Juice (3/4 cup)
        Coffee (1 cup)
                Milk, skim (1 oz)

Lunch

        Minestrone Soup, canned, low sodium (1 1/2 cups)
        Roast Beef Sandwich
                Whole Wheat Bread (2 slices)
                *Lean Roast Beef, unseasoned (2 oz)
                American Cheese, low-fat and low sodium (3/4 oz)
                Lettuce (1 leaf)
                Tomato (3 slices)
                Margarine (2 tsp)
        Fruit and Cottage Cheese Salad
                Cottage Cheese, 1% and low sodium (1/2 cup)
                Peaches, canned in juice (1/2 cup)
                Apple Juice, unsweetened (1 cup)

Dinner

        *Flounder (3 oz)
                Vegetable Oil (1 tsp)
        *Baked Potato (1 medium)
                Margarine (2 tsp)
        *Green Beans (1/2 cup), seasoned with margarine (1/2 tsp)
        *Carrots (1/2 cup), seasoned with margarine (1/2 tsp)
        White Dinner Roll (1 medium)
                Margarine (1 tsp)
        Frozen Yogurt (1 cup)
        Iced Tea, unsweetened (1 cup)

Snack

        *Popcorn (3 cups)
                Margarine (1 T)

Calories	2,533	Total Carb, % kcals:	55
Total Fat, % kcals:	28	Simple Carb, % Carb:	36
SFA, % kcals:	6.6	Complex Carb, % Carb:	64
Cholesterol, mg:	150	*Sodium, mg:	1,803
Protein, % kcals:	17		

100% RDA met for all nutrients except: Zinc 90%
*No salt is added in recipe preparation or as seasoning. All margarine is low sodium.
From National Cholesterol Education Program. Second Report of the Expert Panel on Detection, Evaluation, and Treatment of High Blood Cholesterol in Adults (Adult Treatment Panel II). National Heart, Lung, and Blood Institute; September 1993. Publication NIH 93–3095.

Table 6.3. Step II Sample Menus: Traditional American Cuisine, Females 25–49 Years

Breakfast
- Bagel, plain (1/2 medium)
  - Margarine (1 tsp)
  - Jelly (1 tsp)
- Cereal, shredded wheat (1 cup)
- Banana (1 small)
- Milk, skim (1 cup)
- Orange Juice (1 cup)
- Coffee (1 cup)
  - Milk, skim (1 oz)

Lunch
- Minestrone Soup, canned, low sodium (1/2 cup)
- Roast Beef Sandwich
  - Whole Wheat Bread (2 slices)
  - *Lean Roast Beef, unseasoned (2 oz)
  - American Cheese, low-fat and low sodium (3/4 oz)
  - Lettuce (1 leaf)
  - Tomato (3 slices)
  - Margarine (2 tsp)
- Apple (1 medium)
- Water (1 cup)

Dinner
- *Flounder (3 oz)
  - Vegetable Oil (1 tsp)
- *Baked Potato (1/2 medium)
  - Margarine (1 tsp)
- *Green Beans (1/2 cup), seasoned with margarine (1/2 tsp)
- *Carrots (1/2 cup), seasoned with margarine (1/2 tsp)
- White Dinner Roll (1 medium)
  - Margarine (1 tsp)
- Frozen Yogurt (1/2 cup)
- Iced Tea, unsweetened (1 cup)

Snack
- *Popcorn (3 cups)
  - Margarine (2 tsp)

Calories	1,867	Total Carb, % kcals:	55
Total Fat, % kcals:	29	Simple Carb, % Carb:	38
SFA, % kcals:	6.8	Complex Carb, % Carb:	62
Cholesterol, mg:	134	*Sodium, mg:	1,417
Protein, % kcals:	16		

100% RDA met for all nutrients except: Zinc 90%
*No salt is added in recipe preparation or as seasoning. All margarine is low sodium.
From National Cholesterol Education Program. Second Report of the Expert Panel on Detection, Evaluation, and Treatment of High Blood Cholesterol in Adults (Adult Treatment Panel II). National Heart, Lung, and Blood Institute; September 1993. Publication NIH 93–3095.

Table 6.4. Best of the Catch

Eating fish rich in omega-3 fatty acids might help prevent heart disease. Omega-3 amounts are for a 100-gram (3.5-ounce) portion. A fish-oil capsule has up to .5 gram.

Omega-3s (grams)

Norway sardines*.	2.9
Atlantic mackerel.	2.6
Lake trout	2.0
Atlantic herring.	1.7
Albacore tuna	1.5
Anchovy.	1.4
Atlantic salmon.	1.4
Bluefish.	1.2
Pink salmon	1.0
Greenland halibut	9

Sources: U.S. Department of Agriculture. *William Connor, Oregon Health Sciences University. From Monmaney T. Fish oil and cholesterol: A megadose of hype?   Newsweek, April 13, 1987:67–68. Copyright 1987, Newsweek, Inc. All rights reserved. Reprinted by permission.

Table 6.5. Indications for Drug Therapy for Elevated Triglycerides

Diabetic dyslipidemia
Established CAD
Family history of premature CAD
Total cholesterol >240 mg/dL and HDL <35 mg/dL
Type IIB familial combined hyperlipidemia
HyperapoB
Type III familial dysbetalipoproteinemia
Type IV familial hypertriglyceridemia

adipocytes. Reductions in plasma TG levels (20–50%) have been reported with relatively low daily doses (1 to 1.5 g daily). The fibric acid derivatives are similarly effective in reducing plasma TG. These medications stimulate LPL activity and enhance the catabolism of TG-rich particles. Two other fibric acid derivatives currently used in Europe, bezafibrate and fenofibrate, have not yet been approved by the FDA.

RECOMMENDATIONS

The following recommendations are provided by the Adult Treatment Panel of the NCEP. Patients with elevated TG (higher than 200 mg/dL) should be counseled on conservative measures, such as weight loss, low total and saturated fat diet, exercise, smoking cessation, and alcohol restriction. Pharmacologic therapy (Table 6.5) should be considered in patients with TG greater than 200 mg/dL. Fish-oil therapy is reserved for subjects with very high TG (greater than 1,000 mg/dL).

Suggested Readings

Abrams JJ, Grundy SM, Ginsberg H. Metabolism of plasma triglyceride in hypothyroidism and hyperthyroidism in man. J Lipid Res 1981;22:307–322.

Appel GB, Blum C, Chien S, Kunis CL, Appel AS. The hyperlipidemia of the nephrotic syndrome. N Engl J Med 1985;312: 1544–1548.

Assmann G, Schulte H. Triglycerides and atherosclerosis: Results from the Prospective Cardiovascular Münster Study. Atherosclerosis Reviews 1991;22:51–57.

Austin MA. Plasma triglyceride as a risk factor for coronary heart disease. Am J Epidemiol 1989;129:249–259.

Bainton D, Miller NE, Bolton CH, et al. Plasma triglyceride and high density lipoprotein cholesterol as predictors of ischaemic heart disease in British men: The Caerphilly and Speedwell Collaborative Heart Disease Studies. Br Heart J 1992; 68:60–66.

Bass KM, Newschaffer CJ, Klag MJ, Bush TL. Plasma lipoprotein levels as predictors of cardiovascular death in women. Arch Intern Med 1993;153:2209–2216.

Brown AJ, Roberts DCK. The effect of fasting triacylglyceride concentration and apolipoprotein E polymorphism on postprandial lipemia. Arterioscler Thromb 1991;11:1737–1744.

Cambien F, Jacqueson A, Richard JL, Warnet JM, Ducimetiere P, Claude JR. Is the level of serum triglyceride a significant predictor of coronary death in "normocholesterolemic" subjects? The Paris prospective study. Am J Epidemiol 1986;124:624–632.

Carlson LA, Böttinger LE. Risk factors for ischaemic heart disease in men and women: Results of the 19-year follow-up of the Stockholm Prospective Study. Acta Med Scand 1985;218:207–211.

Castelli WP. The triglycerides issue: A view from Framingham. Am Heart J 1986; 112:432–437.

Cohn JS, McNamara JR, Schaefer EJ. Lipoprotein cholesterol concentrations in the plasma of human subjects as measured in the fed and fasted states. Clin Chem 1988;34:2456–2459.

Criqui MH, Heiss G, Cohn R, et al. Plasma triglyceride level and mortality from coronary heart disease. N Engl J Med 1993; 328:1220–1225.

Fontbonne A, Eschwège E, Cambien F, et al. Hypertriglyceridaemia as a risk factor of coronary heart disease mortality in subjects with impaired glucose tolerance or diabetes. Diabetologia 1989;32:300–304.

Glueck CJ, Levy RI, Gueck HI, Gralnick HR, Greten H, Frederickson DS. Acquired type I hyperlipoproteinemia with systemic lupus erythematosus, dysglobulinemia and heparin resistance. Am J Med 1969;47 :318–324.

Goldstein JL, Schrott HG, Hazzard WR, Bierman EL, Motulsky AG. Hyperlipidemia in coronary artery disease. II. Genetic analysis of lipid levels in 176 families and delineation of a new inherited disorder, combined hyperlipidemia. J Clin Invest 1973;2: 1544–1568.

Grundy SM, Vega GL. Two different views of the relationship of hypertriglyceridemia to coronary heart disease. Arch Intern Med 1992;152:28–34.

Hamsten A, Walldius G, Szamosi A, Blombäck M, de Faire U, Dahlén G, Landou C, Wiman B. Plasminogen activator inhibitor in plasma: Risk factor for recurrent myocardial infarction. Lancet 1987;2(8549):3–9.

Hamsten A, Wiman B, de Faire U, Blombäck M. Increased plasma levels of a rapid inhibitor of tissue plasminogen activator in young survivors of myocardial infarction. N Engl J Med 1985;313:1557–1563.

Hulley SB, Roseman RH, Bawol RD, Brand RJ. Epidemiology as a guide to clinical decisions. The association between triglycerides and coronary heart disease. N Engl J Med 1980;302:1383–1389.

Johnson C, Greenland P. Effects of exercise, dietary cholesterol, and dietary fat on blood lipids. Arch Intern Med 1990;150:137–141.

Joven J, Villabona C, Vilella E, Masana L, Alberti R, Valles M. Abnormalities of lipoprotein metabolism in patients with nephrotic syndrome. N Engl J Med 1990;323:579–584.

Kwiterovich PO Jr, Smith HH, Bachorik PS, Derby CA, Pearson TA. Comparison of the plasma levels of apolipoproteins B and A-1, and other risk factors in men and women with premature coronary artery disease. Am J Cardiol 1992 (Apr 15);69:1015–1021.

Lardinois CK. The effects of antihypertensive agents on serum lipids and lipoproteins. Arch Intern Med 1988;148:1280–1288.

Manninen V, Tenkanen L, Koskinen P, et al. Joint effects of serum triglyceride and LDL cholesterol and HDL cholesterol concentrations on coronary heart disease risk in the Helsinki Heart Study. Circulation 1992; 85:37–45.

Meade TW, Brozovic M, Chakrabarti RR, et al. Haemostatic function and ischaemic heart disease: Principal results of the Northwick Park Heart Study. Lancet 1986;2(8506): 533–537.

Miller M, Bachorik PS, Cloey TA. Normal variation of plasma lipoproteins: Postural effects on plasma concentrations of lipids, lipoproteins, and apolipoproteins. Clin Chem 1992;38:569–574.

Miller M, Kwiterovich PO Jr, Bachorik PS, Georgopoulos A. Decreased postprandial response to a fat meal in normotriglyceridemic men with hypoalphalipoproteinemia. Arterioscler Thromb 1993;13:385–392.

Nestel PJ, Connor WE, Reardon MF, Connor S, Wong S, Boston R. Suppression by diets rich in fish oil of very low density lipoprotein production in man. J Clin Invest 1984;74:82–89.

NIH Consensus Development Panel on Triglyceride, High-Density Lipoprotein, and Coronary Heart Disease. Triglyceride, high-density lipoprotein, and coronary heart disease. JAMA 1993;269:505–510.

Patsch JR, Karlin JB, Scott LW, Gotto AM Jr. Inverse relationship between blood levels of high density lipoprotein subfraction 2 and magnitude of postprandial lipemia. Proc Natl Acad Sci USA 1983;80:1449–1453.

Patsch JR, Miesenböck G, Hopferwieser T, et al. Relation of triglyceride metabolism and coronary artery disease. Arterioscler Thromb 1992;12:1336–1345.

Phillipson BE, Rothrock DW, Connor WE, Harris WS, Illingworth DR. Reduction of plasma lipids, lipoproteins, and apoproteins by dietary fish oils in patients with hypertriglyceridemia. N Engl J Med 1985; 312:1210–1216.

Reymer PWA, Gagne E, Groenemeyer BE, Zhang H, Forsyth I, et al. A lipoprotein lipase mutation (Asn291Ser) is associated with reduced HDL cholesterol levels in premature atherosclerosis. Nature Genetics 1995;10:28–34.

Simpson HCR, Meade TW, Stirling Y, Mann JI, Chakrabarti R, Woolf L. Hypertriglyceridaemia and hypercoagulability. Lancet 1983;1(8328):786–790.

Sniderman A, Shapiro S, Marpole D, Skinner B, Teng B, Kwiterovich PO Jr. Association of coronary atherosclerosis with hyperapobetalipoproteinemia: Increased protein but normal cholesterol levels in human plasma low density (beta lipoprotein). Proc Natl Acad Sci USA 1980;77:604–608.

Sniderman AD, Wolfson C, Teng B, Franklin FA, Bachorik PS, Kwiterovich PO Jr. Association of hyperapobetalipoproteinemia with endogenous hypertriglyceridemia and atherosclerosis. Ann Intern Med 1982;97:833–839.

Tenkanen L, Pietilä K, Manninen V, Mänttäri M. The triglyceride issue revisited. Arch Intern Med 1994;154:2714–2720.

Tverdal A, Foss OP, Leren P, Holme I, Lund-Larsen PG, Bjartveit K. Serum triglycerides as an independent risk factor for death from coronary heart disease in middle-aged Norwegian men. Am J Epidemiol 1989; 129:458–465.

Uiterwaal CSPM, Grobbee DE, Witteman JCM, et al. Postprandial triglyceride response in young adult men and familial risk for coronary atherosclerosis. Ann Intern Med 1994;121:576–583.

von Schacky C. Prophylaxis of atherosclerosis with marine omega-3 fatty acids. Ann Intern Med 1987;107:890–899.

Weintraub MS, Eisenberg S, Breslow JL. Dietary fat clearance in normal subjects is regulated by genetic variation in apolipoprotein E. J Clin Invest 1987;80: 1571–1577.

Zilversmit DB. Atherosclerosis: A postprandial phenomenon. Circulation 1979;60: 473–485.

7/ Hypertension

Although arterial (systemic) hypertension was identified as a coronary risk factor nearly four decades ago, it was not until the 1970s that the National Institutes of Health (NIH) launched a vigorous campaign designed to identify the nearly 60 million affected Americans. Randomized controlled clinical trials have unequivocally demonstrated the beneficial effect of blood pressure (BP) lowering on cerebrovascular events, nephrosclerosis, and CHF. This chapter will highlight some of the more recent advances, including treatment of systolic hypertension in the elderly and the recommendations in the Fifth Report of the Joint National Committee on Detection, Evaluation, and Treatment of High Blood Pressure (JNC V).

PATHOPHYSIOLOGY

Elevations in BP are injurious to the vascular endothelium and initiate a cascade of reactions resembling that described for hyperlipidemia. Specifically, there is enhanced transcytosis of atherogenic elements, including lipoproteins (e.g., LDL) and monocyte-macrophages. The increased fluid shear stresses affect ion fluxes and enhance proteoglycan production and smooth muscle cell proliferation and accumulation. While hyperlipidemia accelerates this process, endothelial damage induced by chronic elevations in BP is sufficient to cause intimal thickening without elevations in cholesterol (Fig. 7.1).

As a result of endothelial injury, there is an associated reduction in the synthesis of the potent vasodilator EDRF-NO. Conversely, when EDRF-NO is inhibited by L-arginine analogues, BP increases. Depression in renal production of EDRF-NO may also cause sodium retention and hypertension.

GENETIC STUDIES

The genetics of essential hypertension are considerably more complex than the genetics of monogenic disorders such as familial hypercholesterolemia. While essential hypertension has been seen as a polygenic disorder, other causes of hypertension (e.g., glucocorticoid remediable aldosteronism) are inherited by Mendelian transmission. Nevertheless, studies in sib pairs have disclosed evidence of linkage between the angiotensinogen gene located on chromosome 1 and diastolic hypertension DBP >100 mm Hg). The higher prevalence of similar HLA haplotypes among hypertensive siblings suggests a second important locus on chromosome 6. Other postulated loci, including those for ACE and renin, do not appear to play an important role in the genetics of essential hypertension.

DIFFERENTIAL DIAGNOSIS

Essential hypertension comprises more than 90% of all cases of hypertension. Table 7.1 lists the estimated frequency of secondary causes of hypertension.

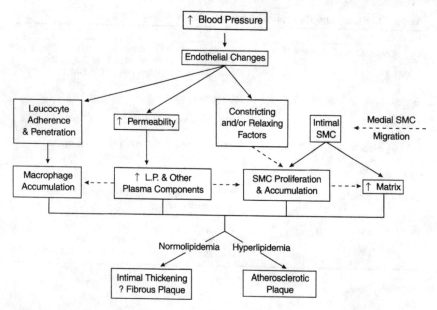

Figure 7.1. Diagram summarizing the effects of hypertension (HBP) on the arterial intima. SMC = smooth muscle cell; L.P. = lipoprotein. From Chobanian AV. 1989 Corcoran Lecture: Adaptive and maladaptive responses of the arterial wall to hypertension. Hypertension 1990;15:666–674. Reproduced with permission. Hypertension Copyright © 1990 American Heart Association.

EPIDEMIOLOGY

Although the intensive campaign in the U.S. during the 1970s increased public awareness of hypertension as a major modifiable cardiovascular risk factor, certain segments of our society (e.g., lower SES) remain unidentified or inadequately treated. Based on the National Health and Nutrition Examination Survey (NHANES), it is estimated that approximately 50 million American adults are hypertensive. The incidence of hypertension increases with age (Fig. 7.2) and the prevalence is highest among African-Americans (Table 7.2).

The classification of hypertension is illustrated in Table 7.3. The incidence of CAD events increases with elevation in systolic or diastolic BP (Fig. 7.3). Cardiovascular event rate increases as the diastolic BP exceeds 90 mm Hg; a diastolic BP of 105 mm Hg or greater doubles the rate of coronary events and nearly quadruples the risk of stroke compared with DBP <80 mm Hg (Fig. 7.4).

Table 7.1. Secondary Causes of Hypertension

Disorder (Frequency)	Diagnostic Tests
Renal parenchymal disease (5%)	Spot urine to R/O glomerulonephritis (RBC casts); ultrasound to R/O polycystic disease; renin levels reduced in DM
Renovascular disease (4%)	Captopril challenge
Coarctation of the aorta (1%)	2-D echocardiography, aortography
Primary aldosteronism (0.5%)	24-hour urine (>100 mEq Na+), computed tomography (CT) to differentiate adenoma/hyperplasia
Cushing's syndrome (0.2%)	24-hour urine (free cortisol), dexamethasone suppression test
Pheochromocytoma (0.2%)	24-hour urine (metanephrines), plasma catecholamines, CT scan ^{131}I-MIBG (metaiodobenzylguanidine) for localization

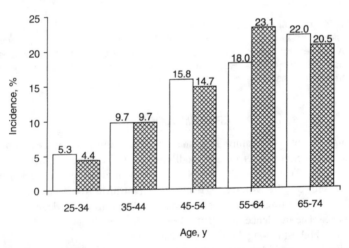

Figure 7.2. Incidence rates of hypertension for white men (*open bars*) and women (*cross-hatched bars*) with average followup of 9.5 years (National Health Epidemiologic Follow-up Study (NHEFS)). From Cornoni-Huntley J, LaCroix AZ, Havlik RJ. Race and sex differentials in the impact of hypertension in the United States: The National Health and Nutrition Examination Survey I. Epidemiologic Follow-up Study. Arch Intern Med 1989;149:780–788.

Table 7.2. Hypertensive Category at Follow-up by Age, Race, and Sex Among Participants Normal at Baseline

Sex, Race, and Age, y	No. of Persons	% of Participants		
			Hypertension	
		Normal	Borderline	Definite
White, men				
25–34	548	88.1	6.6	5.3
35–54	725	73.2	14.3	12.4
55+	442	58.1	21.7	20.1
Total	1715	74.1	13.8	12.1
White, women				
25–34	1260	91.8	3.7	4.4
35–54	1486	78.5	10.2	11.3
55+	477	56.6	21.6	21.8
Total	3223	80.4	9.4	10.2
Black, men				
25–34	55	72.7	16.4	10.9
35–54	69	59.4	10.1	30.4
55+	48	54.2	18.8	27.1
Total	172	62.2	14.5	23.3
Black, women				
25–34	174	76.4	6.9	16.7
35–54	174	60.9	15.5	23.6
55+	39	56.4	5.1	38.5
Total	387	67.4	10.6	22.0

From Cornoni-Huntley J, LaCroix AZ, Havlik RJ. Race and sex differentials in the impact of hypertension in the United States: the National Health and Nutrition Examination Survey I. Epidemiologic Follow-up Study. Arch Intern Med 1989;149:780–788.

Table 7.3. Classification of Blood Pressure for Adults Aged 18 Years and Older*

Category	Systolic, mm Hg	Diastolic, mm Hg
Normal†	<130	<85
High normal	130–139	85–89
Hypertension‡		
Stage 1 (mild)	140–159	90–99
Stage 2 (moderate)	160–179	100–109
Stage 3 (severe)	180–209	110–119
Stage 4 (very severe)	≥210	≥120

*Not taking antihypertensive drugs and not acutely ill. When systolic and diastolic pressures fall into different categories, the higher category should be selected to classify the individual's BP status. For instance, 160/92 mm Hg should be classified as stage 2, and 180/120 mm Hg should be classified as stage 4. Isolated systolic hypertension is defined as a systolic BP of 140 mm Hg or more and a diastolic BP of less than 90 mm Hg and staged appropriately (e.g., 170/85 mm Hg is defined as stage 2 isolated systolic hypertension).
In addition to classifying stages of hypertension on the basis of average BP levels, the clinician should specify presence or absence of target-organ disease and additional risk factors. For example, a patient with diabetes and a BP of 142/94 mm Hg, plus left ventricular hypertrophy, should be classified as having "stage 1 hypertension with target-organ disease (left ventricular hypertrophy) and with another major risk factor (diabetes)." This specificity is important for risk classification and management.
†Optimal BP with respect to cardiovascular risk is less than 120 mm Hg systolic and less than 80 mm Hg diastolic. However, unusually low readings should be evaluated for clinical significance.
‡Based on the average of two or more readings taken at each of two or more visits after an initial screening.
From The Fifth Report of the Joint National Committee on Detection, Evaluation, and Treatment of High Blood Pressure (JNC V). Arch Intern Med 1993;153:154–183.

Important contributors to BP elevation are described below.

Abdominal Obesity

Overweight individuals have a two- to sixfold increased risk of developing hypertension. At particular risk are subjects with abdominal obesity (as measured by the waist:hip circumference). Obesity promotes peripheral insulin resistance leading to hyperinsulinemia. Hyperinsulinemia may promote hypertension by one of the mechanisms illustrated in Figure 7.5.

Alcohol Consumption

Consumption of alcohol enhances sympathetic CNS activity. With excessive consumption there may also be an increase in cortisol production. There is a J-shaped association between alcohol intake and prevalence of hypertension with the lowest prevalence observed among occasional or light consumers (Fig. 7.6).

Renin Levels

Laragh and colleagues reported that plasma renin levels were associated with an increased risk of CAD in hypertensive patients. An 8-year followup study by

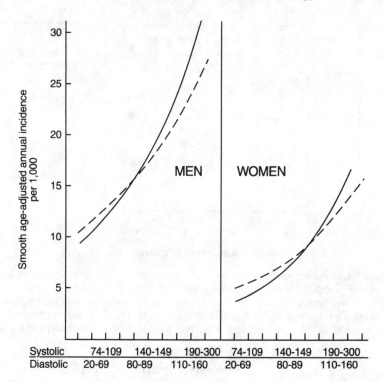

Figure 7.3. Incidence of CAD according to systolic (*solid lines*) compared with diastolic (*broken lines*) BP in men and women aged 47 to 74 years (Framingham). From Kannel WB. Hypertension, blood lipids, and cigarette smoking as co-risk factors for coronary heart disease. Ann N Y Acad Sci 1978;304:128–139. Used with permission.

Alderman et al. disclosed that subjects with the highest baseline renin levels had the greatest risk of MI. This effect was accentuated in the presence of other CAD risk factors (Fig. 7.7). High renin levels in the absence of other cardiac risk factors enhanced the risk of MI sevenfold. Conversely, there were no reported MIs among 241 subjects with low renin levels and no cardiac risk factors. Renin stimulates secretion of angiotensin, which has been shown to induce smooth muscle migration. High renin levels are most prevalent among Caucasian hypertensive males, in whom pharmacologic treatment with renin lowering agents such as β-blockers and ACE inhibitors has been advocated.

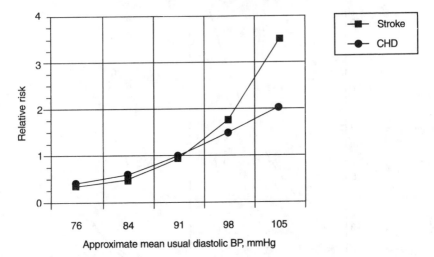

Figure 7.4. Increasing relative 10-year risk of stroke and CHD at increasing usual diastolic BP in nine studies of untreated subjects. Adapted from MacMahon S, Peto R, Cutler J, et al. Blood pressure, stroke, and coronary heart disease. Part 1, prolonged differences in blood pressure: Prospective observational studies corrected for the regression dilution bias. Lancet 1990;335:765–774. Copyright © by The Lancet Ltd. 1990. Used with permission.

Sedentary Lifestyle

A study by Paffenbarger and associates revealed a 35% increased risk of developing hypertension among sedentary (vs physically active) Harvard alumni males. Similar results were subsequently confirmed in another long-term prospective observational study (see Blair et al.).

Sodium Intake

The average American diet includes 4,000 to 7,000 mg sodium daily. In the INTERSALT study of 10,000 subjects representing 32 countries, a positive association was observed between sodium intake and BP; with a low BMI, the prevalence of hypertension was nearly sixfold higher among high vs. low sodium consumers (11.9% vs 1.7%).

RANDOMIZED TRIALS

A meta-analysis of the major randomized trials of antihypertensive therapy, including the Hypertension Detection and Followup Program (HDFP; United States) and Medical Research Council (MRC; United Kingdom) demonstrated a 42% reduction in the incidence of stroke and a 14% reduction in CAD events (Fig. 7.8) (see Collins et al.).

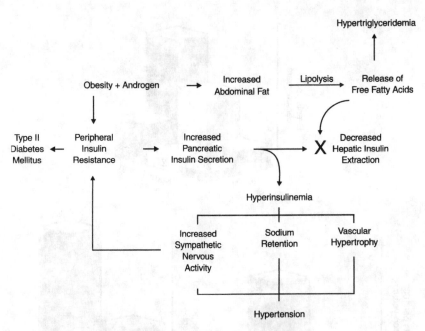

Figure 7.5. An overall scheme for the mechanism by which upper-body obesity could promote glucose intolerance, hypertriglyceridemia, and hypertension via hyperinsulinemia. From Kaplan NM. The deadly quartet: Upper-body obesity, glucose intolerance, hypertriglyceridemia, and hypertension. Arch Intern Med 1989;149:1514–1520. Copyright © 1989, American Medical Association. Used with permission.

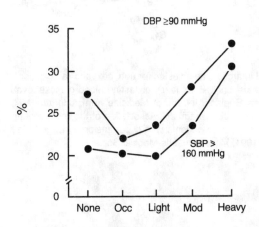

Figure 7.6. Age-adjusted prevalence rates (%) of measured systolic and diastolic hypertension by levels of alcohol intake in drinks: Occasional (Occ), light (one to two daily), moderate (Mod) (three to six daily), and heavy (more than six daily). From Shaper AG, Wannamethee G, Whincup P. Alcohol and blood pressure in middle-aged British men. J Hum Hypertens 1988; 2:71–78S. Used with permission.

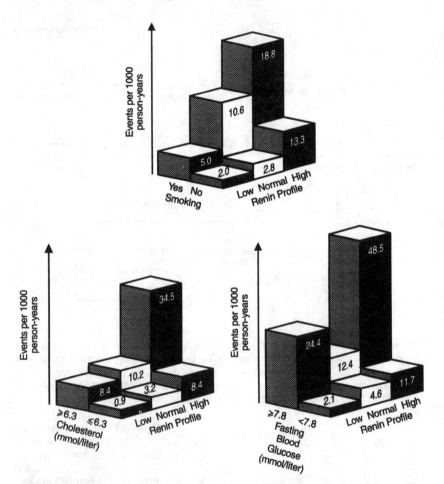

Figure 7.7. Incidence of myocardial infarction, as adjusted for age, sex, and race, according to renin profile and smoking status, cholesterol level, or fasting blood glucose level. Reprinted by permission of the New England Journal of Medicine from Alderman MH, Madhavan S, Ooi WL, Cohen H, Sealey JE, Laragh JH. Association of the renin-sodium profile with the risk of myocardial infarction in patients with hypertension. N Engl J Med 1991;324:1098–1104, Copyright © 1991, Massachusetts Medical Society.

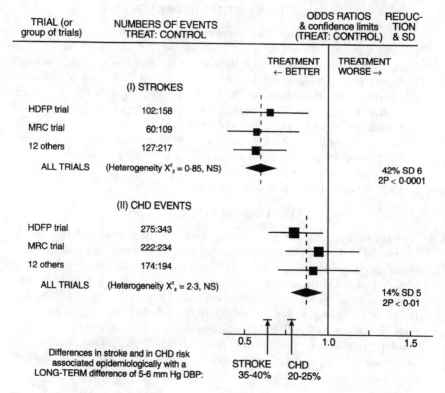

Figure 7.8. Reduction in the odds of stroke and of CHD in the HDFP trial, the MRC trial, and in all 12 other smaller unconfounded randomized trials of antihypertensive therapy (mean diastolic BP (DBP) difference 5 to 6 mm Hg for 5 years).

Solid squares represent the simple odds ratio for the two larger trials and the properly stratified odds ratio for the combination of the 12 smaller trials. From Collins R, Peto R, MacMahon S, et al. Blood pressure, stroke, and coronary heart disease. Part 2, short-term reductions in blood pressure: Overview of randomised drug trials in their epidemiological context. Lancet 1990;335:827–838. Copyright © by The Lancet Ltd. 1990. Used with permission.

ISOLATED SYSTOLIC HYPERTENSION

Isolated systolic hypertension is common in men and women over age 65, with an estimated prevalence of 15% and is an independent risk factor for CAD. In younger subjects, the differential diagnosis of isolated systolic hypertension includes high output states such as anemia, aortic insufficiency, arteriovenous fistula, beriberi, hyperthyroidism, and Paget's disease. In the Systolic Hypertension in the Elderly Program (SHEP) of nearly 5,000 subjects over age 60 yrs, there was a 36% reduction in stroke and a 25% reduction in CAD events in treated subjects (mean followup 4.5 yrs). A recent meta-analysis by Mulrow and colleagues disclosed that one coronary or cerebrovascular event would be prevented for every 18 patients treated (>60 years). Thus, antihypertensive treatment in the elderly is effective, and the benefits extend to octogenarians.

THE J CURVE PHENOMENON

A key issue in antihypertensive management is the degree to which DBP should be reduced. A J curve phenomenon (as reported for TC) has been observed with overall mortality increasing with DBP <90 mm Hg as illustrated in Fig. 7.9. In addition, there was a U-shaped curve among the nontreated subjects. Coinciding with increased mortality rates were reductions in overall health characterized by reduced body weight and hemoglobin concentrations. Overall, these data suggest an association between reduced DBP and increased mortality rather than a cause-effect relationship. With CAD, however, marked reduction in DBP may impact negatively on an already compromised coronary circulation. Thus, it is reasonable to maintain DBP between 80 and 85 mm Hg in hypertensive patients with CAD.

TREATMENT

Nonpharmacologic

WEIGHT REDUCTION

Many studies have demonstrated that weight loss in obese subjects is associated with reduction in both SBP and DBP. The results of BP reduction in three major trials are noted in Table 7.4. The fall in BP is believed to be mediated in part by reduction in plasma insulin levels.

DIET

Sodium Restriction

In an analysis of 20 randomized controlled trials, (see Cutler et al. 1991) it was reported that with modest reduction of sodium intake (approximately 2,000

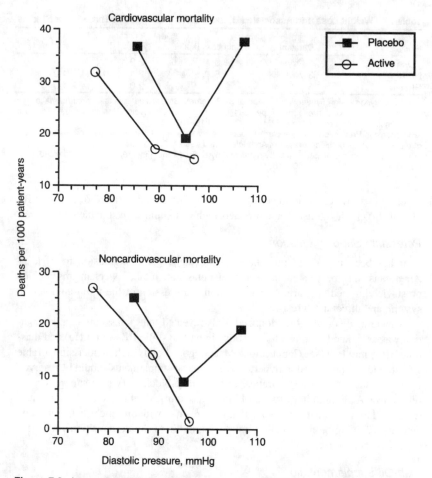

Figure 7.9. J curve in treated and placebo groups. From Staessen J, Bulpitt C, Clement D, et al. Relation between mortality and treated blood pressure in elderly patients with hypertension: Report of the European Working Party on High Blood Pressure in the Elderly. Br Med J 1989;298:1552–1556. Published by BMJ Publishing Group. Used with permission.

Table 7.4. Weight Loss and Associated Blood Pressure Changes in Three Major Studies

Study	Duration	Weight Loss (kg)	Reduction in BP (mm Hg)	
			Systolic	Diastolic
TOHP[1]	18 mo	3.9	2.9	2.3
HPT[2]	3 yr	1.6	2.4	1.8
PPH[3]	5 yr	2.7	2.0	1.9

[1]Trials of Hypertension Prevention Collaborative Research Group. The effects of nonpharmacologic interventions on blood pressure of persons with high normal levels: Results of the Trials of Hypertension Prevention, Phase I. JAMA 1992;267:1213–1220.
[2]Hypertension Prevention Trial Research Group. The Hypertension Prevention Trial: three-year effects of dietary changes on blood pressure. Arch Intern Med 1990;150:153–162.
[3]Primary prevention of hypertension by nutritional-hygienic means. Final report of a randomized, controlled trial. JAMA 1989;262:1801–1807.

mg/day) there was a mean lowering of systolic BP (5 mm Hg) and of diastolic BP (3 mm Hg). Table 7.5 lists some products high in sodium with suitable alternatives.

Potassium Supplementation

It has been postulated that the high prevalence of hypertension in African-Americans may be related to decreased potassium intake. Mechanisms include prostaglandin-mediated arterial vasodilation, suppression of the renin-angiotensin system, and direct natriuresis.

A meta-analysis of 19 randomized trials revealed that potassium supplementation was associated with mean reductions in both systolic BP (8 mm Hg) and diastolic BP (5 mm Hg) (see Cappuccio & MacGregor). Foods high in potassium (Table 7.6) should be considered in hypertensive subjects; supplements should be reserved for non-potassium sparing diuretics. The use of β-blockers (which suppress renin release) or ACE inhibitors (which blunt potassium excretion) elevate potassium levels and may attenuate the hypokalemia associated with diuretic use. Conversely, patients receiving both β-blockers and ACE inhibitors should have potassium levels closely monitored.

Fish-Oil Supplementation

The ω-3 fatty acids contained in fish oils are believed to reduce BP, in part, by stimulating PGI_2 secretion and reducing the vascular response to norepinephrine. Daily supplementation >200 g cold-water fish (see also Chapter 6) or 6 to 10 fish-oil capsules has resulted in mean reduction of systolic BP (6 mm Hg) and diastolic BP (4 mm Hg) in hypertensive subjects.

Calcium Supplementation

The effect of calcium supplementation on BP has been inconsistent. While one large study of approximately 6,600 men and women reported a 12% reduction in

Table 7.5.   Fifteen High-Sodium Foods With Lower-Sodium Alternatives

High-Sodium Product (Serving Size)	Na+ (mg)/Serving	Lower-Sodium Alternative (Serving Size)	Na+ (mg)/Serving
Bachman Stix Pretzels (1 oz)	1460	Snyder's Old Fashioned Pretzels (1 oz)	590
Bacon, uncooked (3 oz)	1400	Pork, uncooked (3 oz)	65
La Choy Soy Sauce (1 tbsp)	1380	Angostura Low Sodium Soy Sauce (1 tbsp)	390
Corn flakes (4 oz)	1220	Shredded wheat (4 oz)	1
Hardee's Chicken Fillet Sandwich	1100	McDonald's McGrilled Chicken Sandwich	680
Colonel's Chicken Sandwich	1060		
Arby's Chicken Breast	1019		
Celeste pizza for one, cheese (6.5 oz)	1070	Weight Watchers Three Cheese Pizza (6 oz)	350
Frankfurter (2)	850	Ground beef (3 oz)	170
Chef Boyardee spaghetti sauce with mushrooms (1/2 cup)	843	Healthy Choice spaghetti sauce with mushrooms (1/2 cup)	350
Stouffer's lasagna	840	Stouffer's Lean Cuisine lasagna with meat sauce	560
Campbell's Vegetarian Vegetable Soup (8 oz)	790	Campbell's Healthy Request Vegetable Soup (8 oz)	500
Oscar Mayer Deli Thin Roast Turkey (2 oz)	687	Tyson or Weaver turkey breast (2 oz)	272
Green beans (canned)	686	Green beans (fresh)	5
Tomato juice (1 cup)	640	Orange juice (1 cup)	2
Rice-A-Roni, chicken flavor (1/2 cup)	520	Brown or enriched white rice (1/2 cup)	3
Alka-Seltzer/Bromo Seltzer (tab)	550–1540	Tums/Maalox Plus	1–2

Table 7.6. Foods High in Potassium

Foods	Serving Size	Potassium (mg)/Serving
Apricots, dried	5	235
Apricots, fresh	3 medium	300
Banana	1 medium	440
Broccoli	4 oz	430
Cantaloupe	1/2, 5" diameter	680
Carrot	1 medium	245
Cod	3 oz	345
Flounder	3 oz	500
Halibut	3 oz	450
Honeydew	1/2, 6 1/2" diameter	1880
Lettuce, iceberg	1/2 head	450
Lima beans	4 oz	500
Milk, evaporated	1 cup	760
Milk, skim	1 cup	355
Orange	1 medium	290
Potato, baked	1 medium	780
Salmon	3 oz	380
Sweet potato	1 medium	370
Tomato	1 medium	300
Yogurt, plain	1 cup	325

the incidence of hypertension with 1,000 mg of calcium daily, other large trials have recorded no benefit. Subjects most responsive to calcium supplementation appear to be hyporeninemic and sodium sensitive with compensatory secondary hyperparathyroidism (Fig. 7.10). In view of the lack of consistent positive data, there are presently no specific recommendations for calcium supplementation. The RDA is 800 to 1,200 mg/day.

Magnesium Supplementation

As with calcium supplementation, the majority of trials employing magnesium supplementation have been negative. Therefore, routine use of magnesium supplements as a BP lowering aid is not advocated.

Alcohol

While alcohol use has been associated with BP elevation (see above), reduction in consumption has produced favorable BP decreases in both light and moderate drinkers. The cardioprotective benefit of alcohol appears to be maximal at one to two drinks daily (see also Chapter 5).

EXERCISE

Aerobic exercise reduces BP in hypertensive subjects by blunting sympathetic activity (e.g., reduction in norepinephrine levels). In both normotensive and hyper-

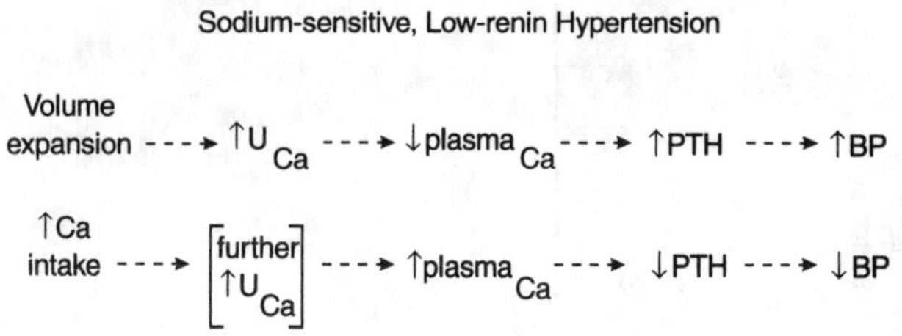

Sodium-sensitive, Low-renin Hypertension

$$\text{Volume expansion} \dashrightarrow \uparrow U_{Ca} \dashrightarrow \downarrow \text{plasma}_{Ca} \dashrightarrow \uparrow PTH \dashrightarrow \uparrow BP$$

$$\uparrow Ca \text{ intake} \dashrightarrow \begin{bmatrix} \text{further} \\ \uparrow U_{Ca} \end{bmatrix} \dashrightarrow \uparrow \text{plasma}_{Ca} \dashrightarrow \downarrow PTH \dashrightarrow \downarrow BP$$

Figure 7.10. A potential explanation for a hypotensive action of increased dietary calcium intake. From Kaplan NM. Calcium and potassium in the treatment of essential hypertension. Semin Nephrol 1988;8:176–184. Used with permission.

tensive subjects, aerobic exercise leads to a mean reduction in systolic BP (6 mm Hg) and diastolic BP (6 mm Hg). Low- to moderate-intensity workouts such as brisk walking, cycling, and dancing are also effective in lowering BP.

Pharmacologic

Antihypertensive drugs can be grouped into the following three classes: diuretics, adrenergic blockers, and vasodilators.

DIURETICS

Diuretics (Table 7.7) continue to be the most prescribed antihypertensive agents (40 million prescriptions in 1992). Their sites of action in the nephron are depicted in Figure 7.11. Decisions regarding agent selection are predicated on renal function; thiazides are useful with normal or mildly impaired renal function (creatinine less than 2.0 mg/dL). On further renal deterioration, loop agents are the diuretics of choice. With enhanced sodium excretion, extracellular volume depletion occurs, resulting in stimulation of the renin-angiotensin system. Subjects with endogenous hyporeninemia (e.g., African-Americans and the elderly) tend to have a better response to diuretic therapy than subjects with elevated renin activity. Side effects such as hypokalemia and hypomagnesemia (except with potassium-sparing diuretics) may produce fatal cardiac arrhythmias. This side effect is believed to have contributed to the increased rate of sudden cardiac death in a subset of hypertensive men in the MRFIT study. Importantly, earlier studies employed large doses of diuretics (e.g., 50 to 100 mg/day). Fortunately, with the institution of lower dosages of diuretics (e.g., 6.25 to 12.5 mg hydrochlorothiazide), metabolic side effects are much less frequent and antihypertensive efficacy is preserved. Although hyperuricemia is reported in approximately one-third of patients, gout is rare. Because urinary calcium excretion is reduced, hypercalcemia may occur. However, this side

Table 7.7. Diuretics

Thiazides	Nonthiazides (Sulfonamides)	Loop Diuretics	Potassium-Sparing
Benzthiazide (Exna)	Chlorthalidone (Hygroton)	Bumetanide (Bumex)	Amiloride (Midamor)
Chlorothiazide (Diuril)	Indapamide (Lozol)	Ethacrynic Acid	Spironolactone
		(Edecrin)	(Aldactone)
Hydrochlorothiazide	Metolazone (Zaroxolyn)	Furosemide (Lasix)	Triamterene (Dyrenium)
(Esidrix, HydroDIURIL,			
Oretic)			
Methyclothiazide (Enduron,			
Aquatensen)			
Polythiazide (Minizide)			

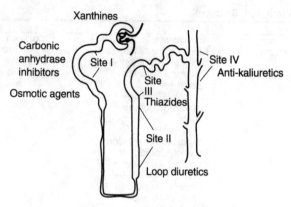

Figure 7.11. Diagrammatic representation of the nephron showing the four main tubular sites where diuretics interfere with sodium reabsorption. The main action of xanthines on the kidney is on vascular perfusion of the glomerulus, though some effect on sodium reabsorption at site I also is likely. From Lant A. Diuretic drugs: Progress in clinical pharmacology. Drugs. 1986;31(Suppl 4):40–55. Used with permission.

effect is most often observed with pre-existing hyperparathyroidism. Hyperlipidemia, characterized by elevation in TC, LDL-C and TG, is observed during the initial months of therapy and usually abates within 1 year of continued use. Thiazide use is also associated with hyperglycemia due to insulin resistance, and is more likely to occur with central adiposity. As with other antihypertensive agents, impotence is a common side effect. Diuretics may be used in combination with other antihypertensive medications (e.g., ACE inhibitors, β-blockers) often attenuating metabolic side effects such as hypokalemia. Other combinations (e.g., diuretics and calcium channel blockers), are less efficacious, owing in part to similar vasodilatory properties.

ADRENERGIC BLOCKERS

α_1-Blockers

α_1-Blockers (Table 7.8) prevent catecholamine-mediated vasoconstriction by inhibiting norepinephrine activation on postsynaptic receptor sites (Fig. 7.12). As a result of vasodilation and excessive initial venous pooling, there is an increased propensity for first-dose syncope as is particularly noteworthy of prazosin. Therefore, the initial dose should be given at bedtime. In addition to first-dose syncope, side effects include fatigue and sedation, both of which often dissipate over time. Side effects that occur with diuretic use (e.g., hyperglycemia, hyperlipidemia)

Table 7.8. Adrenergic Blockers

α_1-Blockers	β-Blockers	Central α_2 Agonists
Doxazosin (Cardura)	Acebutolol (Sectral)[a,c,e,f]	Clonidine (Catapres)
Prazosin (Minipress)	Atenolol (Tenormin)[b,d,e]	Guanabenz (Wytensin)
Terazosin (Hytrin)	Betaxolol (Kerlone)[b,c,e]	Guanfacine (Tenex)
	Bisoprolol (Zebeta, Ziac)[a,c,d,e]	Methyldopa (Aldomet)
	Carteolol (Cartrol)[b,d,f]	
	Carvedilol (Coreg)[a,c,g]	
	Labetalol (Normodyne, Trandate)[a,c,g]	
	Metoprolol (Lopressor)[a,c,e]	
	Nadolol (Corgard)[b,d]	
	Penbutolol (Levatol)[a,c,d,f]	
	Pindolol (Visken)[a,c,d,f]	
	Propranolol (Inderal)[a,c]	
	Sotalol (Betapace)[b,d]	
	Timolol (Blocadren)[a,c]	

a = lipid soluble, b = water soluble, c = hepatic excretion, d = renal excretion, e = β_1 selectivity, f = intrinsic sympathomimetic activity, g = combined α- and β-blocker.

have not been observed with these agents. α_1-blockers are effective in combination with diuretics, β-blockers, or calcium blockers.

β-Blockers

β-Blockers lower BP by reducing catecholamine release. They also attenuate the release of renin from juxtaglomerular cells, thereby lowering renin levels. These agents are classified based on solubility, route of excretion, cardioselectivity (β_1 receptors), and intrinsic sympathomimetic activity (ISA). Water soluble, β-blockers (e.g., atenolol) do not cross the blood-brain barrier and hence are less likely to cause CNS side effects. Nonselective β-blockers may raise TG levels 15–30% and reduce HDL-C by approximately 10–20% (see also Chapter 10). With resting bradycardia, β-blockers with ISA are the preferred agents. The combined α- and β-blocking agent, labetalol, reduces coronary blood flow to a lower extent than other conventional β-blockers and is a useful antihypertensive agent in patients with stable angina. It is also effective in patients with renal insufficiency and in the management of hypertensive emergencies. Carvedilol, another antihypertensive agent with combined α- and β-blocker activity, may soon also be approved by the FDA for the treatment of CHF.

As with thiazides, low doses of β-blockers (e.g., atenolol 25 mg/day) are as effective as high doses with less untoward side effects. Side effects occur more frequently with certain agents. CNS effects such as depression and nightmares are more common with lipid soluble agents. Unfortunately, impotence may occur with either selective or nonselective agents. It is critical that in CAD patients, β-blockers should never be abruptly discontinued, but rather tapered. Tapering of β-blockers should be performed gradually over a 1- to 2-week interval; the dose may be reduced by 50% every 3 to 4 days. Abrupt discontinuation results in rebound sympathetic activity, which may result in unstable angina, MI, pulmonary edema, or sudden cardiac death. The substitution of a calcium blocker for a β-blocker has not been shown to prevent this potentially devastating rebound effect.

Central α_2 Agonists

Central α_2 agonists inhibit norepinephrine release from presynaptic terminals (see Fig. 7.12). These agents also decrease sympathetic outflow to the CNS. The hypotensive effect of these agents is rapid. They are effective in patients with diabetes mellitus and pulmonary disorders (e.g., asthma, chronic obstructive pulmonary disease). The most common side effects include dry mouth and sedation. The use of methyldopa is often accompanied by fluid retention. Rarely, agranulocytosis or hepatitis may occur. A rebound catecholaminergic surge has been observed with abrupt discontinuation of these agents; treatment includes either the agent's reinitiation or labetalol. Guanfacine, the newest agent, appears to have fewer side effects and may be the agent of choice in this class.

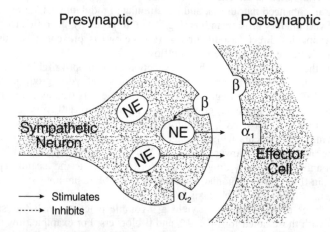

Figure 7.12. Simplified schematic view of the adrenergic nerve ending showing that norepinephrine (NE) is released from the storage granules when the nerve is stimulated and enters the synaptic cleft to bind to α_1 and β receptors on the effector cell (postsynaptic). In addition, a short feedback loop exists, in which NE binds to α_2 and β receptors on the neuron (presynaptic), either to inhibit or to stimulate further release. From Kaplan NM. Clinical Hypertension. 6th ed. Baltimore, MD: Williams & Wilkins, 1994. Used with permission.

Table 7.9. Vasodilators

ACE Inhibitors	Calcium Channel Blockers	Direct Vasodilators
Benazepril (Lotensin)	Amlodipine (Norvasc)	Hydralazine (Apresoline)
Captopril (Capoten)	Diltiazem (Cardizem)	Minoxidil (Loniten)
Enalapril (Vasotec)	Felodipine (Plendil)	
Fosinopril (Monopril)	Isradipine (DynaCirc)	
Lisinopril (Prinivil, Zestril)	Nicardipine (Cardene)	
Quinapril (Accupril)	Nifedipine (Adalat, Procardia)	
Ramipril (Altace)	Verapamil (Calan, Isoptin, Verelan)	

VASODILATORS

The agents in this class include ACE inhibitors, calcium channel blockers, and direct vasodilators (Table 7.9). These antihypertensive agents exhibit their primary vasodilatory action on arteries. Other agents, such as nitroprusside and α-blockers, maintain a balanced vasodilating effect on arteries and veins, while nitroglycerin exerts its actions on the venous system.

ACE Inhibitors

The ACE inhibitors block the conversion of angiotensin I to the potent vaso-constrictor angiotensin II. These agents also (1) reduce secretion of aldosterone, resulting in enhanced natriuresis, and (2) stimulate bradykinin activation and synthesis of vasodilatory prostaglandins (Fig. 7.13). Importantly, the reflex tachycardia that accompanies direct vasodilator use (see below) is prevented because ACE inhibitors decrease sympathetic CNS outflow.

All of the ACE inhibitors with the exception of fosinopril (Table 7.9) are primarily eliminated by the kidneys. The presence of a sulfhydryl group in captopril may afford some desirable (e.g., antioxidant properties) as well as untoward (e.g., taste disturbances, leukopenia) effects compared to the nonsulfhydryl agents. Side effects common to most ACE inhibitors include a nonproductive cough (up to 20%), which often occurs with prolonged use and reflects kininogen stimulation. One may attempt to (1) lower the dose, (2) switch to fosinopril, (3) use a non-steroidal anti-inflammatory drug (NSAID), or (4) switch to the recently approved angiotensin II receptor antagonist, losartan (cozaar). More ominous side effects are angioedema (0.2%) and anaphylaxis.

Low doses of ACE inhibitors yield a favorable outcome on BP as similarly reported with those noted for thiazides and β-blockers. For example, low doses of captopril (12.5 mg TID) and enalapril (10 mg/d) appear to be as effective as higher doses.

Subjects displaying the best response to ACE inhibitors often have high plasma renin levels. Included are patients with renovascular hypertension and renal parenchymal disease. Conversely, these medications are less effective in subjects (e.g., African-Americans) with hyporeninemia. In diabetics, ACE inhibitors may be

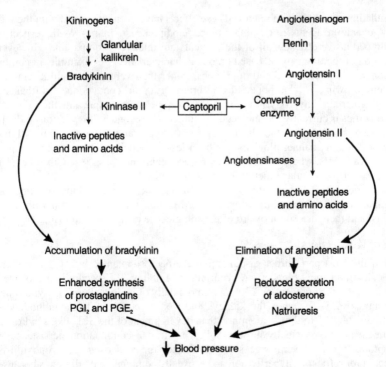

Figure 7.13. Mechanisms by which captopril may lower BP. From Kaplan NM. Clinical Hypertension. 6th ed. Baltimore, MD: Williams & Wilkins, 1994. Used with permission.

particularly valuable because (1) they reduce plasma insulin levels, thereby improving glucose sensitivity, and (2) they improve renal blood flow by selective vasodilation of efferent arterioles. This latter effect has been shown to retard the progression of glomerular disease. In addition to demonstrated antihypertensive efficacy, ACE inhibitors have also been shown to reduce cardiovascular mortality following MI in patients with reduced left ventricular ejection fraction (less than 40%) (see Pfeffer et al.).

Calcium Channel Blockers

Since their introduction as antihypertensive agents during the 1980s, there has been a linear growth in calcium channel blocker use; they presently rank second only to diuretics in the number of prescriptions written in the U.S. Diltiazem and verapamil are negative chronotropic agents. On the other hand, the first-generation dihydropyridines (e.g., nicardipine and nifedipine) produce a reflex tachycardia by stimulating catecholamine release. These effects have been attenuated with the second-generation agents (e.g., amlodipine, felodipine, isradipine). With respect to antihypertensive efficacy, all of these agents are relatively comparable. However, selection of therapy may be based on other characteristics. For example, in combination with β-blockers, dihydropyridines, rather than verapamil or diltiazem, are preferred owing to the potential for bradycardia or conduction disturbances. Whether certain dihydropyridines (e.g., amlodipine) bear unique antiatherosclerotic properties is currently the subject of a multicenter secondary prevention study. In contrast to β-blockers, which have been shown to be cardioprotective post MI, the role of calcium channel blockers has been less convincing. The one exception is non-Q wave MIs, where diltiazem may reduce recurrent events (see Gibson et al.), provided left ventricular function is not compromised.

Common side effects with calcium channel blocker use include constipation (verapamil) and edema (dihydropyridines). Impotence is less common with these agents, and there are no untoward effects on glucose or lipid metabolism.

Direct Vasodilators

For the most part, direct vasodilators have been supplanted by ACE inhibitors and calcium channel blockers. A syndrome resembling SLE occurs in 5% of men and 20% of women receiving 200 mg or more daily of hydralazine. This syndrome, in contrast to SLE, spares the kidneys and CNS. Detection of autoantibodies is approximately 15-fold more common than development of the SLE-like syndrome. While the syndrome usually subsides following drug discontinuation, persistence of symptoms beyond several weeks is an indicator for corticosteroids. Minoxidil is reserved for refractory hypertension and is usually combined with diuretics because of associated fluid retention. Pericardial effusions have been reported and are most commonly observed in renal dialysis patients. Hirsutism is the most disconcerting side effect of this medication.

RECOMMENDATIONS

Recommendations derived from JNC V are summarized in Figure 7.14. As with hyperlipidemia, the cornerstone of therapy is lifestyle modification. Diuretics and β-blockers are the preferred pharmacologic agents with proven efficacy and associated reduction in cardiovascular mortality rates. Diuretics were particularly beneficial in the SHEP trial. While the other agents listed were equally efficacious, there have been no long-term data assessing BP control and associated mortality rates. Nevertheless, many hypertension experts believe that the pharmacologic armamentarium should be individualized based on demographic characteristics. Table 7.10 provides several examples. If a single agent does not produce the desired response, then low-dose combination therapy should be employed. Most antihypertensive agents, and in particular, ACE inhibitors, have been shown to cause regression of left ventricular hypertrophy.

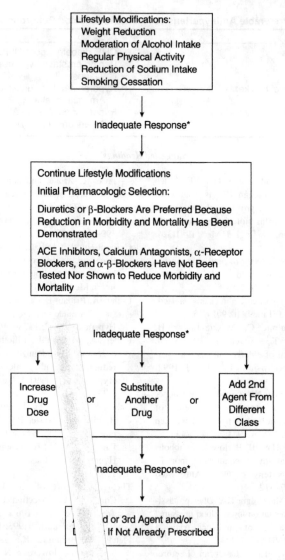

Figure 7.14. Treatment algori...   ...\sterisk indicates that response means the patient achieved goal BP or is makin...   ...siderable progress toward this goal. From the fifth report of the Joint National Co...   ...e on Detection, Evaluation, and Treatment of High Blood Pressure (JNC V). Arch I...   ...Med 1993;153:154–183.

Table 7.10. Preferable Antihypertensive Agents in Selected Subgroups

Class of Agents	Subgroup
ACE inhibitors	CHF, diabetes, post-MI (EF <40%)
α-Blocker	Benign prostatic hypertrophy
β-Blocker	CAD, post MI
Calcium channel blocker	Hyporeninemic (e.g., African-Americans, elderly)
Diuretic	Hyporeninemic (e.g., African-Americans, elderly)

Suggested Readings

Alderman MH, Madhavan S, Ooi WL, Cohen H, Sealey JE, Laragh JH. Association of the renin-sodium profile with the risk of myocardial infarction in patients with hypertension. N Engl J Med 1991;324:1098–1104.

Ames RP. The effects of antihypertensive drugs on serum lipids and lipoproteins. Drugs 1986;32:260–278.

Applegate WB. Hypertension in elderly pa-tients. Ann Intern Med 1989;110: 901–915.

Beard K, Culpitt C, Mascie-Taylor H, O'Malley K, Sever P, Webb S. Management of elderly patients with sustained hypertension. Br Med J 1992; 304:412–416.

Blair SN, Goodyear NN, Gibbons LW, Cooper KH. Physical fitness and incidence of hypertension in healthy normotensive men and women. JAMA 1984;252:487–490.

Blair SN, Kohl HW III, Barlow CE, Gibbons LW. Physical fitness and all-cause mortality in hypertensive men. Ann Med 1991;23:307–312.

Cappuccio FP, MacGregor GA. Does po-tassium supplementation lower blood pressure? A meta-analysis of published trials. J Hypertens 1991;9:465–473.

Chobanian AV. 1989 Corcoran Lecture: Adaptive and maladaptive responses of the arterial wall to hypertension. Hypertension 1990;15:666–674.

Collins R, Peto R, MacMahon S, et al. Blood pressure, stroke, and coronary heart disease. Part 2, short-term reductions in blood pressure: Overview of randomised drug trials in their epidemiological context. Lancet 1990;335: 827–838.

Cornoni-Huntley J, LaCroix AZ, Havlik RJ. Race and sex differentials in the impact of hypertension in the United States. Arch Intern Med 1989;149:780–788.

Cutler JA, Brittain E. Calcium and blood pressure: An epidemiologic perspective. Am J Hypertens 1990;3: 137S–146S.

Cutler JA, Follman D, Elliott P, Suh I. An overview of randomized trials of sodium reduction and blood pressure. Hypertension 1991;17(suppl I):I–27—I–33.

Dahlöf B, Lindholm L, Hansson L, Scherstén B, Ekbom T, Wester P-O. Morbidity and mortality in the Swedish Trial in Old Patients with Hypertension (STOP-Hypertension). Lancet 1991; 338:1281–1285.

The fifth report of the Joint National Committee on Detection, Evaluation, and Treatment of High Blood Pressure (JNC V). Arch Intern Med 1993; 153:154–183.

Fletcher AE, Bulpitt CJ. How far should blood pressure be lowered? N Engl J Med 1992;326:251–254.

Gibson RS, Boden WE, Theroux P, et al. Diltiazem and reinfarction in patients with non-Q-wave myocardial infarction: Results of double-blind, randomized, multicenter trial. N Engl J Med 1986; 315:423–9.

Groppelli A, Giorgi DMA, Omboni S, Parati G, Mancia G. Persistent blood pressure increase induced by heavy smoking. J Hypertens 1992;10:495–499.

Hypertension Prevention Trial Research Group. The Hypertension Prevention Trial: Three-year effects of dietary changes on blood pressure. Arch Intern Med 1990; 150:153–162.

Intersalt Cooperative Research Group: Intersalt: An international study of electrolyte excretion and blood pressure. Results for 24 hour urinary sodium and potassium excretion. BMJ 1988; 297: 319–328.

Kannel WB. Hypertension, blood lipids, and cigarette smoking as co-risk factors for coronary heart disease. Ann N Y Acad Sci 1978;304:128–139.

Kaplan NM. Clinical hypertension. 6th ed. Baltimore, MD: Williams & Wilkins, 1994.

Kaplan NM. Maximally reducing cardiovascular risk in the treatment of hypertension. Ann Intern Med 1988; 109:36–40.

Kaplan NM. Calcium and potassium in the treatment of essential hypertension. Semin Nephrol 1988;8:176–184.

Krishna GG, Kapoor SC. Potassium depletion exacerbates essential hypertension. Ann Intern Med 1991; 115:77–83.

Kurtz TW, Spence MA. Genetics of essential hypertension. Am J Med 1993; 94:77–84.

Lant A. Diuretic drugs. Progress in clinical pharmacology. Drugs 1986;31:40–55.

Lardinois CK, Neuman SL. The effects of antihypertensive agents on serum lipids and lipoproteins. Arch Intern Med 1988;148:1280–1288.

MacMahon S. Alcohol consumption and hypertension. Hypertension 1987; 9:111–121.

MacMahon S, Peto R, Cutler J, et al. Blood pressure, stroke, and coronary heart disease. Part 1, prolonged differences in blood pressure: Prospective observational studies corrected for the regression dilution bias. Lancet 1990;335:765–774.

Miller M. Antihypertensive management of the patient with hyperlipidemia. Prev Cardio Rep 1989;3(3):1–5.

MRC Working Party. Medical Research Council trial of treatment of hypertension in older adults: Principal results. Br Med J 1992;304:405–412.

Mulrow CD, Cornell JA, Herrera CR, Kadri A, Farnett L, Aguilar C. Hypertension in the elderly: Implications and generalizability of randomized trials. JAMA 1994;272: 1932–1938.

Paffenbarger RS Jr, Wing AL, Hyde RT, Jung DL. Physical activity and incidence of hypertension in college alumni. Am J Epidemiol 1983;117:245–257.

Pfeffer MA, Braunwald E, Moyé LA, Basta L, et al. Effect of captopril on mortality and morbidity in patients with left ventricular dysfunction after myocardial infarction. Results of the Survival and Ventricular Enlargement Trial. N Engl J Med 1992;327:669–677.

Primary prevention of hypertension by nutritional-hygienic means. Final report of a randomized controlled trial. JAMA 1989;262:1801–1807.

Samani NJ. Molecular genetics of susceptibility to the development of hypertension. Br Med Bull 1994;50:260–271.

Schulman SP, Weiss JL, Becker LC, et al. The effects of antihypertensive therapy on left ventricular mass in elderly patients. N Engl J Med 1990;322: 1350–1356.

Shaper AG, Wannamethee G, Whincup P. Alcohol and blood pressure in middle-aged British men. J Hum Hypertens 1988; 2:71–78.

SHEP Cooperative Research Group. Prevention of stroke by antihypertensive drug treatment in older persons with isolated systolic hypertension: Final results of the Systolic Hypertension in the Elderly Program (SHEP). JAMA 1991;265: 3255-3264.

Siani A, Strazzullo P, Giacco A, Pacioni D, Celentano E, Mancini M. Increasing the dietary potassium intake reduces the need for antihypertensive medication. Ann Intern Med 1991;115: 753-759.

Siscovick DS, Raghunathan TE, Psaty BM, et al. Diuretic therapy for hypertension and the risk of primary cardiac arrest. N Engl J Med 1994;330: 1852-1857.

Sowers JR, Standley PR, Ram JL, Zemel MB, Resnick LM. Insulin resistance, carbohydrate metabolism, and hypertension. Am J Hypertens 1991;4: 466S-472S.

Staessen J, Bulpitt C, Clement D, et al. Relation between mortality and treated blood pressure in elderly patients with hypertension: Report of the European Working Party on High Blood Pressure in the Elderly. Br Med J 1989; 298:1552-1556.

Stamler R, Stamler J, Gosch FC, Civinelli J, et al. Primary prevention of hypertension by nutritional-hygienic means. Final report of a randomized, controlled trial. JAMA 1989;262:1801-7.

Treatment of Mild Hypertension Research Group. The Treatment of Mild Hypertension Study: A randomized, placebo-controlled trial of a nutritional-hygienic regimen along with various drug monotherapies. Arch Intern Med 1991; 151:1413-1423.

Trials of Hypertension Prevention Collaborative Research Group. The effects of nonpharmacologic interventions on blood pressure of persons with high normal levels: Results of the Trials of Hypertension Prevention, Phase I. JAMA 1992; 267:1213-1220.

Weinberger MH. Antihypertensive therapy and lipids: Evidence, mechanisms, and implications. Arch Intern Med 1985; 145:1102-1105.

Weinberger MH. Do no harm: Antihypertensive therapy and the 'J'curve. Arch Intern Med 1992;152: 473-476.

Williams RR, Hunt SC, Hopkins PN, Hastedt SJ, Wu LL, Lalouel JM. Tabulations and expectations regarding the genetics of human hypertension. Kidney Int 1994;45:S-57—S-64.

8/ Diabetes Mellitus

Ten million Americans have diabetes mellitus (DM), and an additional seven million have impaired glucose tolerance. Diabetes is a major risk factor for all cardiovascular diseases, especially in women. The broad term diabetes covers a wide range of insulin and glucose disorders which frequently cluster with other CAD risk factors. Both focal large-vessel atherosclerosis and small-vessel disease are closely associated with diabetes. Diabetes includes three major subgroups: insulin-dependent diabetes mellitus (IDDM), which is generally considered an autoimmune disease leading to insulin deficiency; non-insulin-dependent diabetes mellitus (NIDDM), which makes up the largest fraction and is associated with low, normal, or high insulin concentrations; and glucose intolerance, which is often associated with hyperinsulinemia and obesity. In the simplest fashion, DM is diagnosed by the presence of multiple fasting glucose determinations greater than 140 mg/dL. A more definitive diagnosis is made by oral glucose tolerance testing. After a 75-g glucose load, a 2-hour blood glucose greater than 200 mg/dL is diagnostic of DM, and a value between 140 and 200 mg/dL signifies impaired glucose tolerance. Alternatively, elevated glycohemoglobin (hemoglobin A_{1C}) is indicative of protracted blood glucose elevation. The measurement of glycohemoglobin is especially helpful in evaluating diabetic control.

PATHOPHYSIOLOGY

Several studies, including the Framingham Heart Study (see Abbott et al., Kannel and McGee) have demonstrated an increased rate of CAD and cerebrovascular and peripheral vascular diseases in diabetics. Women with DM completely lose their gender-related protection from CAD, and nearly 50% of all limb amputations for peripheral arterial disease are accounted for by the diabetic population. Data from the 360,000 men screened in MRFIT found that diabetics were at two to five times greater risk for CAD than normoglycemic subjects, independent of cholesterol levels. The relative risk of CAD rose with increasing cholesterol in both diabetic and nondiabetic subjects. Other studies, such as the Rancho Bernardo Study (see Wingard et al.), suggested that diabetic individuals were more likely to have other cardiovascular risk factors, including hypertension (HTN), lipid abnormalities, and central obesity (see Syndrome X, below).

Diabetes mellitus is associated with decreases in HDL-C and increases in VLDL-C and TG. This appears to be especially true in women which may in part explain their loss of gender-related protection. Diabetic patients have decreased LPL activity, leading to decreased catabolism of chylomicrons and VLDL-C particles (see Chapter 6). These are thought to be especially atherogenic in diabetic individuals. High-density lipoprotein cholesterol levels are indirectly reduced because of the reciprocal interaction between HDL-C and TG. Additionally, LDL-C is increased due to decreased receptor activity. LDL-C is generally not markedly elevated in diabetic patients and may be difficult to calculate especially when TG exceeds 400 mg/dL. HDL-C levels less than 50 mg/dL and VLDL-C levels greater than 20 mg/dL appear to predict CAD mortality in women. In addition to glycohemoglobin, TG levels can be used as an index of diabetic control. In the Paris Heart Study (see Eschwège et al.), TG levels were the strongest lipid predictor of CAD mortality, particularly with elevated fasting insulin levels.

High insulin concentrations, found with all three subgroups of DM, have been shown to be associated with CAD independent of other risk factors. NIDDM patients often have high insulin concentrations because of peripheral insulin resistance, and IDDM is subjected to high concentrations of exogenous insulin. Moreover, insulin resistance is associated with central adiposity (increased waist:hip ratio), which is an additional marker of enhanced CAD risk. As a vascular smooth muscle cell growth factor, insulin is believed to contribute to atherogenic risk by stimulating subintimal cellular proliferation. Elevated glucose levels also lead to increased modified (glycosylated) LDL-C, resulting in enhanced uptake and incorporation by scavenger cells (see Chapter 4). Postangioplasty restenosis is also increased in diabetic patients. The restenotic process is generally considered to result from excess growth factor stimulation. In addition to lipid abnormalities, DM has been reported to be associated with altered platelet function, including increased platelet aggregability, increased fibrinogen levels, and decreased serum fibrinolytic activity.

SYNDROME X

Several epidemiological studies have demonstrated a clustering of insulin resistance, HTN, dyslipidemia, and central obesity. The prevalence of HTN is increased in patients with DM (50%) or glucose intolerance (15–18%). The presence of both DM and HTN is also common in obese individuals. Moreover, the risk of HTN in obese individuals is doubled by the presence of glucose intolerance. The common defect in this risk factor clustering, termed Syndrome X, is insulin resistance. Hyperinsulinemia stimulates hepatic production of VLDL-C and may lead to HTN via a variety of mechanisms, including sodium-water retention, sympathetic nerve stimulation, changes in transmembrane ion traffic, and direct stimulation of smooth muscle cell growth (see also Chapter 7). As noted above, insulin is directly atherogenic.

DIABETIC CONTROL

Considerable debate has focused on the value of aggressive diabetic control in retarding the associated devastating sequelae. In a study of 1441 patients with IDDM, the Diabetes Control and Complications Trial (DCCT), demonstrated that intensive therapy, (e.g., external insulin pump, frequent insulin injections) and frequent blood glucose monitoring resulted in less progression of retinopathy compared with standard management. Retinopathy was reduced by 76% in a primary prevention cohort and by 54% with established retinopathy (Fig. 8.1). Intensive therapy also reduced the occurrence of albuminuria by 39% in the two groups combined (Fig. 8.2). Neuropathy was reduced by 69% (Fig. 8.3). Although the DCCT was not primarily an event trial, intensive therapy reduced major cardiovascular events by 41%. Hypercholesterolemia (LDL-C greater than 160 mg/dL) was reduced by 34%. The major adverse effect associated with intensive therapy was a two- to threefold increase in severe hypoglycemia. Overall, these findings suggest that intensive diabetic control reduces the sequelae of the disease. In the DCCT, the goals of intensive therapy included preprandial blood glucose concentrations between 70 and 120 mg/dL, postprandial concentrations of less than 180 mg/dL, and glycohemoglobin (hemoglobin A_{1C}) of approximately 6%.

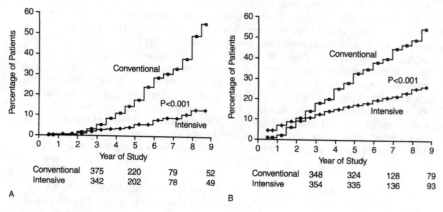

Figure 8.1. Cumulative incidence of a sustained change in retinopathy in patients with IDDM receiving intensive or conventional therapy. A sustained change in the severity of retinopathy was defined as a change observed by fundus photography of at least three steps from baseline that was sustained for at least six months. In the primary-prevention cohort (**Panel A**), intensive therapy reduced the adjusted mean risk of the onset of retinopathy by 76% during the course of the study, as compared with conventional therapy (P<0.001). In the secondary-intervention cohort (**Panel B**), intensive therapy reduced the adjusted mean risk of progression of retinopathy by 54% as compared with conventional therapy (P<0.001). The numbers of patients in each therapy group who were evaluated at years 3, 5, 7, and 9 are shown below the graphs. Reprinted by permission of The New England Journal of Medicine from The Diabetes Control and Complications Trial Research Group. The effect of intensive treatment of diabetes on the development and progression of long-term complications in insulin-dependent diabetes mellitus. N Engl J Med 1993;329:977–986, Copyright © 1993, Massachusetts Medical Society.

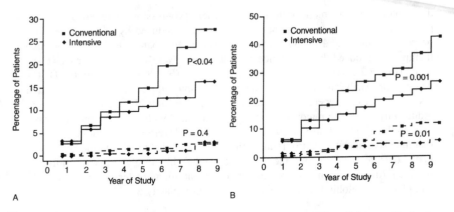

Figure 8.2. Cumulative incidence of urinary albumin excretion ≥300 mg/24 hours (dashed line) and ≥40 mg/24 hours (solid line) in patients with insulin-dependent diabetes mellitus receiving intensive or conventional therapy. In the primary-prevention cohort (**Panel A**), intensive therapy reduced the adjusted mean risk of microalbuminuria by 34% (P<0.04). In the secondary-intervention cohort (**Panel B**), patients with urinary albumin excretion of ≥40 mg/24 hours at baseline were excluded from the analysis of the development of microalbuminuria. Intensive therapy reduced the adjusted mean risk of albuminuria by 56% (P = 0.01) and the risk of microalbuminuria by 43% (P = 0.001), as compared with conventional therapy. Reprinted by permission of The New England Journal of Medicine from The Diabetes Control and Complications Trial Research Group. The effect of intensive treatment of diabetes on the development and progression of long-term complications in insulin-dependent diabetes mellitus. N Engl J Med 1993;329:977–986, Copyright © 1993, Massachusetts Medical Society.

In addition to insulin therapy, diet is a major factor in the management of diabetes. Weight loss improves insulin sensitivity and lowers TG levels. The American Diabetes Association recommends a diet low in total fat (less than 30% of calories), saturated fat (less than 10%), and cholesterol (less than 300 mg/day). Monounsaturated fat predominance has replaced the high fat and protein recommendations of the past. There is continuing debate on the impact of the high carbohydrate diet on insulin resistance, but the high prevalence of dyslipidemias and CAD reinforce its use. Fish-oil supplements rich in ω-3 fatty acids are also effective in lowering TG but may raise LDL-C; routine use is not recommended, except with markedly elevated TG (see Chapter 6).

LIPID MANAGEMENT

Diabetic patients commonly have elevations of TG, decreases in HDL-C, and mild elevations of LDL-C. The use of hypolipidemic drugs in diabetics presents

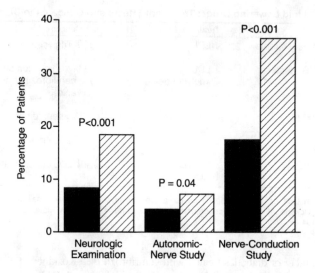

Figure 8.3. Prevalence of abnormal clinical neurologic examinations, abnormal results of nerve-conduction studies, and abnormal autonomic-nerve studies at 5 years in patients receiving intensive (solid bars) or conventional (hatched bars) therapy. Abnormal results of nerve-conduction studies were defined as abnormal results of neurophysiologic tests in at least two peripheral nerves. The analysis included all patients from either cohort who did not have the abnormality in question at baseline. Reprinted by permission of The New England Journal of Medicine from The Diabetes Control and Complications Trial Research Group. The effect of intensive treatment of diabetes on the development and progression of long-term complications in insulin-dependent diabetes mellitus. N Engl J Med 1993; 329:977–986, Copyright © 1993, Massachusetts Medical Society.

specific problems. Bile acid sequestrants such as cholestyramine reduce LDL-C but may induce hypertriglyceridemia and should generally not be used with fasting TG levels above 200 mg/dL (Table 8.1). To reduce LDL-C, the HMG-CoA reductase inhibitors are better suited to diabetic management. Caution must be taken when combining these agents with either gemfibrozil or nicotinic acid because of a higher frequency of myositis and rhabdomyolysis (see Chapter 4).

Nicotinic acid would be an ideal drug for dyslipidemic diabetic patients because it lowers TG and raises HDL-C. Unfortunately, nicotinic acid may worsen glycemic control. This medication may be attempted with NIDDM, but close monitoring is required. Gemfibrozil has beneficial effects on TG and HDL-C with modest effects on LDL-C. It is particularly efficacious with NIDDM and elevated TG (see Vinik et al.). In the Helsinki Heart Study, there was a trend towards reduced CAD events in

Table 8.1. Lipid Lowering Drugs: Treatment Effects and Concerns in Diabetes

Drug	Treatment Effect	Concerns
Bile Acid Sequestrants	↓ LDL	↑ Triglycerides
HMG-CoA Reductase Inhibitors	↓ LDL ↓ Triglycerides	Myositis if combined with gemfibrozil or nicotinic acid
Nicotinic Acid	↓ Triglycerides ↑ HDL ↓ LDL	Worsens diabetic control ↑ Uric Acid
Gemfibrozil	↓ Triglycerides ↑ HDL	↓ LDL effect small

Adapted from Orchard TJ. Intervention for the prevention of coronary heart disease in diabetes. In: Ockene IS, Ockene JK, eds. Prevention of coronary heart disease. Boston, Mass: Little, Brown & Co, 1992:383–404.

a small number of diabetics treated with gemfibrozil (see Koskinen et al.). As most angiographic and event rate trials have excluded patients with DM, little information is available regarding optimal management of dyslipidemia. Previously, lipoprotein disorders were rarely treated in diabetics. Today, emphasis is placed on controlling both the underlying systemic disorder *and* associated dyslipidemia. In view of the very high incidence of cardiovascular complications associated with DM, it appears prudent to manage dyslipidemias aggressively in this high-risk subgroup.

MANAGEMENT OF HYPERTENSION

Hypertension is also prevalent in DM and, in addition to CAD, is a risk factor for the development of nephropathy, retinopathy, and neuropathy. As with lipid managements, antihypertensive drugs pose special problems in diabetic individuals. Thiazides elevate LDL-C and TG and worsen glycemic control (see also Chapter 7). β-Blockers may mask the symptoms of hypoglycemia, but would still be selected in the post-MI diabetic. In contrast, ACE inhibitors do not affect glucose control or lipoproteins. Due to their ability to reduce intraglomerular hypertension, ACE inhibitors reduce albuminuria and retard progression of renal disease. This effect has been documented in diabetics with normal BP. ACE inhibitors are, thus, currently recommended for the primary prevention of diabetes-associated nephropathy.

Suggested Readings

Abbott RD, Donahue RP, Kannel WB, et al. The impact of diabetes on survival following myocardial infarction in men vs. women. The Framingham study. JAMA 1988;260:3456–3460.

American Diabetes Association. Position statement: Screening for diabetes. Diabetes Care 1989;12:588–590.

Brenner BM, Meyer TW, Hostetter TH. Dietary protein intake and the progressive nature of kidney disease: The role of hemodynamically mediated glomerular injury in the pathogenesis of progressive glomerular sclerosis in aging, renal ablation, and intrinsic renal disease. N Engl J Med 1982; 307:652–959.

Diabetes Control and Complications Trial Research Group. The effect of intensive treatment of diabetes on the development and progression of long-term complication in insulin-dependent diabetes mellitus. N Engl J Med 1993;329:977–986.

Ducimetière P, Eschwège E, Papoz L, et al. Relationship of plasma insulin levels to the incidence of myocardial infarction and coronary heart disease mortality in a middle-aged population. Diabetologia 1980;19:205–210.

Eschwège E, Richard JL, Thibult N, et al. Coronary heart disease mortality in relation with diabetes, blood glucose and plasma insulin levels. The Paris Prospective Study, ten years later. Horm Metab Res Suppl 1985; 15: 41–46.

Feldt-Rasmussen B, Mathiesen ER, Deckert T. Effect of two years strict metabolic control on the progression of incipient nephropathy in insulin-dependent diabetes. Lancet 1986;2: 1300–1304.

Garg A, Bonanome A, Grundy SM, et al. Comparison of a high-carbohydrate diet with a high-monounsaturated-fat diet in patients with non-insulin-dependent diabetes mellitus. N Engl J Med 1988;319:829–834.

Garg A, Grundy SM. Lovastatin for lowering cholesterol levels in non-insulin-dependent diabetes mellitus. N Engl J Med 1988;318:81–86.

Garg A, Grundy SM. Gemfibrozil alone and in combination with lovastatin for treatment of hypertriglyceridemia in NIDDM. Diabetes 1989;38:364–372.

Goldschmid MG, Barrett-Connor E, Edelstein SL, et al. Dyslipidemia and ischemic heart disease mortality among men and women with heart disease. Circulation 1994;89:991–997.

Howard BV. Lipoprotein metabolism in diabetes mellitus. J Lipid Res 1987; 28:613–628.

Kannel WB, McGee DL. Diabetes and cardiovascular disease. The Framingham study. JAMA 1979;241:2035–2038.

Konttinen A, Juisma I, Ralli R, et al. The effect of gemfibrozil on serum lipids in diabetic patients. Ann Clin Res 1979;11:240–245.

Koskinen P, Mänttäri M, Manninen V, Huttunen JK, et al. Coronary heart disease incidence in NIDDM patients in The Helsinki Heart Study. Diabetes Care 1992;15:820–825.

Lapidus L, Bengtsson C, Larsson B, et al. Distribution of adipose tissue and risk of cardiovascular disease and death: A 12 year follow-up of participants in the population study of women in Gothenburg, Sweden. Br Med J 1984; 289:1257–1261.

Leaf A, Weber PC. Cardiovascular effects of n-3 fatty acids. N Engl J Med 1988;318:549–557.

Liu GC, Coulston AM, Reaven GM. Effects of high-carbohydrate-low-fat diets on plasma glucose, insulin and lipid responses in hypertriglyceridemic humans. Metabolism 1983;32:750–753.

Multiple Risk Factor Intervention Trial Research Group: Multiple Risk Factor Intervention Trial: Risk factor changes and mortality results. JAMA 1982; 248:1465–1477.

Orchard TJ. Intervention for the prevention of coronary heart disease in diabetes. In: Ockene IS, Ockene JK, eds. Prevention of Coronary Heart Disease. Boston, Mass: Little, Brown & Co, 1992:383–404.

Phillips A, Shaper AG, Winchup PH. Association between serum albumin and mortality from cardiovascular disease, cancer and other causes. Lancet 1989;2:1434–1436.

Reaven GM. Non-insulin-dependent diabetes mellitus, abnormal lipoprotein metabolism and atherosclerosis. Metabolism 1987;36:1–8.

Reaven GM. Insulin resistance and compensatory hyperinsulinemia: Role in hypertension, dyslipidemia and coronary heart disease. Am Heart J 1991;121:1283–1288.

Simpson RW, Mann JI, Eaton J, et al. Improved glucose control in maturity-onset diabetes treated with high-carbohydrate modified fat diet. Br Med J 1979;1:1753–1756.

Vinik AI, Colwell JA. Effects of gemfibrozil on triglyceride levels in patients with NIDDM. Diabetes Care 1993;16: 37–44.

Waller BJ, Palumbo PJ, Lie JT, et al. Status of the coronary arteries at necropsy in diabetes mellitus with onset after age 30 years. Analysis of 229 diabetic patients with and without clinical evidence of coronary heart disease and comparison to 183 control subjects. Am J Med 1980;69:498–506.

Wingard DL, Barrett-Connor E, Criqui MH, et al. Clustering of heart disease risk factors in diabetic compared to nondiabetic adults. Am J Epidemiol 1983; 117:19–26.

The working group on hypertension in diabetes: Statement on hypertension in diabetes mellitus. Final report. Arch Intern Med 1987;147:830–842.

9/ Cigarette Smoking

Cigarette smoking is the most preventable cause of death in the United States. It claims the life of one out of every six individuals and is responsible for two out of every five cardiovascular deaths. When the Surgeon General's report documenting the hazards of cigarette smoking was released in 1964, nearly half of all U.S. adults smoked. Despite the antismoking fervor that has penetrated our society, it is estimated (based on actual deaths in 1990, Table 9.1) that more than 400,000 Americans will die of cigarette-smoking-related causes. The economic burden due to smoking-related illnesses is indeed staggering; an estimated $50 to $100 billion yearly will be spent in direct health care costs and lost productivity. Some sobering statistics regarding life expectancy are shown in Table 9.2.

Nearly 40% of cardiovascular deaths (21% of CAD and 18% of cerebrovascular disease) are attributable to smoking. Cigarette smokers have twice the risk of developing CAD and a two- to fourfold increased risk of sudden cardiac death. Middle-aged male smokers (ages 55 to 59) face a 45% increased risk of death during the ensuing 15 years (Fig. 9.1). Equally distressing are the rates of death among nonsmokers exposed to passive smoke; an estimated 37,000 will succumb to a cardiovascular event as a result of environmental toxins produced by cigarettes. The statistics in Table 9.3 point to the prevalence of this addiction. These ratios, although trending downward, are not expected to be substantially altered as we

Table 9.1. Actual Causes of Death in the United States in 1990

| | Deaths | |
Causes	Estimated No.*	Percentage of Total Deaths
Tobacco	400,000	19
Diet/activity patterns	300,000	14
Alcohol	100,000	5
Microbial agents	90,000	4
Toxic agents	60,000	3
Firearms	35,000	2
Sexual behavior	30,000	1
Motor vehicles	25,000	1
Illicit use of drugs	20,000	<1
Total	1,060,000	50

*Composite approximation drawn from studies that use different approaches to derive estimates, ranging from actual counts (e.g., firearms) to population attributable risk calculations (e.g., tobacco). Numbers over 100,000 rounded to the nearest 100,000; over 50,000, rounded to the nearest 10,000; below 50,000, rounded to the nearest 5,000.
From McGinnis JM, Foege WH. Actual causes of death in the United States. JAMA 1993;270:2207–2212.

Table 9.2. **Life Expectancy Lost Based on Cigarette Smoking in a 25-Year-Old Man**

Amount	Time Lost
1 cigarette	5.5 minutes
1 pack/day	4.6 years
2 packs/day	8.3 years

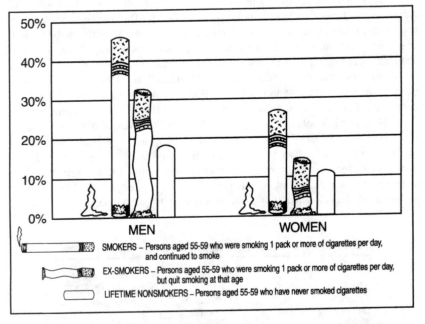

Figure 9.1. Chance of dying in next 15 years, smokers vs ex-smokers vs lifetime non-smokers. Data from American Cancer Society, Cancer Prevention Study II (1982–1986). Graphics from US Department of Health and Human Services.

enter the next millennium; at least one in five adults will continue to smoke. There is a particularly alarming prevalence among African-Americans, blue-collar workers, and persons without a high school education. In addition to the nearly 50 million adult smokers in the United States, 2.2 million teenagers have initiated the habit. Education is inversely proportional to smoking status; smoking is approximately one-third as prevalent among the college educated as among those lacking a high school diploma (Fig. 9.2).

Table 9.3. Smoking Prevalence in the United States (%)

	1974	1984	1994
Men	43.4	33.5	28.1
Women	31.2	27.6	23.5
Caucasian	36.1	29.4	25.6
African-Americans	44.0	35.4	29.7

Data from Cox JL. How to help your patients stop smoking. J Am Acad Physician Assist 1990;3:600–606.

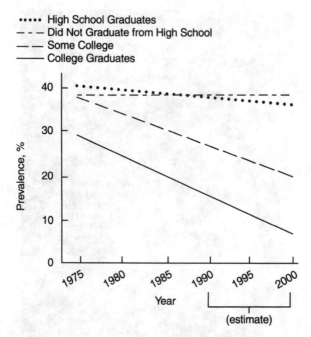

Figure 9.2. Smoking prevalence by educational status. From Pierce JP, Fiore MC, Novotny TE, Hatziandreu EJ, Davis RM. Trends in cigarette smoking in the United States: Projections to the year 2000. JAMA 1989;261:61–65.

During the 1950s, when cigarette smoking was fashionable and the hazards less well established, physicians were primary endorsers of certain brands (Figs. 9.3 and 9.4). Not surprisingly, the rates of smoking within the allied health fields have dropped as well between 1974 and 1991. The one exception are LPNs whose high prevalence of cigarette smoking, approximates that of the general population (Table 9.4).

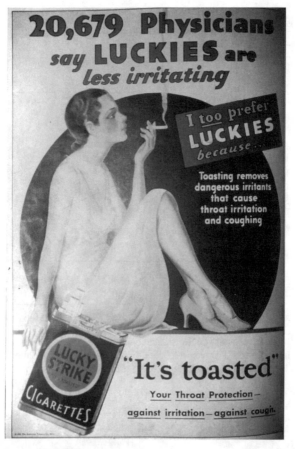

Figure 9.3. Smoking advertisement from the 1950s, courtesy of Office on Smoking and Health, Centers for Disease Control and Prevention, Atlanta, Ga.

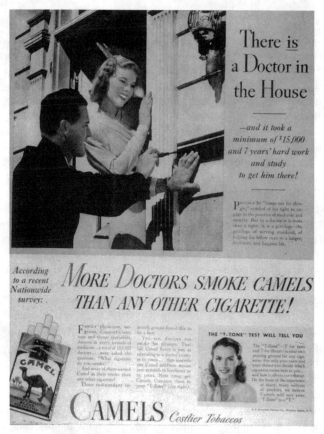

Figure 9.4. Smoking advertisement from the 1950s, courtesy of Office on Smoking and Health, Centers for Disease Control and Prevention, Atlanta, Ga.

Table 9.4. Prevalence of Smokers Within the Medical Profession (%)

	1974	1991
MDs	18.8	3.3
RNs	31.7	18.3
LPNs	37.1	27.2

BIOCHEMISTRY AND PATHOPHYSIOLOGY

Enhanced thrombogenicity results from impairment of endothelial function due to inhibition in prostacyclin (PGI_2) synthesis. Smoking one cigarette enhances platelet adhesion to the endothelial lining (Fig. 9.5). Persistent smoking results in enhanced platelet aggregability and release of potent mediators (e.g., platelet-derived growth factor), stimulating smooth muscle cell proliferation and migration to the intimal surface.

Of the more than 4,000 chemicals released from cigarette smoke, carbon monoxide and nicotine have been the most widely studied; both exert toxic effects on the endothelium. Carbon monoxide causes hypoxia and loss of endothelial cell integrity, thereby facilitating transport of atherogenic lipoproteins and scavenger cells across the endothelial barrier with penetration into the subintimal layer. Carbon monoxide also has a very high affinity for hemoglobin; smokers experience an estimated 15% reduction in O_2-carrying capacity leading to an increased risk of angina and arrhythmogenic events. In addition to its cellular effects, nicotine stimulates catecholamine release, acute increases in heart rate, BP, and peripheral vascular resistance. In the Metoprolol And Propranolol Hypertension Trial (MAPHY) (Wikstrand et al.), CAD mortality was lower in smokers who received β-blockers vs. diuretics.

Cigarette smokers have an increased production of fibrinogen (see Chapter 11) and reduced fibrinolytic activity owing to low endogenous production of TPA. Smoking also appears to have a direct effect on plasma lipids and lipoproteins (Fig. 9.6). Nicotine stimulates catecholamine release, which mediates lipolysis, enhancing FFA mobilization and elevating plasma TG (see Craig et al.).

EPIDEMIOLOGY

The effect of cigarette smoking on coronary atherosclerosis is related to both quantity and duration of usage. Within a given age group, the percentage of raised coronary artery lesions is lowest in nonsmokers and highest in heavy smokers (more than 25 cigarettes daily: Fig. 9.7).

Patients with CAD who continue to smoke suffer severe consequences. Data obtained from the Coronary Artery Surgery Study (CASS) revealed that compared to quitters, persistent smokers evidenced a 32% increase in 5-year mortality. Myocardial infarction survivors who receive thrombolytic therapy have an approximately fourfold increased risk of reinfarction within 1 year if they resume smoking (see Rivers et al.). Importantly, the efficacy of antianginal therapy (e.g., β-blockers, calcium blockers) and aspirin may be attenuated in CAD patients who continue to smoke (see Deanfield et al.). Among patients surviving a sudden cardiac arrest, 27% of habitual smokers (compared to 19% of reformed smokers) suffered a recurrent arrest during a 3-year followup period (see Hallstrom et al.).

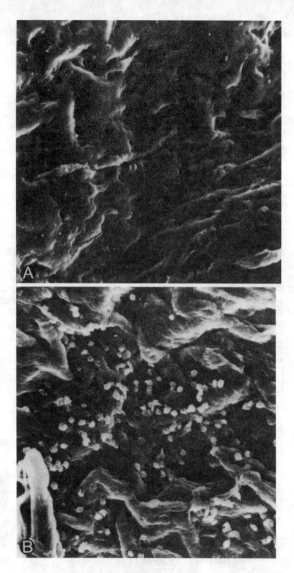

Figure 9.5. A, Rabbit endothelium after being exposed in vitro for 10 minutes to presmoke blood. No adhering platelets can be seen in this micrograph. × 1200. **B,** Rabbit endothelium after being exposed in vitro for 10 minutes to postsmoking blood. Many activated platelets adhere to the endothelial surface. × 1200. From Pittilo RM, Clarke JMF, Harris D, et al. Cigarette smoking and platelet adhesion. Brit J Haematol 1984;58:627–632. Blackwell Science Ltd. Used with permission.

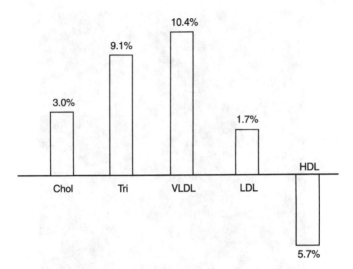

Figure 9.6. Percentage increase or decrease in lipid levels in smokers, compared with non-smokers. Chol = cholesterol; Tri = triglycerides. Adapted with permission from Craig WY, Palomaki GE, Haddow JE. Cigarette smoking and serum lipid and lipoprotein concentrations: An analysis of published data. Br Med J 1989;298:784–788. Published by BMJ Publishing Group.

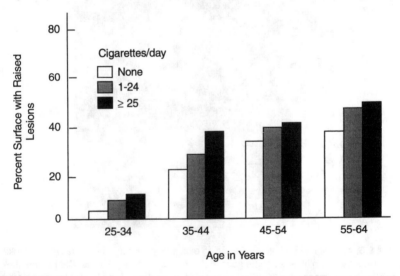

Figure 9.7. Coronary artery raised lesions (fibrous plaques and complicated lesions) by age and degree of smoking in 553 white men. From McGill HC Jr. The cardiovascular pathology of smoking. Am Heart J 1988;115:250–257. Used with permission. (Drawn from data in Strong JP, Richards MS. Cigarette smoking and atherosclerosis in autopsied men. Atherosclerosis 1976;23:451–476.)

In addition to the higher CAD rate, cigarette smoking has also been associated with diffuse ventricular hypokinesis and dilated cardiomyopathy resulting from intramural coronary vessel obstruction. Smoking induces coronary vasoconstriction and enhances myocardial ischemia in patients with CAD; these effects may be partially ameliorated with nitroglycerin or calcium antagonists (see Winniford et al.). Cigarette smoking also increases the risk of cerebral infarction nearly threefold in one-pack-per-day smokers. The prevalence of aortoiliac and femoropopliteal disease is markedly enhanced with cigarette use; abdominal aortic aneurysms are twice as likely to occur in smokers as in nonsmokers.

The deleterious effects of cigarette smoking are particularly noteworthy in the young. Among MI survivors below the age of 40, the most common accompanying risk factor was cigarette smoking. Although heavily advertised by the cigarette industry, "low yield" cigarettes (e.g., reduced nicotine and carbon monoxide) have not been demonstrated to lower MI risk. In fact, smokers tend to inhale more deeply, resulting in greater exposure to these noxious elements.

As reported in men, women who smoke are also at increased risk for CAD. In the Nurses Health Study, Willett and associates reported a twofold increased risk of cardiovascular events (e.g., fatal CAD and nonfatal MI) among women smoking as few as one to four cigarettes per day; an approximately 11-fold increased risk was observed when smoking exceeded 45 cigarettes per day. The addition of a second risk factor (e.g., HTN, hyperlipidemia, or DM) enhanced CAD risk nearly 20-fold. The presence of DM-enhanced CAD risk was noteworthy among smokers of 15 or more cigarettes daily (Fig. 9.8). Similarly, the combination of cigarette smoking and use of oral contraceptives has been shown to elevate CAD mortality by 10-fold. Compared with nonsmoking women not receiving oral contraceptives, the relative risk of stroke (hemorrhagic and thrombotic) was increased more than 20-fold. Cigarette smoking also appears to exert an antiestrogenic effect, characterized by premature menopause, decreased endometrial carcinoma, and increased osteoporosis. Increased oxidation of estradiol to 2-hydroxyestrone, a metabolite lacking estrogenic activity, has been the proposed mechanism (see Michnovica et al.).

Fortunately, smoking cessation yields a favorable impact on initial and recurrent CAD event rate. On average, the rate may be reduced by 50% within 1 year of cessation. In men who quit smoking, the risk of an initial nonfatal MI approximated that of a nonsmoker after 2 years of abstention. These results were unaffected by either intensity or duration of smoking. With arteriographically documented CAD, smoking cessation led to reduced anginal episodes and improvement in ST segment during exercise stress testing, as well as reduced MIs and cardiovascular death in both younger (less than 40 years) and older (more than 65 years) patients. In post-MI patients, there is a reduction of approximately 50% in reinfarction rates and cardiovascular mortality: Table 9.5). Smoking cessation also reduces extracranial carotid lesions and retards the progression of aortoiliac and femoropopliteal disease.

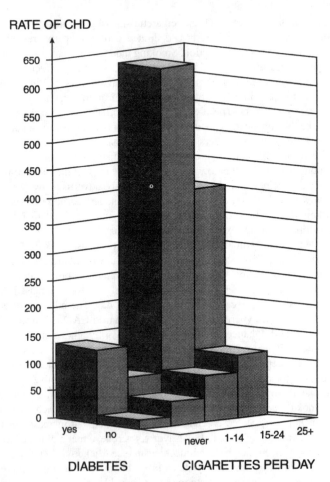

RATE OF CHD

DIABETES   CIGARETTES PER DAY

Figure 9.8. Age-standardized rates of CHD per 100,000 person-years (vertical scale) among women, according to cigarette use and history of diabetes. Reprinted by permission of The New England Journal of Medicine from Willett WC, Green A, Stampfer MJ, et al. Relative and absolute excess risks of coronary heart disease among women who smoke cigarettes. N Engl J Med 1987;317:1303–1309, Copyright © 1987, Massachusetts Medical Society.

Table 9.5. Smoking Cessation After MI

Study location and publications	N	Followup period (year)	Mortality reduction (%)
Göteborg Wilhelmsson et al., 1975[1] Åberg et al., 1983[2]	938	10	38
Dublin Mulcahy et al., 1975[3] Mulcahy, 1983[4]	374	13	55
Framingham Sparrow et al., 1978[5]	202	6	60
Helsinki Pohjola et al., 1979[6]	648	5	60
North Karelia Salonen et al., 1980[7]	523	3	40

[1]Wilhelmsson C, Elmfeldt D, Vedin JA, Tibblin G, Wilhelmsen L. Smoking and myocardial infarction. Lancet 1975;1:415–420.
[2]Åberg A, Bergstrand R, Johansson S, et al. Cessation of smoking after myocardial infarction— effects on mortality after 10 years. Br Heart J 1983;49:416–422.
[3]Mulcahy R, Hickey N, Graham I, McKenzie G. Factors influencing long-term prognosis in male patients surviving a first coronary attack. Br Heart J 1975;37:158–165.
[4]Mulcahy R. Influence of cigarette smoking on morbidity and mortality after myocardial infarction. Br Heart J 1983;49:410–415.
[5]Sparrow D, Dawber TR, Colton T. The influence of cigarette smoking on prognosis after a first myocardial infarction. J Chronic Dis 1978;31:425–432.
[6]Pohjola S, Siltanen P, Romo M, et al. Effect of quitting smoking on the long-term survival after myocardial infarction [Abstract] Trans Eur Soc Cardiol 1979;1:2.
[7]Salonen JT. Stopping smoking and long-term mortality after acute myocardial infarction. Br Heart J 1980;43:463–469.

From Wilhelmsen L. Coronary heart disease: Epidemiology of smoking and intervention studies of smoking. Am Heart J 1988;115:242–249. Adapted with permission.

Passive Smoking

It has been estimated that nearly 50 million nonsmoking adults are exposed to environmental tobacco on a regular basis, accounting for more than 50,000 deaths yearly (Fig. 9.9). Passive smoking represents the third most preventable cause of death in the U.S., following active smoking and alcohol abuse.

Environmental tobacco smoke consists of "mainstream," or exhaled, smoke and "sidestream" smoke, or smoke released into the atmosphere between puffs. Sidestream smoke releases a higher concentration of noxious elements (e.g., carbon monoxide, benzopyrene) than smoke ordinarily filtered during inhalation. As with

Deaths from Passive Smoking
Total Deaths: 53,000

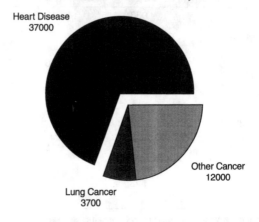

Heart Disease
37000

Other Cancer
12000

Lung Cancer
3700

Figure 9.9. US deaths from environmental tobacco smoke. The majority of annual deaths are attributed to heart disease. From Glantz SA, Parmley WW. Passive smoking and heart disease: Epidemiology, physiology, and biochemistry. Circulation 1991;83:1–12. Reproduced with permission. Circulation Copyright © 1991 American Heart Association.

active smoking, passive smoking has been shown to enhance platelet aggregation, and chemicals such as benzopyrene are directly injurious to endothelial cells.

Exposure to environmental tobacco smoke leads to increased heart rate, BP, and blood carboxyhemoglobin levels. With reduction in maximum oxygen uptake, exercise performance is impaired in both healthy and CAD subjects. Male and female nonsmokers exposed to environmental tobacco smoke have a 30% increased risk of death from MI or CAD, translating into nearly 40,000 cardiovascular deaths yearly.

RECOMMENDATIONS

Smoking Cessation: Overview

The average nicotine content of a cigarette is 10 mg, of which approximately 1 to 2 mg are effectively delivered to the lungs and distributed to the brain within 7 seconds. Nicotine is the most addictive chemical present in cigarette smoke; its withdrawal signals a syndrome marked by anxiety, irritability, and difficulty concentrating. These physiological effects peak within the first 72 to 96 hours (Table 9.6) and may persist for approximately 3 weeks. The psychological urge for nico-

Table 9.6. Tobacco Withdrawal Symptoms Reported During the First Week of Untreated Tobacco Deprivation

Symptom	% Reporting
Anxiety	87
Inadequate sleep	84
Irritability	80
Impatience	76
Difficulty concentrating	73
Restlessness	71
Craving tobacco	62
Hunger	53
Gastrointestinal problems	33
Headaches	24
Drowsiness	22

Data from Hughes JR, Hatsukami D. Signs and symptoms of tobacco withdrawal. Arch Gen Psychiatry 1986;43:289–294.
From Fiore MC, Jorenby DE, Baker TB, Kenford SL. Tobacco dependence and the nicotine patch: Clinical guidelines for effective use. JAMA 1992;268:2687–2694. Copyright © 1992, American Medical Association. Used with permission.

tine may last for several months. Thus, it is not surprising that smoking cessation is an enormously difficult challenge. It is estimated that 70% of smokers in the United States desire to quit smoking. Of the 17 million Americans who attempt smoking cessation each year, however, only 8% are successful. The relapse rate within the first 3 months of smoking cessation may be as high as 80%, and even with the various methods described below, the overall success rate after 1 year is a dismal 10%. On average, three to five attempts are made during a 7-year period before successful cessation is accomplished. Moreover, a 5–10 lb weight gain is anticipated. The role of the physician in promoting cessation efforts is essential, as exemplified by the 10-fold increase in success rate among those counseled during their office visits. Among those who were initially successful in their bid to quit, the most important predictors of relapse are

1. high level of postcessation craving
2. low level of confidence in maintaining abstinence
3. insufficient extent of social support systems
4. high degree of alcohol consumption.

Nonpharmacologic Intervention

The American Heart Association, American Cancer Society, and American Lung Association sponsor smoking cessation programs emphasizing behavioral changes, including stress reduction, meditation, and relaxation exercises.

Behavioral self-monitoring techniques are also useful and can be supervised by the family physician or internist. Patients maintain a diary and record the triggering event (e.g., coffee consumption). Following identification of these triggering events, appropriate substitutive behaviors may be promoted (e.g., tea consumption) to alter the conditioned response. Other techniques, including hypnosis, have been reported to be useful in selected individuals. Aversive conditioning techniques (e.g., blowing cigarette smoke in the face) have been employed in smoking cessation clinics.

Pharmacologic Intervention

NICOTINE GUM

Nicotine gum (nicotine polacrilex) is another useful aid for patients attempting to quit smoking. Each piece contains 2 mg nicotine, and the nicotine level is one-third that of cigarette smoke. Recently, a 4 mg dose of nicotine per piece (Nicorette DS) has become available. Patients are asked to chew the gum slowly (10 to 20 seconds), then place the gum in the buccal cavity for mucosal absorption (1 to 2 minutes), and repeat the procedure. When rapidly chewed, nicotine is primarily absorbed within the gastrointestinal (GI) tract, and may produce gastric distress. One piece of gum, the equivalent of 2 cigarettes smoked, has a duration of action lasting 15–30 minutes. The maximum daily allotment is 30 pieces. It is important that subjects not consume acidic beverages (e.g., coffee, citrus juices) while chewing, because absorption of nicotine may be hindered. Although there is often mild improvement in smoking abstinence, the use of nicotine gum has not been shown to be statistically superior to placebo gum in studies extending from 6 months to 1 year (see Lee and D'Alonzo). A meta-analysis revealed that in medical practices, there was an 11% abstinence rate on average; these rates were considerably higher in smoking cessation clinics (23%), which employ behavioral methods (e.g., physician advice, educational materials). In general, the duration of therapy varies between 3 and 6 months; thereafter, gradual weaning is recommended. Contraindications to the use of nicotine gum are outlined in Table 9.7.

NICOTINE PATCH

In its introductory year of 1992, more than 5 million patients at a cost of $1 billion subscribed to the nicotine patch for smoking cessation. The average cost per patient is $25 to $30 weekly, or upwards of $360 for a 3-month course of therapy.

There are potential advantages of nicotine patches over nicotine gum. First, the nicotine patch is not associated with temporomandibular fatigue and gastrointestinal distress is unusual. Second, and perhaps more importantly, transdermal preparations provide a fixed dose of nicotine and steady state response, which provides relief from both withdrawal and craving sensations. The patch is placed on a hairless portion of the upper trunk or arm (absorption is decreased if directly applied to

Table 9.7. Recommended Exclusion Criteria for Nicotine Gum

Postmyocardial infarction
Peripheral vascular disease
Serious cardiac arrhythmias
Systemic hypertension
Vasospastic disease
Active peptic ulcer disease
Active esophagitis
Oral or pharyngeal inflammation
Pheochromocytoma
Hyperthyroidism
Insulin-dependent diabetes mellitus
Pregnancy
Breast feeding
Active temporomandibular joint disease
Extensive dental work

From Lee EW, D'Alonzo GE. Cigarette smoking, nicotine addiction, and its pharmacologic treatment. Arch Intern Med 1993;153:34–48. Copyright 1993, American Medical Association. Used with permission.

hairy surfaces) and provides approximately 50% absorption of the nicotine level generally found in cigarette smokers. The major side effects include mild skin irritation (such as itching and burning) at the patch site and local erythema (Table 9.8); these may respond to rotation of the daily patch site. If side effects persist following patch removal, 1% hydrocortisone cream or ointment should be applied to the area. In cases of heightened craving, the use of nicotine gum may either supplement patch therapy or serve as a substitute following patch discontinuation. In concert with behavioral modification, 1-year cessation rates as high as 35% have been reported.

The various nicotine patch products are illustrated in Table 9.9. The 21 mg/day patch is the most commonly used and should be initiated in heavy smokers (more than one pack daily). Patients with CAD or light smokers (less than one-half pack daily) may begin with a lower dose patch (e.g., 10 to 14 mg/day). The patch is worn daily at the same dose for 6 to 8 weeks and then titrated down to the next lower dose. The 24-hour patch delivers a steady-state concentration of plasma nicotine after 72 hours. The 16-hour patch is worn during waking hours only; no differences between the 16- and 24-hour patches have been observed with respect to smoking cessation rates. Importantly, active patch users have a two-fold increased rate of successful smoking cessation compared with placebo patch users (see Fiore et al., 1994). The combination of the patch tailored with behavioral therapy appears to maximize abstinence rates. Randomized, controlled studies have demonstrated a 25–35% abstinence rate at 1 year with this combination, compared to 9-17% without adjuvant therapy.

Table 9.8. Side-Effect Profile for the Nicotine Patch[1-4]

Effect	Reported Frequency %
Short-lived erythema, pruritus, or burning	35–54
Local erythema	7–22
Local edema	3–8
Cutaneous hypersensitivity	2–3
Mild to moderate insomnia	1–23
Diarrhea	1–9
Dyspepsia	1–9
Myalgia	3–9
Nervousness	3–9
Somnolence	1–9
Abnormal dreams	1–9
Arthralgia	1–9
Abdominal pain	1–3
Dry mouth	1–3
Sweating	1–3

[1]CIBA-GEIGY Corp. Habitrol (nicotine transdermal therapeutic system) prescribing information. Edison, NJ: CIBA-GEIGY Corp, 1992.
[2]Marion Merrell Dow Inc. Nicoderm (nicotine transdermal system) prescribing information. Kansas City, Mo: Marion Merrell Dow Inc, 1991.
[3]Lederle Laboratories. PROSTEP (nicotine transdermal system) prescribing information. Wayne, NJ: Lederle Laboratories, 1992.
[4]Parke-Davis. Nicotrol (nicotine transdermal system) prescribing information. Morris Plains, NJ: Parke-Davis, 1992.
From Fiore MC, Jorenby DE, Baker TB, Kenford SL. Tobacco dependence and the nicotine patch: clinical guidelines for effective use. JAMA 1992;268:2687–2694. Copyright © 1992, American Medical Association. Adapted with permission.

Table 9.9. Dosage of Four Transdermal Nicotine Systems

Product (manufacturer)	Dose length	Regimen
Habitrol (Ciba-Geigy)	24 hours	21 mg/day for 6 weeks, 14 mg/day for 2 weeks, 7 mg/day for 2 weeks
Nicoderm (Marion Merrell Dow)	24 hours	21 mg/day for 6 weeks, 14 mg/day for 2 weeks, 7 mg/day for 2 weeks
Nicotrol (Parke-Davis)	daytime (16 hours)	15 mg/day for 4–12 weeks, 10 mg/day for 2–4 weeks, 5 mg/day for 2-4 weeks
ProStep (Lederle)	24 hours	22 mg/day for 4 to 8 weeks, 11 mg/day for 2 to 4 weeks

From DeNelsky GY. Transdermal nicotine patches: How effective are they? Cleve Clin J Med 1993;60:252–253. Used with permission.

Caution must be exercised in patients with CAD. It is extremely important to emphasize that complete abstention from cigarette smoking is required, as there have been reports of acute MIs with patch use and concurrent smoking. The patches are safe with lower doses initiated (14 mg) and have been shown in a 5-week study to result in abstinence rates of 36%.

NICOTINE NASAL SPRAY

As with nicotine gum, there is a variable-dose delivery system for nicotine nasal spray. The nasal spray produces a higher peak plasma nicotine concentration within 10 minutes of administering 1 mg, whereas the gum and patch take 4 to 10 hours. A 1-year abstinence rate of 26% was reported in subjects receiving the nasal spray, compared with 10% in the placebo (see Sutherland et al.).

Interestingly, the nasal spray prevented the weight gain that often accompanies smoking cessation, perhaps reflecting higher plasma nicotine levels. Unfortunately, nasal and ocular irritation have been commonly reported. The nasal spray is not presently approved for use in the United States.

NICOTINE INHALER

Recently a nicotine inhaler was introduced as the fourth nicotine preparation for smoking cessation. Compared with the nasal spray, the nicotine inhaler produces lower plasma nicotine levels. In a Danish study assessing the sole effects of a nicotine inhaler on smoking cessation rates at the end of 1 year, there were significantly improved abstinence rates among inhaler users (15%) compared to placebo users (5%) ($P = 0.001$) (see Tønnesen et al.). The inhaler was well tolerated; the most common side effects were irritation (mouth and throat) and coughing. In contrast to the nasal spray, the nicotine inhaler did not prevent weight gain. Further studies are pending, and the inhaler has not been approved by the FDA at the time of this writing.

CLONIDINE PATCH

As a central α-agonist and inhibitor of catecholamine release, clonidine has been useful in alcohol and opiate withdrawal syndromes. Although withdrawal and nicotine craving were reduced in small studies, these results were not confirmed in others. Smoking cessation rates appear to be slightly higher in clonidine-treated groups, although the clinical implications remain to be established. The doses employed have been 0.2 to 0.4 mg/day. Side effects include dry mouth and sedative effects, but hypotension is not a prominent feature. The FDA has not approved the clonidine patch for smoking cessation. It may be considered when other therapies (e.g., nicotine preparations) have failed.

Suggested Readings

Åberg A, Bergstrand R, Johansson S, et al. Cessation of smoking after myocardial infarction—effects on mortality after 10 years. Br Heart J 1983;49:416–422.

Adams KF, Koch G, Chatterjee B, et al. Acute elevation of blood carboxyhemoglobin to 6% impairs exercise performance and aggravates symptoms in patients with ischemic heart disease. J Am Coll Cardiol 1988;12:900–909.

Allen RA, Kluft C, Brommer EJP. Effect of chronic smoking on fibrinolysis. Arteriosclerosis 1985;5:443–450.

CIBA-GEIGY Corp. Habitrol (nicotine transdermal therapeutic system) prescribing information. Edison, NJ: CIBA-GEIGY Corp, 1992.

Cox JL. How to help your patients stop smoking. J Am Acad Physician Assist 1990; 3:600–606.

Craig WY, Palomaki GE, Haddow JE. Cigarette smoking and serum lipid and lipoprotein concentrations: An analysis of published data. Br Med J 1989;298:784–788.

Curry SJ, McBride CM. Relapse prevention for smoking cessation: Review and evaluation of concepts and interventions. Annu Rev Public Health 1994;15:345–366.

Davis JW, Hartman CR, Lewis HD Jr, et al. Cigarette smoking-induced enhancement of platelet function: Lack of prevention by aspirin in men with coronary artery disease. J Lab Clin Med 1985;105:479–483.

Davis JW, Shelton L, Watanabe IS, Arnold J. Passive smoking affects endothelium and platelets. Arch Intern Med 1989;149:386–389.

Deanfield J, Wright C, Krikler S, Ribeiro P, Fox K. Cigarette smoking and the treatment of angina with propranolol, atenolol, and nifedipine. N Engl J Med 1984;310:951–954.

DeNelsky GY. Transdermal nicotine patches: How effective are they? Cleve Clin J Med 1993;60:252–253.

Fiore MC, Smith SS, Jorenby DE, Baker TB. The effectiveness of the nicotine patch for smoking cessation. JAMA 1994;271: 1940–1947.

Fiore MC, Jorenby ED, Baker TB, Kenford SL. Tobacco dependence and the nicotine patch: Clinical guidelines for effective use. JAMA 1992;268:2687–2694.

Fiore MC, Novotny TE, Pierce JP, Hatziandreu EJ, Patel KM, Davis RM. Trends in cigarette smoking in the United States: The changing influence of gender and race. JAMA 1989;261:49–55.

Friedman GD, Dales LG, Ury HK. Mortality in middle-aged smokers and nonsmokers. N Engl J Med 1979;300:213–217.

Gill JS, Shipley MJ, Tsementzis SA, et al. Cigarette smoking: A risk factor for hemorrhagic and nonhemorrhagic stroke. Arch Intern Med 1989;149:2053–2057.

Glantz SA, Parmley WW. Passive smoking and heart disease: Epidemiology, physiology, and biochemistry. Circulation 1991; 83:1–12.

Hajek P, Jackson P, Belcher M. Long-term use of nicotine chewing gum: Occurrence, determinants, and effect on weight gain. JAMA 1988;260:1593–1596.

Hallstrom AP, Cobb LA, Ray R. Smoking as a risk factor for recurrence of sudden cardiac arrest. N Engl J Med 1986;314:271–275.

Hartz AJ, Anderson AJ, Brooks HL, Manley JC, Parent GT, Barboriak JJ. The association of smoking with cardiomyopathy. N Engl J Med 1984;311:1201–1206.

Hermanson B, Omenn GS, Kronmal RA, et al. Beneficial six-year outcome of smoking cessation in older men and women with coronary artery disease: Results from the CASS Registry. N Engl J Med 1988; 319:1365–1369.

Holbrook JH, Grundy SM, Hennekens CH, Kannel WB, Strong JP. Cigarette smoking and cardiovascular diseases: A statement for health professionals by a task force appointed by the Steering Committee of the American Heart Association. Circulation 1984;70:1114A–1117A.

Hughes JR, Hatsukami D. Signs and symptoms of tobacco withdrawal. Arch Gen Psychiatry 1986;43:289–294.

Jonason T, Bergström R. Cessation of smoking in patients with intermittent claudication: Effects on the risk of peripheral vascular complications, myocardial infarction and mortality. Acta Med Scand 1987;221: 253–260.

Klaiber EL, Broverman DM, Dalen JE. Serum estradiol levels in male cigarette smokers. Am J Med 1984;77:858–862.

Kottke TE, Battista RN, DeFriese GH, Brekke ML. Attributes of successful smoking cessation interventions in medical practice: A meta-analysis of 39 controlled trials. JAMA 1988;259:2882–2889.

Lederle Laboratories. PROSTEP (nicotine transdermal system) prescribing information. Wayne, NJ: Lederle Laboratories, 1992.

Lee EW, D'Alonzo GE. Cigarette smoking, nicotine addiction, and its pharmacologic treatment. Arch Intern Med 1993;153: 34–48.

Marion Merrell Dow Inc. Nicoderm (nicotine transdermal system) prescribing information. Kansas City, Mo: Marion Merrell Dow Inc, 1991.

McGill HC Jr. Potential mechanisms for the augmentation of atherosclerosis and atherosclerotic disease by cigarette smoking. Prev Med 1979;8:390–403.

McGill HC Jr. The cardiovascular pathology of smoking. Am Heart J 1988;115:250.

McGinnis JM, Foege WH. Actual causes of death in the United States. JAMA 1993; 270:2207–2212.

Michnovica JJ, Hershcopf RJ, Naganuma H, Bradlow HL, Fishman J. Increased 2-hydroxylation of estradiol as a possible mechanism for the anti-estrogenic effect of cigarette smoking. N Engl J Med 1986;315:1305–1309.

Mjøs OD. Lipid effects of smoking. Am Heart J 1988;115:272–275.

Mulcahy R, Hickey N, Graham I, McKenzie G. Factors influencing long-term prognosis in male patients surviving a first coronary attack. Br Heart J 1975;37:158–165.

Mulcahy R. Influence of cigarette smoking on morbidity and mortality after myocardial infarction. Br Heart J 1983;49: 410–415.

Nyboe J, Jensen G, Appleyard M, Schnohr P. Smoking and the risk of first acute myocardial infarction. Am Heart J 1991; 122:438–447.

Palmer JR, Rosenberg L, Shapiro S. "Low yield" cigarettes and the risk of nonfatal myocardial infarction in women. N Engl J Med 1989;320:1569–1573.

Parke-Davis. Nicotrol (nicotine transdermal system) prescribing information. Morris Plains, NJ: Parke-Davis, 1992.

Petitti DB, Wingerd J. Use of oral contraceptives, cigarette smoking, and risk of subarachnoid hœmorrhage. Lancet 1978;2 (8083):234–235.

Pierce JP, Fiore MC, Novotny TE, Hatziandreu EJ, Davis RM. Trends in cigarette smoking in the United States: Projections to the year 2000. JAMA 1989;261:61–65.

Pittilo RM, Clarke JMF, Harris D, et al. Cigarette smoking and platelet adhesion. Br J Haematol 1984;58:627–632.

Pohjola S, Siltanen P, Romo M, et al. Effect of quitting smoking on the long-term survival after myocardial infarction. [Abstract] Trans Eur Soc Cardiol 1979;1:2.

Prochazka AV, Petty TL, Nett L, et al. Transdermal clonidine reduced some withdrawal symptoms but did not increase smoking cessation. Arch Intern Med 1992;152:2065–2069.

Reinders JH, Brinkman H-J, van Mourik JA, de Groot PG. Cigarette smoke impairs endothelial cell prostacyclin production. Arteriosclerosis 1986;6:15–23.

Rivers JT, White HD, Cross DB, Williams BF, Norris RM. Reinfarction after thrombolytic therapy for acute myocardial infarction followed by conservative management: Incidence and effect of smoking. J Am Coll Cardiol 1990;16:340–348.

Rosenberg L, Kaufman DW, Helmrich SP, Shapiro S. The risk of myocardial infarction after quitting smoking in men under 55 years of age. N Engl J Med 1985; 313:1511–1514.

Sachs DPL, Säwe U, Leischow SJ. Effectiveness of a 16-hour transdermal nicotine patch in a medical practice setting, without intensive group counseling. Arch Intern Med 1993;153:1881–1890.

Salonen JT. Stopping smoking and long-term mortality after acute myocardial infarction. Br Heart J 1980;43:463–469.

Sparrow D, Dawber TR, Colton T. The influence of cigarette smoking on prognosis after a first myocardial infarction. J Chronic Dis 1978;31:425–432.

Steenland K. Passive smoking and the risk of heart disease. JAMA 1992;267:94–99.

Sutherland G, Stapleton JA, Russell MAH, Jarvis MJ, et al. Randomised controlled trial of nasal nicotine spray in smoking cessation. Lancet 1992;340:324–329.

Taylor AE, Johnson DC, Kazemi H. Environmental tobacco smoke and cardiovascular disease: A position paper from the Council on Cardiopulmonary and Critical Care, American Heart Association. Circulation 1992;86:1–4.

Tell GS, Howard G, McKinney WM, Toole JF. Cigarette smoking cessation and extracranial carotid atherosclerosis. JAMA 1989;261:1178–1180.

Tønnesen P, Nørregaard J, Mikkelsen K, Jørgensen S, Nilsson F. A double-blind trial of a nicotine inhaler for smoking cessation. JAMA 1993;269:1268–1271.

Turner DM. Carbon monoxide, tobacco smoking, and the pathogenesis of atherosclerosis. Prev Med 1979;8:303–309.

Vlietstra RE, Kronmal RA, Oberman A, Frye RL, Killip T III. Effect of cigarette smoking on survival of patients with angiographically documented coronary artery disease. Report from the CASS Registry. JAMA 1986;255:1023–1027.

Wells A. An estimate of adult mortality in the United States from passive smoking: A response to criticism. Environ Int 1990;16:187–193.

Wikstrand J, Berglund G, Tuomilehto J. Beta-blockade in the primary prevention of coronary heart disease in hypertensive patients. Review of present evidence. Circulation 1991;84:VI93–100.

Wilhelmsen L. Coronary heart disease: Epidemiology of smoking and intervention studies of smoking. Am Heart J 1988; 115:242–249.

Wilhelmsson C, Elmfeldt D, Vedin JA, Tibblin G, Wilhelmsen L. Smoking and myocardial infarction. Lancet 1975;1:415–420.

Willett WC, Green A, Stampfer MJ, et al. Relative and absolute excess risks of coronary heart disease among women who smoke cigarettes. N Engl J Med 1987; 317:1303–1309.

Winniford MD, Jansen DE, Reynolds GA, Apprill P, Black WH, Hillis LD. Cigarette smoking-induced coronary vasoconstriction in atherosclerotic coronary artery disease and prevention by calcium antagonists and nitroglycerin. Am J Cardiol 1987;59:203–207.

Winniford MD, Wheelan KR, Kremers MS, et al. Smoking-induced coronary vasoconstriction in patients with atherosclerotic coronary artery disease: Evidence for adrenergically mediated alterations in coronary artery tone. Circulation 1986; 73:662–667.

10/ Comprehensive Preventive Cardiology: Vasoprotective Drugs and Rehabilitation

Whether as part of primary or secondary prevention, comprehensive preventive cardiology should be directed toward the major goals of reducing coronary ischemia, nonfatal cardiovascular events, and mortality (Table 10.1). Clinically, ischemia is manifest as angina pectoris, transient left ventricular dysfunction, and arrhythmias. Cardiovascular events include acute MI, unstable angina, need for coronary revascularization, decompensated CHF, and syncope. From the viewpoint of therapy, these clinical goals can be achieved by reducing the progression of coronary atherosclerosis, thrombosis, inappropriate vasoconstriction, and arrhythmogenicity. These pathophysiological processes can be effectively managed through risk-factor modification, the use of vasoprotective drugs, and rehabilitation. The probable mechanisms of vasoprotection afforded by these preventive measures are summarized in Table 10.2. The major modifiable risk factors of hypercholes-

Table 10.1. Treatment Goals in Coronary Artery Disease

Clinical	Pathophysiologic
↓ Ischemia	↓ Atherosclerosis
↓ Nonfatal CVEs	↓ Thrombosis
↓ Mortality	↓ Vasoconstriction
	↓ Arrhythmogenicity

CVE = cardiovascular event

Table 10.2. Mechanisms of Vasoprotection

	Atherosclerosis	Thrombosis	Vasoactivity	Arrhythmias
Cholesterol Lowering	+	+	+	0
Smoking Cessation	+	+	+	+
Hypertension Control	+	0	+	+
Aspirin	0	+	0	0
β-Blocker	−	+	−	+
ACE Inhibitor	0	0	+	0
Hormone Replacement	+	±	+	0
Exercise	+	+	0	+

+ = Improves
0 = No Effect
− = Worsens

terolemia, hypertension, and smoking adversely affect multiple pathophysiological processes; therefore, they are of central importance in the genesis of CAD. Detailed discussions of these key risk factors are provided in Chapters 4, 7, and 9. Comprehensive preventive cardiology should also provide patients with drugs proven to be cardioprotective and should encourage physical activity. Major drug classes which have been proven to be vasoprotective include aspirin, β-blockers, ACE inhibitors, and hormone replacement therapy. This chapter focuses on these agents and the use of rehabilitation.

ASPIRIN

The anti-inflammatory, antipyretic, and analgesic effects of willow bark have been known for several centuries. Sodium salicylate was isolated by Laroux in 1829 and acetylsalicylic acid introduced by Hoffman under the name "aspirin" at the turn of this century. Aspirin was recognized as a platelet inhibitor in the late 1960s. The mechanism of action, the irreversible inhibition of the cyclooxygenase enzyme, was identified approximately a decade later. Aspirin permanently inactivates the conversion of arachidonate to prostaglandins G and H, resulting in decreased thromboxane A_2 in platelets and prostacyclin in vascular endothelial cells. The former action results in inhibition of platelet aggregation, but the latter may actually increase platelet aggregation. In the lower antiplatelet doses, aspirin is predominately antithrombotic.

Dramatic vasoprotective benefits of aspirin have been demonstrated in patients with acute MI, unstable angina, and proven CAD, i.e., secondary prevention. The second International Study of Infarct Survival (ISIS-II), which enrolled 17,187 patients with suspected acute MI, demonstrated that aspirin was roughly equivalent to thrombolytic therapy in reducing short-term mortality (23%). Reinfarction was reduced by 44% and stroke by 46%. Although the rate of minor bleeding increased (32%), major bleeds requiring transfusion actually declined (–6%). These facts have been substantiated by other trials, and prompt aspirin administration is recommended to all patients with suspected acute MI. Unfortunately, recent practice surveys have found that only approximately 70% of patients diagnosed with acute MI receive aspirin, and only about 30% receive it within 1 day of the diagnosis. Currently, following the diagnosis of MI, one patient in four is not continued on the drug at home.

Three trials have demonstrated that aspirin reduces MI and mortality rates in patients presenting with unstable angina. Aspirin doses have ranged from 75 to 1300 mg/day, and long-term reduction of death or acute MI from 30–48%. There appears to be no additional benefit for more than 324 mg/day (see below).

The value of antiplatelet therapy in secondary prevention was documented in an extensive meta-analysis by the Antiplatelet Trialists' Collaboration (Fig. 10.1). Eleven randomized trials consisting of nearly 20,000 patients with CAD prior to MI

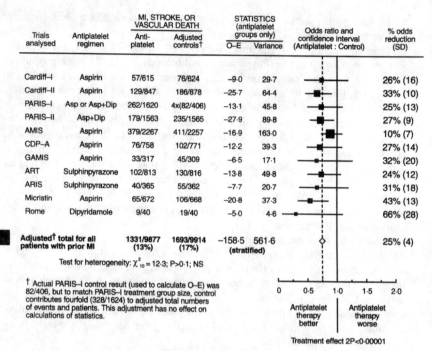

Trials analysed	Antiplatelet regimen	MI, STROKE, OR VASCULAR DEATH		STATISTICS (antiplatelet groups only)		Odds ratio and confidence interval (Antiplatelet : Control)	% odds reduction (SD)
		Anti-platelet	Adjusted controls†	O–E	Variance		
Cardiff–I	Aspirin	57/615	76/624	–9.0	29.7		26% (16)
Cardiff–II	Aspirin	129/847	186/878	–25.7	64.4		33% (10)
PARIS–I	Asp or Asp+Dip	262/1620	4x(82/406)	–13.1	45.8		25% (13)
PARIS–II	Asp+Dip	179/1563	235/1565	–27.9	89.8		27% (9)
AMIS	Aspirin	379/2267	411/2257	–16.9	163.0		10% (7)
CDP–A	Aspirin	76/758	102/771	–12.2	39.3		27% (14)
GAMIS	Aspirin	33/317	45/309	–6.5	17.1		32% (20)
ART	Sulphinpyrazone	102/813	130/816	–13.8	49.8		24% (12)
ARIS	Sulphinpyrazone	40/365	55/362	–7.7	20.7		31% (18)
Micristin	Aspirin	65/672	106/668	–20.8	37.3		43% (13)
Rome	Dipyridamole	9/40	19/40	–5.0	4.6		66% (28)
Adjusted† total for all patients with prior MI		**1331/9877 (13%)**	**1693/9914 (17%)**	**–158.5 (stratified)**	**561.6**		**25% (4)**

Test for heterogeneity: $\chi^2_{10} = 12.3$; P>0.1; NS

† Actual PARIS–I control result (used to calculate O–E) was 82/406, but to match PARIS–I treatment group size, control contributes fourfold (328/1624) to adjusted total numbers of events and patients. This adjustment has no effect on calculations of statistics.

0   0.5   1.0   1.5   2.0

Antiplatelet therapy better   Antiplatelet therapy worse

Treatment effect 2P<0·00001

Figure 10.1. Proportional effects on vascular events (MI, stroke, or vascular death) in 11 randomized trials of prolonged antiplatelet therapy (for 1 month or more) vs control in patients with prior MI. O-E = Observed minus expected. Asp = Aspirin. Dip = Dipyridamole. From Antiplatelet Trialists' Collaboration. Collaborative overview of randomized trials of antiplatelet therapy—I: Prevention of death, myocardial infarction, and stroke by prolonged antiplatelet therapy in various categories of patients. Br Med J 1994;308:81–106. Published by BMJ Publishing Group. Used with permission.

were reviewed. Overall, there was a 25% reduction in the incidence of subsequent vascular events. Importantly, one vascular event was prevented for every 25 patients treated with antiplatelet therapy. No significant differences were noted between higher (500–1500 mg/day) and lower doses (75–325 mg/day) or between aspirin monotherapy and adjunctive use of sulfinpyrazone or dipyridamole. The benefit of antiplatelet use was observed within the first year of institution and continues to be protective for at least three years with continued use. The cardiac benefits of treating patients presenting with cerebral occlusive disease appear to be the same as in those with known CAD. Taken together, these data strongly suggest that all patients with established CAD or cerebral occlusive disease should receive chronic aspirin therapy.

The value of aspirin for primary prevention, especially in low-risk subjects, is more controversial. The Physicians' Health Study of 22,071 male physicians aged 40 to 84 years, randomized to 325 mg aspirin every other day or placebo for 5 years, found a 44% reduction in the incidence of MI in the aspirin group. Aspirin-treated men had a slight but insignificant increase in hemorrhagic stroke, and no effect on overall cardiovascular mortality was observed. The British Doctors Trial of 5,139 male physicians aged 50 to 78 years, randomized to 500 mg aspirin daily or placebo, found no difference in the combined endpoint of important cardiovascular events, MI, stroke, and total cardiovascular mortality between the groups. For primary prevention, chronic aspirin administration appears to have some benefit for healthy individuals at higher cardiovascular risk, including those over the age of 50, but appears to be of limited benefit for healthy, low-risk individuals.

Aspirin dosage remains controversial. Equivalent benefit appears to exist over the 75 to 324 mg/day range, with little evidence for additional benefit at higher doses. Gastrointestinal side effects, including bleeding, increase with higher aspirin dosage, but the risk does not disappear at even the lower dose levels. Although possibly beneficial for cerebral vascular disease, doses higher than 324 mg/day for primary or secondary CAD prevention are not recommended. Little data exists differentiating daily doses within the 75 to 324 mg range or between daily and every-other-day administration.

β-ADRENERGIC BLOCKING AGENTS

β-blockers reduce oxygen demand by lowering heart rate, BP, and contractility. They also oppose the direct effects of catecholamines and therefore have antiarrhythmic properties. β-blockers have diverging effects on the four atherophysiologic mechanisms determining vasoprotection. Small prospective angiographic trials have demonstrated greater progression of existing coronary disease and appearance of new lesions associated with β-blocker use compared with patients receiving either long-term nitrates or calcium channel blockers. The proatherosclerotic effect of β-blockers may in part be due to adverse effects on lipids. Nonselective β-blockers decrease HDL 10–20% and increase TG 15–30% by impairing LPL activity, a byproduct of unopposed α-adrenergic stimulation. Therefore, β-blockers with ISA or combined α- and β-blockade (see Table 7.8) are less likely to adversely alter HDL-C and TG. Selective $β_1$-blockers exert an intermediate effect with average HDL-C reductions of 5–10% and TG elevations of 10–20% (see Frishman et al). Unopposed α-adrenergic stimulation may also enhance vasoconstriction. This effect is clinically observed in patients with Prinzmetal's (variant) angina. As can be seen in Table 10.2, the adverse effects of β-blockers are opposed by the beneficial effects on thrombosis and arrhythmogenicity. Platelet aggregability is decreased by this class of agents, as are ventricular fibrillation thresholds and complex ventricular arrhythmias. In selected patients such as those with recent Q wave MI, the beneficial vasoprotective effects of β-blockers appear to outweigh the adverse effects.

In the prethrombolytic era, several studies of patients with acute Q wave MI demonstrated reductions in mortality with β-blocker use, mostly due to decreases in sudden death. Meta-analysis from 28 randomized trials including approximately 27,500 patients demonstrates a 14% mortality reduction in the first week following acute MI (Table 10.3). Even within the first week, most of the benefit appeared to occur within the first 2 days and was chiefly due to prevention of cardiac rupture and ventricular fibrillation. Nonfatal cardiovascular events are also reduced about 20% with β-blocker use. No significant reduction in mortality with β-blocker use has been found in studies of non-Q wave MI. Patients predominantly benefited from β-blocker use appear to be those with higher risks such as tachycardia on presentation and those with poor ventricular function. Early postinfarction administration is recommended in these hyperadrenergic individuals. In Q wave MI, the value of β-blockers appears to be cardioprotective for at least one year.

Less data is available on the use of β-blockers in the thrombolytic era. The Thrombolysis in Myocardial Infarction (TIMI)-IIB Study randomized immediate and delayed use of β-blocker therapy in patients receiving thrombolytic therapy additionally randomized to invasive and conservative strategies. Whereas short-term ventricular function was not improved by immediate use of a β-blocker, there were lower instances of reinfarction and recurrent chest pain in low-risk patients randomized to immediate administration, and 6-week mortality was reduced. These data support the continued acute and chronic use of β-blockers in patients experiencing Q wave MI for about a year, whether they receive thrombolytic therapy or

Table 10.3. One-Week Mortality in Trials of β-Blockers for Acute Myocardial Infarction

Trial	Deaths	
	β-B	Control
ISIS-1	317	367
MIAMI	79	93
26 Small Trials	117	126
Total Mortality	513	586
Total Patients	13,815	13,721
Mortality Reduction	14%	

Adapted from Yusuf S, Sleight P, Helf P, et al. Routine medical management of acute myocardial infarction: Lessons from overviews of recently randomized controlled trials. Circulation 1990;82(suppl II):II-117—II-134. Used with permission. Circulation Copyright © 1990 American Heart Association.

not. Presently, only about 40% of non-Q risk patients with Q wave infarction without relative or absolute contraindications receive β-blocker therapy.

ACE INHIBITORS

ACE inhibitors represent an important class of drugs for preventive cardiology, as they are primary agents in the management of hypertension, improve symptoms and survival in patients with CHF and left ventricular dysfunction, reduce cardiovascular events in patients with left ventricular dysfunction, and decrease the progression of diabetic nephropathy. By inhibiting ACE, circulating and tissue levels of angiotensin II are reduced and levels of bradykinin are increased. This results in a decrement in generalized vasoconstriction. In animal experiments, ACE inhibitors have been shown to retard the development of atherosclerosis and post-injury intimal hyperplasia. It is not clear, however, that clinically utilized doses of ACE inhibitors affect the progression of atherosclerosis in humans.

Patients with CHF have shown improved survival in controlled trials of ACE inhibitors, as well as in comparison with hydralazine-isosorbide dinitrate vasodilator therapy. In addition to providing beneficial effects on mortality, ACE inhibitors have reduced MI and rehospitalization rates for CHF exacerbation. CAD events in asymptomatic patients with left ventricular dysfunction have also been reduced.

In post-MI patients with LVEF <40%, the Survival and Ventricular Enlargement (SAVE) Trial demonstrated a 19% reduction in mortality in patients assigned to ACE inhibitor therapy (Fig. 10.2) (see Pfeffer et al.). Progressive left ventricular dilatation was reduced due to more favorable postinfarction ventricular remodeling. Nonfatal cardiovascular events and rehospitalization were also significantly decreased. A recent large postinfarction trial demonstrated improved survival with ACE inhibitor use irrespective of ventricular function, although the major benefit occurred in patients with ventricular dysfunction. Controversy continues regarding the optimum time for initiation of therapy. Angiotensin-converting enzyme inhibition begun within 24 hours of the onset of acute MI did not improve 6-month survival in a 6,000-patient study (CONSENSUS II). At the present time, the initiation of ACE inhibitors following MI is recommended after 1 to 2 days. Patients with anterior and/or large MIs appear to derive the greatest benefit.

The above-mentioned data have been obtained from studies using captopril 25 mg t.i.d., enalapril 10 mg b.i.d., or equivalent doses. The beneficial cardioprotective effects of ACE inhibitors can be verified only at these clinical doses. Whereas patients with CHF and/or left ventricular dysfunction often have lower BP, it is important to titrate these individuals up to full therapeutic ACE-inhibitor doses, if tolerated. Dry cough can occur as a side effect of all ACE inhibitors; switching to another agent may be warranted. Renal dysfunction is also associated with ACE-inhibitor use, especially in hypovolemic individuals. Current recommendations are for use of full-dose ACE inhibitors in all patients with left ventricular dysfunction, whether associated with clinical CHF or not, to be initiated 1 to 2 days following the onset of acute MI, especially if ventricular dysfunction is present. As with other

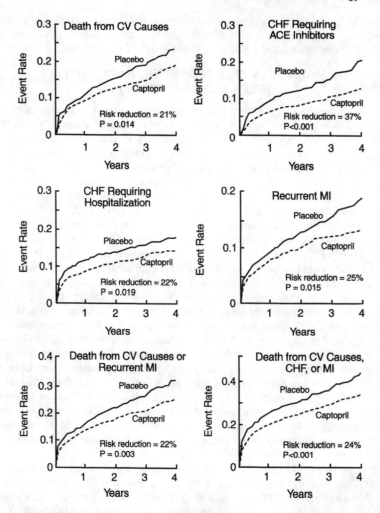

Figure 10.2. Life tables for cumulative fatal and nonfatal cardiovascular events. Reprinted by permission of The New England Journal of Medicine from Pfeffer MA, Braunwald E, Moyé LA, et al. Effect of captopril on mortality and morbidity in patients with left ventricular dysfunction after myocardial infarction. Results of the survival and ventricular enlargement trial. N Engl J Med 1992;327:669–677. Copyright © 1992, Massachusetts Medical Society.

agents, ACE inhibitors are not uniformly administered to patients potentially bene-fitting from them. It is estimated that 40–60% of appropriate patients currently receive ACE inhibitors, and a smaller number receive full therapeutic doses.

HORMONE REPLACEMENT THERAPY [HRT]
(SEE ALSO CHAPTER 13)

Premenopausal women have a low incidence of clinical CAD compared with men of the same age unless major risk factors, such as diabetes or smoking, are present. In general, women present with CAD about 8 to 10 years later than men. One exception to this rule is diabetic women, who lose their gender-related protection. After menopause the vasoprotective effect of endogenous estrogen is rapidly lost, and CAD rates between the sexes are similar over age 70 years. As in men, CAD remains the leading source of mortality in women; approximately five times as many women die of CAD as die of breast cancer (see Figure 13.2).

As seen in Table 10.2, estrogen therapy has several vasoprotective effects. Unopposed oral estrogen raises HDL-C, decreases LDL-C, and has a modest effect on decreasing TC (see also Figure 13.13). Oral estrogen also elevates TG levels, which is not thought to be an important adverse clinical affect. Estrogen adminis-tered through transdermal patch has considerably less effect on lipid metabolism. The addition of progestins tends to attenuate the beneficial lipid effects of estrogen administration, with continuous administration having more deleterious effects than cyclic progestin usage. Hormone replacement therapy has been demonstrated to reduce Lp(a), fibrinogen, factor VII, and fasting insulin levels. These combined effects are believed to be generally antiatherosclerotic. The effects of hormone replacement therapy on thrombogenicity are variable depending upon doses of estrogen and progestin. Contraceptive hormone therapy is associated with increased venous, coronary, and cerebral thrombosis, especially in older smoking women. There is no evidence that postmenopausal HRT produces similar effects. Estrogens favorably affect endothelium-mediated vasoactivity both directly and through lipid alterations. Vasoactive responses to acetylcholine improve within minutes of inter-arterial estrogen administration.

Retrospective evidence from several case-controlled studies support a vasopro-tective effect of hormone replacement therapy in postmenopausal women (Fig. 10.3). Meta-analysis of HRT suggests a 40–50% reduction in cardiovascular events. Ten-year followup of current users of estrogen replacement therapy in the 120,000-patient Nurses' Health Study (NHS) demonstrated a 44% reduction in CAD risk. Some observational studies have demonstrated a reduction in cerebral vascular dis-ease as well, although this was not true for the NHS. Although little controlled data exists, combined estrogen-progestin therapy appears to be as vasoprotective as is estrogen therapy alone.

Unopposed estrogen is associated with endometrial hypertrophy and cancer. This necessitates the use of daily or cyclic adjunctive progestin therapy such as

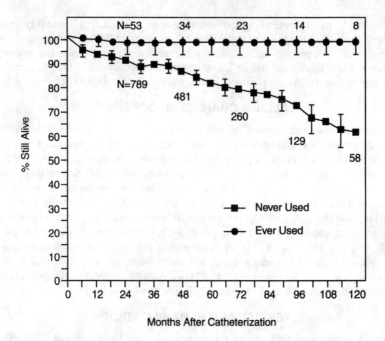

Figure 10.3. Ten-year survival of patients with left main coronary stenosis of 50% or greater or other stenosis of 70% or greater, who used or did not use estrogens. From Sullivan JM, Vander Zwaag R, Hughes JP, et al. Estrogen replacement and coronary artery disease. Effect on survival in postmenopausal women. Arch Intern Med 1990;150:2557–2562. Copyright © 1990, American Medical Association. Used with permission.

medroxyprogesterone acetate either 2.5 mg daily or 5–10 mg cyclically for 10 out of 30 days. Adjunctive progesterone therapy makes clinical administration of HRT more complex because of its adverse psychological effects and cyclic bleeding. The effect of estrogen on breast cancer risk has been a source of concern and controversy in the area of HRT. The NHS found a relative risk of 1.1 for women who have ever used estrogen, 1.0 for current users, and 1.3 for past users. Other observational data suggest a relative risk as high as 1.4 for breast cancer for current estrogen administration. This risk is small compared to the benefit of HRT on CAD risk, but it must be factored into individual patient decisions. Overall, HRT is estimated to provide a 2.4% absolute risk reduction for CAD and at most a 0.3% increase in absolute risk of breast cancer. The increased risk of uterine cancer is small, and most carcinomas are locally invasive. HRT also provides noncardiovascular benefits in the form of protection against osteoporosis, vasoactive instability (hot flashes), urogenital atrophy, and psychological symptoms. HRT appears to be vaso-protective in both primary and secondary prevention. Its use in postmenopausal women without significant risk of breast cancer is generally warranted. Currently, only approximately 15% of postmenopausal women are receiving HRT.

CALCIUM CHANNEL BLOCKERS

Considerable debate remains regarding the effects of calcium channel blockers on CAD progression and post-MI morbidity and mortality. Experimental animal data found reduction in the appearance of new lesions. In contrast, clinical trials have demonstrated no effect on the progression of existing CAD, with a slight but clinically insignificant adverse trend toward higher cardiovascular event rates. Diltiazem has been shown to reduce CAD events in non-Q wave MI patients with-out CHF. This suggests a divergence of clinical benefit which may in part be based upon chronotropic effects of specific calcium channel blockers. Calcium channel blockers appear to be useful in the management of hypertension, and third-genera-tion agents are currently under investigation as vasodilators in patients with CHF. As a class, however, calcium channel blockers cannot be considered vasoprotective in comparison with aspirin, β-blockers, ACE inhibitors, and HRT.

EXERCISE AND REHABILITATION

Increased physical activity has salutary effects on LDL-C, HDL-C, TG, BP, weight, and DM (Table 10.4). Reduced adrenergic drive associated with physical conditioning has a beneficial impact on thrombogenicity and arrhythmogenicity as well. Encouragement of physical activity is an important part of primary and sec-ondary prevention. There is a strong inverse association between the risk of an ini-tial MI and physical activity, independent of other coronary risk factors. A 69% reduction in risk-adjusted MI rate has been demonstrated in subjects exercising more than 2.2 hours per week, compared with inactive individuals (Table 10.5).

In patients with established CAD, the Heidelberg Study verified less progression and more regression of angiographic CAD in patients randomized to combined pru-dent diet and high-level exercise regimens.

A meta-analysis of 22 randomized trials involving nearly 4600 patients demon-strated the benefit of cardiac rehabilitation post-MI; among those assigned to an exercise program, there were significant reductions in reinfarction rate (25%), car-diovascular mortality (22%), and total mortality (20%) (see O'Connor et al.). Conditioning improves aerobic capacity as measured by ventilatory oxygen con-sumption (VO_2). Maximal oxygen consumption, or VO_2 max, reflects utilization by exercising tissues during peak exercise. For every liter of oxygen consumed, there are approximately 5 kcal of energy expended. The most widely used parame-ters of work capacity are metabolic equivalents, or METs. One MET is equal to 3.5

Table 10.4. Effects of Physical Activity

	Low Activity	Medium Activity	High Activity
Body Mass Index	24.2	24.0	23.4
Cholesterol (mg/dL)	220	218	217
Hypertension	39%	36%	33%
Diabetes	15%	13%	11%
CAD Incidence	6.2	6.3	5.2

Adapted from Rodriguez BL, Curb JD, Burchfiel CM, et al. Physical activity and 23-year incidence of coronary heart disease morbidity and mortality among middle-aged men. The Honolulu Heart Program. Circulation 1994;89:2540–2544. Used with permission. Circulation Copyright 1994 American Heart Association.

Table 10.5. Relative Hazards for First Acute Myocardial Infarction by Physical Activity

Conditioning Physical Activity	Normal ECG	Abnormal ECG
(hours/week)	(n = 1166)	(n = 287)
0.7 – 2.2	1.11	0.52
>2.2	0.31	0.19
	P = 0.04	P = 0.03

Adapted from Lakka TA, Venäläinen JM, Rauramaa R. Relationship of leisure-time physical activity and cardiorespiratory fitness to the risk of acute myocardial infarction in men. N Engl J Med 1994;330:1549–1554, Copyright © 1994, Massachusetts Medical Society.

mL of oxygen consumed per kg of body weight per minute at rest. Examples of various activities and their associated METs are listed in Table 10.6. The inability to attain 5 METs during stress testing is associated with poor prognosis. Blair and coworkers observed the lowest mortality rates in the most conditioned or aerobically fit subjects (e.g., capacity greater than 9 METs). The highest METs (greater than 18) are achieved by endurance athletes.

Following an acute MI, convalescent inpatients should participate in a supervised exercise regimen. Phase I cardiac rehabilitation involves performing low-stress activities of 5 METs or less. Post-MI patients able to successfully complete a submaximal stress test (greater than 5 METs) prior to hospital discharge have a mortality rate of 1–2% over the ensuing 12 months. Phase II cardiac rehabilitation

Table 10.6.   Metabolic Equivalents Associated With Various Activities

Activity	METs	Activity	METs
Reading/television	1	Square dancing	5
Walking 1 mph	1	Water-skiing	5
Desk work	1.5	Ballet	6
Bartending	2	Cross-country skiing 3 mph	6
Bathing	2	Snow shoveling	6
Cooking	2	Car washing/waxing	6
Golf (using golf cart)	2	Carrying up to 85 lb	7
Shuffleboard	2	Chopping wood	7
Washing dishes	2	Kayaking	7
Cycling 6 mph	3	Lifting 100 lb	7
Fly-fishing	3	Mountain climbing	7
Gardening	3	Swimming backstroke	7
Housework	3	Cross-country skiing 4 mph	8
Sexual intercourse (old partner)	3	Handball	8
Ballroom dancing	4	Karate	8
Carrying up to 44 lb	4	Racquetball	8
Painting	4	Running 12 minutes/mile	8
Carrying up to 65 lb	5	Swimming breaststroke	8
Cycling 10 mph	5	Cross-country skiing 5 mph	9
Downhill skiing	5	Running 11 minutes/mile	9
Mowing the lawn	5	Wrestling	9
Roller skating	5	Brisk walking for 30 minutes	10
Sexual intercourse (new partner)	5	Running 9 minutes/mile	10
Scuba diving	5	Jumping rope 120–140/min	11

is initiated after hospital discharge and is designed to improve cardiovascular endurance, muscle strength, and work capacity. Supervised sessions are usually conducted three times weekly for 45 to 60 minutes, and patients are monitored by telemetry. The intensity of exercise sessions is gradually increased to achieve the target heart rate (60–85% of age-adjusted maximal rate). In addition to improving self-confidence, patients engaged in these programs are also more likely to be compliant with lifestyle modification. Patients should be encouraged to continue regular exercise after successfully completing cardiac rehabilitation.

COMPREHENSIVE PREVENTIVE CARDIOLOGY

Table 10.7 summarizes the 10 key elements of a comprehensive preventive cardiology program, including control of hypercholesterolemia, HTN, and DM, smoking cessation, and the encouragement of physical activity. Vasoprotective drugs should also be used in specific patient circumstances: aspirin for all individuals with demonstrated CAD, β-blockers within 1 year of Q wave MI, ACE inhibitors for individuals with CHF and/or left ventricular dysfunction, and HRT in post-

Table 10.7. Preventive Cardiology Practice Indexes

Risk Factors	Cardioprotection
Smoking cessation*	Aspirin (CAD)**
LDL <100 mg/dL (CAD)*	ACE inhibitor (left ventricular dysfunction)**
<130 mg/dL (multiple risk factors)**	β-Blocker (post MI)**
HDL >35 mg/dL**	Hormone replacement therapy*
BP <140/90 mm Hg**	
Physically active**	
Hemoglobin A_{1c} <7%**	

* Based on consensus data
**Based on RCT's and consensus data

Table 10.8. Important Factors for Successful Secondary Prevention Programs

1. Physician commitment to preventive measures
2. Cooperation between primary care physicians and subspecialists
3. Formal program including practice documentation
4. Use of support personnel including nurses and dietitians
5. Positive patient reinforcement
6. Involvement of the patient's family
7. Long-term management

menopausal women. Weight reduction is also an integral part of the control of hypercholesterolemia, HTN, and DM. Currently, physicians document the presence of only about 60% of these risk factors for patients with established CAD and effectively treat less than 40%.

Several factors have proven helpful in establishing effective prevention programs (Table 10.8). Whereas physician commitment is essential, the need for support personnel including nurses and dieticians with sufficient time to counsel patients is crucial. Involvement of support personnel has been demonstrated to reduce risk-factor profiles, alter the progression of coronary disease, and decrease cardiovascular events (Table 10.9). Before undertaking comprehensive preventive cardiology programs, a review of current group or individual practice is suggested. This will serve to document the likely level of undertreatment and can be used as a baseline to judge changes in practice. A formal program focusing on both initiation and compliance of preventive measures is recommended. Successful programs involve close cooperation and communication between primary care practitioners

Table 10.9. Effects of Lifestyle Intervention and Drug Treatment on Coronary Disease Progression and Cardiovascular Events

Treatment	Effect on Atherosclerosis Progression	Effect on Cardiovascular Events	Estimated Frequency of Use
Diet	Decrease	Decrease	20%
Exercise	Decrease	Decrease	10%
Smoking Cessation	Possible Decrease	Decrease	20%
ACE Inhibitor	Unknown	Decrease	60%
Aspirin	None	Decrease	70%
β-Blocker	Possible Increase	Decrease	40%
Ca²⁺-Blocker	Possible Decrease	Variable	60%
Cholesterol Lowering Drug	Decrease	Decrease	25%
Hormone Replacement	Decrease	Decrease	15%

UNIVERSITY OF MARYLAND SCHOOL OF MEDICINE
CENTER FOR PREVENTIVE CARDIOLOGY
22 SOUTH GREENE STREET, S3B06
BALTIMORE, MARYLAND 21201-1595
(410) 328-6299

_____, 1995

Dear Dr. _____ :

As you are aware, _____, was recently an inpatient in one of our cardiovascular units. On admission, the following risk factors were noted. The patient received the following cardioprotective medications upon discharge:

RISK FACTORS
___ POSITIVE FAMILY HISTORY
___ HISTORY OF CIGARETTE SMOKING
___ ELEVATED LDL CHOLESTEROL
___ HIGH BLOOD PRESSURE
___ DIABETES
___ LOW HDL
___ SEDENTARY LIFESTYLE
___ PREMATURE MENOPAUSE

MEDICATIONS
___ ASA (CAD)
___ ACE INHIBITOR (CHF)
___ BETA-BLOCKER (POST-MI)
___ ESTROGEN REPLACEMENT THERAPY
___ LIPID-LOWERING THERAPY

	LDL	HDL		TC:HDL
		Men	Women	
DESIRABLE	<100	>45	>50	<4:1
BORDERLINE	101-130	40-45	45-50	4.1:5.4
ABNORMAL	>130	<40	<45	>5.5:1
PATIENT'S VALUE	___	___	___	___

The importance of risk factor modification was emphasized and the patient was informed that aggressive secondary preventive measures would be addressed in follow-up with you. We appreciate the opportunity of having taken care of this patient and if we can assist you in any way in the future regarding risk factor modification, please do not hesitate to contact us.

Sincerely,

Michael Miller, M.D.
Director, Preventive Cardiology
Assistant Professor of Medicine
MM:rgb

Figure 10.4. Letter distributed to the Primary Care Physician outlining risk factors and medications prescribed for their patient(s) discharged from the University of Maryland Medical System.

and specialists. A letter listing CAD risk factors and cardioprotective medication may be effective (Fig 10.4). Involvement of the patient's family has been found helpful, and long-term reinforcement and followup are valuable. From a therapeutic point of view, these preventive measures are among the most effective forms for both preventing and managing CAD.

Suggested Readings

Antiplatelet Trialists' Collaboration. Collaborative overview of randomised trials of antiplatelet therapy—I: Prevention of death, myocardial infarction, and stroke by prolonged antiplatelet therapy in various categories of patients. Br Med J 1994;308: 81–106.

Belchetz PE. Drug therapy: Hormonal treatment of post-menopausal women. N Engl J Med 1994;330:1062–1071.

Blair SN, Kohl HW III, Paffenbarger RS Jr, et al. Physical fitness and all-cause mortality: A prospective study of healthy men and women. JAMA 1989;262:2395–2401.

Bush TL, Barrett-Connor E, Cowan LD, et al. Cardiovascular mortality and noncontraceptive use of estrogen in women: Results from the Lipid Research Clinics Program Follow-up Study. Circulation 1987;75: 1102–1109.

Cohn JN, Johnson G, Ziesche S, et al. A comparison of enalapril with hydralazine-isosorbide dinitrate in the treatment of congestive heart failure. N Engl J Med 1991;325:303–310.

Colditz GA. Epidemiology of breast cancer: Findings from the Nurses' Health Study. Cancer 1993;71(4 suppl):1480–1489.

Colditz GA, Stampfer MJ, Willett WC, et al. Type of postmenopausal hormone use and risk of breast cancer: 12-year follow-up from the Nurses' Health Study. Cancer Causes Control 1992;3:433–439.

Cupples ME, McKnight A. Randomized controlled trial of health promotion in general practice for patients at high cardiovascular risk. Br Med J 1994;309:993–996.

Frishman WH, Johnson BF, Pulos G, Danylchuk MA, et al. The effects of cardiovascular drugs on plasma lipids and lipoproteins. In: Frishman, William H. (ed): Medical Management of Lipid Disorders: Focus on Prevention of Coronary Artery Disease. Mount Kisco, NY: Futura Publishing, 1992

Fuster V, Cohen M, Halperin J. Aspirin in the prevention of coronary disease. N Engl J Med 1989;321:183–185.

Haskell WL, Alderman EL, Fair JM, et al. Effects of intensive multiple risk factor reduction on coronary atherosclerosis and clinical cardiac events in men and women with coronary artery disease: The Stanford Coronary Risk Intervention Project (SCRIP). Circulation 1994;89:975–990.

Hull SS, Vanoli E, Adamson PB, et al. Exercise training confers anticipatory protection from sudden death during acute myocardial infarction. Circulation 1994; 89:548–552.

ISIS-2 (Second International Study of Infarct Survival) Collaborative Group. Morning peak in the incidence of myocardial infarction: Experience in the ISIS-2 trial. Eur Heart J 1992;13:594–598.

Lakka TA, Venäläinen JM, Rauramaa R. Relationship of leisure-time physical activity and cardiorespiratory fitness to the risk of acute myocardial infarction in men. N Engl J Med 1994;330:1549–1554.

Miller M. Maximizing secondary prevention of CAD: A model program. J Myocard Ischemia 1995;7:166–169.

Mittleman MA, Maclure M, Tofler GH, et al. Triggering of acute myocardial infarction by heavy exercise: Protection by regular exercise. N Engl J Med 1993;329:1677–1683.

O'Connor GT, Buring JE, Yusuf S, et al. An overview of randomized trials after rehabilitation with exercise after myocardial infarction. Circulation 1989;80:234–244.

Patrono C. Drug therapy: Aspirin as an antiplatelet drug. N Engl J Med 1994; 330:1287–1294.

Peto R, Gray R, Collins R, et al. Randomized trial of prophylactic aspirin in British male doctors. Br Med J 1988;296:313–316.

Pfeffer MA, Brunweld E, Moye LA, et al. Effect of captopril on mortality and morbidity in patients with left ventricular dysfunction after myocardial infarction: Results of the survival and ventricular enlargement trial. N Engl J Med 1992;327:669–677.

Roberts R, Rogers WJ, Mueller HS, et al. Immediate versus deferred β-blockade following thrombolytic therapy in patients with acute myocardial infarction. Results of the Thrombolysis in Myocardial Infarction (TIMI)II-B Study. Circulation 1991;83:422–437.

Rodriguez BL, Curb JD, Burchfiel CM, et al. Physical activity and 23-year incidence of coronary heart disease morbidity and mortality among middle-aged men: The Honolulu Heart Program. Circulation 1994;89:2540–2544.

The SOLVD Investigators. Effect of enalapril on survival in patients with reduced left ventricular ejection fraction and congestive heart failure. N Engl J Med 1991;325:293–302.

Stampfer MJ, Colditz GA, Willett WC, et al. Postmenopausal estrogen therapy and cardiovascular disease. Ten-year follow-up from the Nurses' Health Study. N Engl J Med 1991;325:756–762.

Steering Committee of the Physicians' Health Study Research Group. Final report on the aspirin component of the ongoing Physicians' Health Study. N Engl J Med 1989;321:129–135.

Sullivan JM, Vander Zwaag R, Hughes JP, et al. Estrogen replacement and coronary artery disease: Effect on survival in postmenopausal women. Arch Intern Med 1990;150:2557–2562.

Swedberg K, Held P, Kjekshus J, et al. Effects of early administration of enalapril on mortality on patients with acute myocardial infarction: Results of the Cooperative New Scandinavian Enalapril Survival Study II (CONSENSUS II). N Engl J Med 1992;327:678–684.

Willich SN, Lewis M, Löwel H, et al. Physical exertion as a trigger of active myocardial infarction. N Engl J Med 1993;329: 1684–1690.

Yusuf S, Sleight P, Held P, et al. Routine medical management of acute myocardial infarction: Lessons from overviews of recently randomized controlled trials. Circulation 1990;82(suppl II):II–117–II–134.

Yusuf S, Wittes J, Friedman L. Overview of results of randomized clinical trials in heart disease. I. Treatment following myocardial infarction. JAMA 1988;260: 2088–2093.

11/ Nontraditional Risk Factors

It has been estimated that 50% of cardiovascular risk cannot be explained by traditional risk factors detailed in previous chapters. In recent years, "nontraditional" risk factors have gained notoriety both in the scientific community and lay public, prompting an inquiry into their relevance as potentially important determinants of CAD.

DEHYDROEPIANDROSTERONE SULFATE

The adrenal steroid, dehydroepiandrosterone sulfate (DHEAS) is the most abundant steroid hormone. Its concentration in plasma is 20-fold greater than any other steroid hormone. Steroid sulfatases convert DHEAS to the active form, DHEA. However, because of significant diurnal variation in DHEA, DHEAS is usually measured in clinical studies.

DHEA inhibits glucose-6-phosphate dehydrogenase hindering processes activated by the pentose phosphate pathway (e.g., fatty acid and cholesterol synthesis) (see Oertel and Benes). DHEA has also been shown to inhibit cell growth and smooth muscle cell proliferation (see Dworkin et al.). Indeed, DHEA supplementation has been shown to prevent obesity (see Yen et al.), lower cholesterol, and indirectly retard the aging process in mice and rats (see Schwartz). Reductions in aortic fatty streaks (see Arad et al.) and atherosclerosis (see Gordon et al.) have also been observed with DHEA supplementation. Eich and colleagues were also able to demonstrate that DHEAS retarded the progression of accelerated atherosclerosis in rabbit recipients of a cardiac transplant.

Increased levels of DHEAS have been found to occur with low-fat, vegetarian diets, weight loss, physical activity and stress reduction (see Psychosocial Factors below). DHEAS levels are inversely related to TG and insulin concentrations in premenopausal women. In general, they are positively correlated with HDL-C.

Although the urinary metabolites (17-ketosteroids) of DHEA and DHEAS were initially observed to be reduced in MI survivors nearly 40 years ago (see Marmorston et al.), the first prospective study examining DHEA as a risk factor for CAD was not published until 1986 (see Barrett-Connor et al.). In a 12-year study, men 50 years of age and older who had baseline DHEAS levels below 140 µg/dL exhibited a three-fold increased rate of cardiovascular death, compared with men whose DHEAS levels were greater than or equal to 140 µg/dL. Baseline DHEAS levels grouped by age and CAD status are shown in Table 11.1. Not only were baseline DHEAS levels reduced in CAD patients, but lower values were observed in the elderly. Peak DHEAS levels occur during the third decade of life and are reduced by 90–95% by the ninth decade. In fact, there is an approximate 6 µg/dL reduction of DHEAS levels per year, believed to reflect decreased activity of the adrenal enzyme, 17,20 desmolase. Studies in male survivors of MI who were younger than 40 years of age also demonstrated a significant inverse correlation between CAD and DHEAS.

Table 11.1 Mean Base-Line DHEAS Levels (±SD) in 242 Men, According to Age Group and History of Heart Disease at Base Line

Age Group	All Subjects		Men with No History of Heart Disease		Men with a History of Heart Disease	
	No.	DHEAS Level	No.	DHEAS Level	No.	DHEAS Level
		µg/dl		µg/dl		µg/dl
50–54	26	270±147	22	265±135	4	298±224
55–59	33	208±111	28	219±112	5	142±80
60–64	49	152±73	40	164±74	9	102±40
65–69	56	142±72	52	143±71	4	126±87
70–74	61	128±78	52	135±81	9	85±42
75–79	17	85±41	14	90±43	3	64±30
Total	242	159	208	164±99	34	126±107
Age-adjusted means			166		124*	

*P = 0.012 for men without a history of heart disease as compared with men with a history of heart disease.

Among patients undergoing diagnostic coronary arteriography at The Johns Hopkins Hospital, Herrington and associates found that both DHEA and DHEAS were inversely correlated with CAD severity in men. In three different age groups, mean DHEAS levels were significantly lower with extensive CAD (Fig. 11.1). However, in women, there was no association between DHEAS levels and CAD as reported previously by Barrett-Connor.

Similarly, LaCroix and associates were unable to find an association between DHEAS and CAD after adjustment for eight coronary risk factors. They postulated that low DHEAS may simply be the consequence of debilitated health. More prospective data are therefore necessary to adjudicate the role of DHEA/DHEAS in the assessment of CAD risk.

FIBRINOGEN

Plasma concentrations of fibrinogen have been shown to correlate with primary cardiovascular events (e.g., MI and stroke), presumably owing to direct enhancement of blood viscosity and accelerated thrombus formation. Fibrinogen is converted into the mitogen fibrin, an essential element in atherothrombosis. Early case-control studies suggesting the link between elevated fibrinogen and CAD (see McDonald and Edgill; Ogston and Ogston) have been confirmed in several prospective trials. In the Framingham Heart Study, mean fibrinogen levels were measured in 1,315 subjects, initially free of cardiovascular disease. Fibrinogen levels increased approximately 0.1 g/L (10 mg/dL) with each decade of advancing age (Table 11.2). Over the ensuing 12 years, the incidence of CAD (117 men and 97 women) was significantly greater with baseline fibrinogen levels exceeding 3.1 g/L

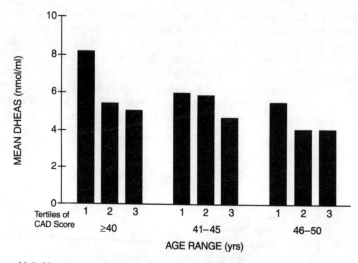

Figure 11.1. Mean plasma DHEAS levels in 98 men according to extent of angiographically defined coronary atherosclerosis; 1 = no CAD, 3 = extensive CAD. Age-adjusted mean level in men with no CAD was significantly higher than that in men with extensive coronary disease (6.5 ± 3.0 versus 4.9 ± 3.3 nmol/mL, p = 0.05).

From Herrington DM, Gordon GB, Achuff SC, et al. Plasma dehydroepiandrosterone and dehydroepiandrosterone sulfate in patients undergoing diagnostic coronary angiography. J Am Coll Cardiol 1990;16:862–870. Reproduced with permission.

Table 11.2 Fibrinogen Level by Age and Sex, Framingham Study

Age, y	No. of Subjects		Mean Fibrinogen Level, g/l (mg/dL)*	
	Men	Women	Men	Women
47–54	201	257	2.8 (278)	2.8 (284)
55–64	229	295	2.9 (287)	3.0 (297)
65–79	124	209	3.0 (295)	3.1 (309)
Total	554	761	2.9 (285)†	3.0 (296)†

*Trends over ages significant for both sexes (P<.05)
†Sexes not significantly different (P>.10)

or 312 mg/dL. Although CAD event rate in men correlated with increases in fibrinogen that were age-related, a similar effect in women was not observed beyond 70 years of age (Fig. 11.2). Nonetheless, fibrinogen was an independent predictor of CAD in both men and women as well as stroke in men.

Wilhelmsen and associates analyzed data from a random sample of nearly 800 Swedish middle-aged men over a 13.5-year follow-up period. At baseline, significantly higher levels of fibrinogen were found in men who later suffered an MI or stroke. Patients with the highest systolic blood pressures (greater than or equal to

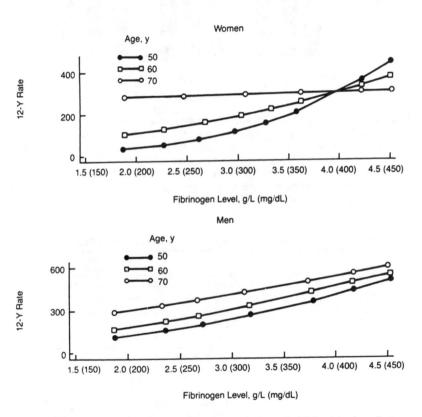

Figure 11.2. Twelve-year follow-up (examinations 10 through 12) for risk of cardiovascular disease by fibrinogen level and age. From Kannel WB, Wolf PA, Castelli WP, D'Agostino RB. Fibrinogen and risk of cardiovascular disease. The Framingham Study. JAMA 1987;258:1183–1186. Reproduced with permission.

180 mm Hg) and fibrinogen concentrations (greater than or equal to 3.5 g/L) posed the highest risk for stroke (Fig. 11.3).

In another longitudinal study of nearly 300 men, Stone and Thorp observed a significant correlation between fibrinogen and MI event rate. With total cholesterol greater than 240 mg/dL or systolic blood pressure greater than 140 mm/Hg, the risk of MI was increased 6-fold and 12-fold respectively, when accompanied by fibrinogen levels greater than 3.5 g/L (Fig. 11.4). The largest of these studies, The Caerphilly and Speedwell Collaborative Heart Disease Studies reported the joint contribution of fibrinogen, viscosity, and WBC count as an important predictor of CAD.

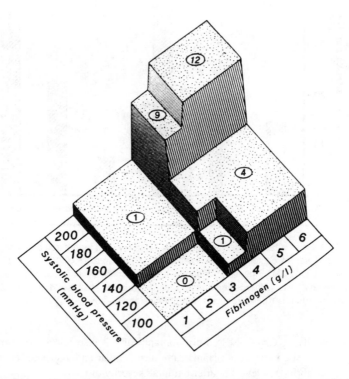

Figure 11.3. Incidence of stroke (circled percentages) according to groups delineated by various combinations of systolic blood-pressure and fibrinogen levels. From Wilhelmsen L, Svärdsudd K, Korsan-Bengtsen K, Larsson B, et al. Fibrinogen as a risk factor for stroke and myocardial infarction. N Engl J Med 1984;311:501–505. Reproduced with permission.

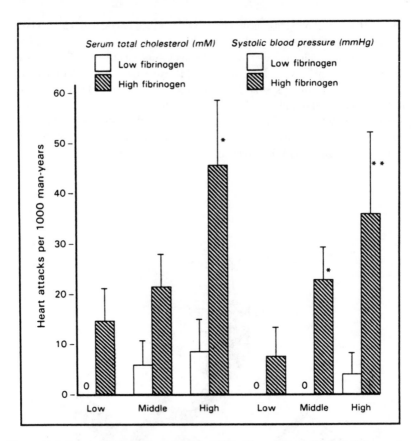

Figure 11.4. Heart attack incidence rates (+ SEM) at low and high thirds of fibrinogen for each third of serum cholesterol and systolic blood pressure. *P<0.05, **P<0.01. From Stone MC, Thorp JM. Plasma fibrinogen—a major coronary risk factor. In: Lenzi S, Descovich GC, eds. Atherosclerosis and cardiovascular disease. Bologna: Editrice Compositori, 1984:3–10. Reproduced with permission.

The severity of CAD assessed arteriographically is also related to fibrinogen concentration (see Lowe et al.; Hamsten et al.). Bolibar and associates correlated increases in fibrinogen levels to arteriographic severity of CAD.

Fibrinogen may also be a determinant of peripheral atherosclerosis (see Joensuu et al.). Sanguigni and colleagues noted progression of carotid atherosclerosis coinciding with elevated fibrinogen and LDL-C. In claudicants, Fowkes and colleagues

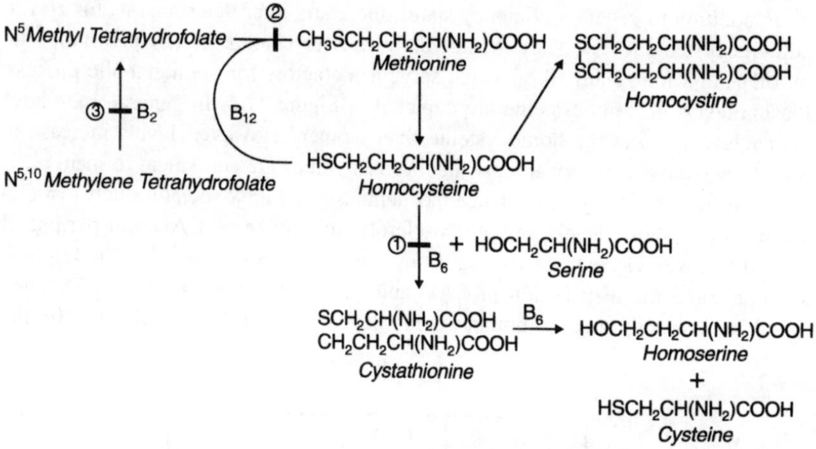

Figure 11.5. Metabolism of homocysteine. 1 = cystathionine β-synthase, 2 = homocysteine methyltransferase, 3 = methylenetetrahydrofolate reductase. From Masser PA, Taylor LM Jr, Porter JM. Importance of elevated plasma homocysteine levels as a risk factor for atherosclerosis. Ann Thorac Surg 1994;58:1240–1246. Reproduced with permission.

observed that in addition to age, plasma fibrinogen levels were the most important predictors of CAD death. Lower levels of fibrinogen have been reported with alcohol (see Meade et al.) and estrogen use (see Nabulsi et al.).

HOMOCYSTEINE

High levels of homocysteine have been shown to be an independent risk factor for premature cardiovascular disease. Accumulation of homocysteine appears to have a direct toxic effect on the endothelium by impairing EDRF-NO production (see Stamler et al.) as well as stimulating smooth muscle cell proliferation (see Tsai et al.). In the homozygous form of homocysteinuria, an autosomal recessive disorder with an incidence of 1:200,000, severe vascular disease begins during childhood. Affected individuals are often tall, with skeletal malformations and ectopia lentis which may resemble Marfan syndrome. Caused by deficiency in cystathionine β-synthase (Fig. 11.5), nearly 2 of every 3 affected patients will develop a thromboembolic event before age 40. The most common causes of death are pulmonary embolism, MI, CVA, and renal or portal vein thrombosis. Pathology often reveals extensive arteriosclerosis throughout the arterial tree (see McCully). Boers and colleagues also observed a predilection for premature arterial occlusive disease in heterozygous subjects. In the general population, the frequency of heterozygosity is estimated to be approximately 1:100.

In addition to genetic deficiency states, there are other determinants for elevated homocysteine levels. They include deficiency in vitamin B_6 (pyridoxine), vitamin B_{12}, and folic acid, all of which serve as cofactors for the metabolic process. Plasma levels of homocysteine are depicted in Figure 11.6. In general, men have higher levels of plasma homocysteine than women. However, levels increase in women beyond age 50; mean post-menopausal values are equivalent to men.

A considerable body of evidence has demonstrated an association between elevated homocysteine levels and atherosclerotic disease (e.g., CAD and peripheral arterial disease). Genest and colleagues measured homocysteine levels in 425 men and compared the distribution in CAD and CAD-free subjects (Fig. 11.7). They found significantly higher homocysteine levels among CAD subjects. In the

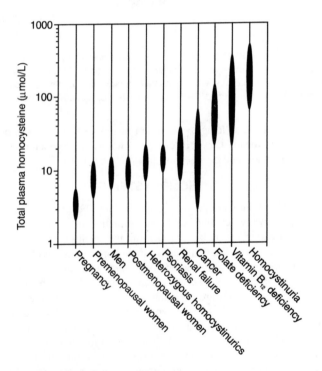

Figure 11.6. Conditions causing elevated plasma homocysteine. From Ueland PM, Refsum H. Plasma homocysteine, a risk factor for vascular disease: Plasma levels in health, disease, and drug therapy. J Lab Clin Med 1989;114:473–501. Reproduced with permission.

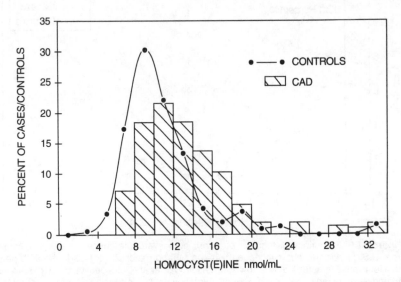

Figure 11.7. Homocyst(e)ine level distribution in 255 control subjects and 170 patients with CAD. From Genest JJ Jr, McNamara JR, Salem DN, Wilson PWF, Schaefer EJ, Malinow MR. Plasma homocyst(e)ine levels in men with premature coronary artery disease. J Am Coll Cardiol 1990;16:1114–1119. Reproduced with permission.

Physicians' Health Study, a threefold increased risk of MI was observed with plasma homocysteine levels above 15.8 nmol/mL representing the 95% percentile (Fig. 11.8) (see Stampfer et al.).

Recently, a cross-sectional analysis was undertaken from the Framingham Heart Study evaluating severity of carotid arterial stenosis with plasma homocysteine levels in subjects greater than 65 years old. Levels of homocysteine greater than 14.4 nmol/mL were associated with a twofold increase in carotid stenosis (Fig. 11.9) and confirmed similar observations by Malinow and O'Leary and their associates. Similarly, elevated levels of homocysteine have been found commonly among patients with aortoiliac occlusive disease (see Brattström et al.). Taken together, these studies suggest that homocysteine is an important independent risk factor for atherosclerotic disease.

In addition to measuring fasting levels of homocysteine, an oral methionine load (0.1 g/kg) may uncover a potential defect in methionine metabolism (Fig. 11.10). Elevated plasma homocysteine may be successfully treated with folate, 1–5 mg/daily (the RDA is 200 and 180 µg/d, for men and women, respectively), vitamin B$_6$ (100–1,000 g/d is successful in approximately 50% with cystathionine β-

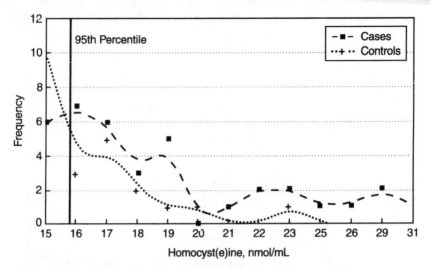

Figure 11.8. Frequency distribution of higher homocyst(e)ine concentrations in plasma from U.S. physicians who subsequently had a MI and matched controls in the 95th percentile. From Stampfer MJ, Malinow RM, Willett WC, et al. A prospective study of plasma homocyst(e)ine and risk of myocardial infarction in US physicians. JAMA 1992;268: 877–881. Reproduced with permission.

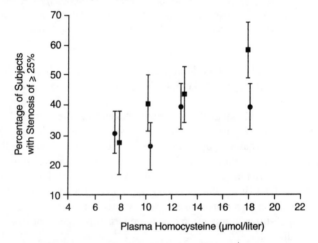

Figure 11.9. Age-adjusted prevalence of maximal extracranial carotid-artery stenosis of greater than or equal to 25% in men ( ) and women ( ) according to quartile of plasma homocysteine concentration. Bars indicate 95% confidence intervals. Quartiles of homocysteine concentrations were less than or equal to 9, 9.2 to 11.3, 11.4 to 14.3, and greater than or equal to 14.4 μmol/L. The prevalence is plotted at the sex-specific median concentration for each quartile. Test for linear trend, P less than 0.001 for men and P=0.03 for women. From Selhub J, Jacques PF, Bostom AG, et al. Association between plasma homocysteine concentrations and extracranial carotid-artery stenosis. N Engl J Med 1995;332:286–291. Reproduced with permission.

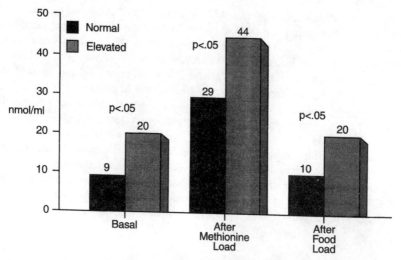

Figure 11.10. Total plasma homocysteine levels in 13 subjects before and after methionine loading, and before and after meals. Numbers at top of bars are mean plasma homocysteine values in nmol/μL. From Taylor LM Jr, Porter JM. Elevated plasma homocysteine as a risk factor for atherosclerosis. Semin Vasc Surg 1993;36–45. Reproduced with permission.

synthase deficiency), betaine, choline, or penicillamine. In general, good nutrition or vitamin supplementation may lower homocysteine levels. Plasma homocysteine levels were normalized within 6 weeks using a daily vitamin supplement consisting of 10 mg pyridoxal, 1 mg folate, and 0.4 mg cyanocobalamin in 44 men with elevated homocysteine levels of greater than 16 nmol/mL (see Ubbink et al.). A recent study found that fish and corn oil supplementation were associated with reduced homocysteine concentrations. Plasma homocysteine may be increased with methotrexate and drugs that interfere with folate metabolism (e.g., anticonvulsants).

While studies linking homocysteine to premature atherosclerosis are provocative, prospective studies assessing the efficacy of reducing homocysteine levels on CAD event rate are lacking. Formal recommendations regarding screening for homocysteinemia/uria and/or vitamin supplementation await the results of randomized trials.

IRON

In the early 1980s, Sullivan speculated that the reduced cardiovascular risk afforded to menstruating women was in large part attributable to reduced iron stores. By enhancing oxidation of LDL-C, atherosclerosis rates would seemingly be enhanced. Although some cardiac implications of iron toxicity (e.g., myocardial ischemia and necrosis) had previously been demonstrated in animal models, little data was available to support the role of iron in promoting CAD until the study by Salonen and coworkers. In the Kuopio Ischaemic Heart Disease Risk Factor Study of 1,931 middle-aged Finnish men, 51 experienced an MI over a 3-year follow-up period. Serum ferritin levels were correlated with increased MI rate; a twofold increased risk was observed with ferritin greater than or equal to 200 µg/L. The most intriguing finding was the markedly higher risk observed in subjects with both elevated LDL-C 5 mM (approximately 190 mg/dL or greater) and ferritin (200 µg/L or greater) (Fig. 11.11).

In addition to the worldwide media attention that accompanied the publication of the Finnish study and suggestions for changes in health care policy vis-á-vis iron supplementation, further validation was necessary. Several studies evaluating iron and CAD risk appeared in 1994. Ascherio and coworkers documented nearly 850 CAD cases from among 45,000 subjects followed for 4 years in The Health

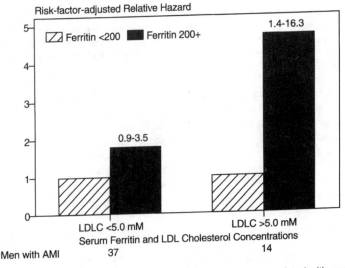

Figure 11.11. Risk factor-adjusted relative hazard of acute MI associated with serum ferritin concentration greater than or equal to 200 µg/L (with 95% confidence intervals) in men with serum LDL cholesterol greater than or equal to 5 mmol/L and those with serum LDL cholesterol less than 5 mmol/L. From Salonen JT, Nyyssönen K, Korpela H, Tuomilehto J, Seppänen R, Salonen R. High stored iron levels are associated with excess risk of myocardial infarction in Eastern Finnish men. Circulation 1992;86:803–811. Reproduced with permission.

Professionals Follow-up Study. They were unable to find an association between dietary iron intake and CAD rate. Total MI rate (which included nonfatal MI and fatal CAD events) was significantly higher among men in the upper quintile of heme iron intake. However, it is not known whether the fatal CAD events were ischemic or arrhythmogenic in origin.

In a prospective Icelandic study of more than 2,000 men and women followed for 8.5 years, iron stores measured by serum ferritin were not an important determinant of CAD. Moreover, Sempos and associates studied 4,500 men and women in the National Health and Nutrition Examination Survey and did not find a relationship between transferrin-saturation levels (an indirect measure of body iron stores) and CAD. Finally, the presence and severity of CAD among autopsied cases of iron overload (e.g., hemochromatosis and hemosiderosis) presenting to The Johns Hopkins Hospital were systematically evaluated. The authors reasoned that if iron were indeed an important risk factor for CAD, then subjects with iron overload might exhibit significant coronary luminal narrowing. What was observed instead was a relative paucity of CAD (Table 11.3). Taken together, these recent studies cast a smoldering effect on the role of iron as an important CAD risk factor.

LIPOPROTEIN(a)

Lipoprotein(a) (Lp[a]) was discovered in the early 1960s at the University of Oslo by Dr. K. Berg. It is composed of a structure resembling LDL-C and an apoB-100 moiety to which another glycoprotein (apolipoprotein or apo[a]) is attached

Table 11.3. Descriptive Postmortem Findings and Prevalence of Coronary Artery Disease in Iron-Overload Cases and Controls at The Johns Hopkins Hospital Between 1898 and 1989

	Iron-Overload Cases		Controls	
	n	Mean±SD	n	Mean±SD
Age, y	41	57.6±13.2	82	57.0±13.8
Body mass index	24	24±7	66	23±6
Heart, g	38	406±112*	78	465±156
Liver, g	39	1930±755	79	1684±547
Coronary artery disease				
None	20†	...	20	...
Mild	16	...	31	...
Advanced	3	...	14	...
Severe	2	...	17	...

*P=.03, †P=.01 by χ^2 analysis.
From Miller M, Hutchins GM. Hemochromatosis, multiorgan hemosiderosis, and coronary artery disease. JAMA 1994;272:231–233. Reproduced with permission.

(Fig. 11.12). Apo(a) consists of a series of repeated domains referred to as kringles (in deference to the Danish pastry). Of great interest was the finding that apo(a) bears structural sequence homology with plasminogen and the cellular mitogen, hepatocyte growth factor, suggesting a link between atherosclerosis and thrombosis.

The distribution of Lp(a) levels in most populations is shown in Figure 11.13. Plasma Lp(a) levels are much lower than LDL-C and account for less than one-sixth of the total plasma cholesterol. The vast majority of the population have Lp(a) levels lower than 0.2 g/L or 20 mg/dL. There is an approximate 2-fold increased risk of CAD with levels exceeding 30 mg/dL. Lp(a) levels are correlated with LDL-C and are threefold higher with familial hypercholesterolemia (FH). As well, there is a particularly high prevalence of CAD among subjects with both elevated Lp(a) (greater than 40 mg/dL) and FH. On average, levels of Lp(a) are higher in African-

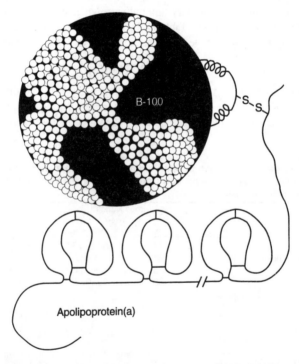

Figure 11.12. Schematic model of lipoprotein(a). From Rader DJ, Brewer HB Jr. Lipoprotein(a). Clinical approach to a unique atherogenic lipoprotein. JAMA 1992;267: 1109–1112. Reproduced with permission.

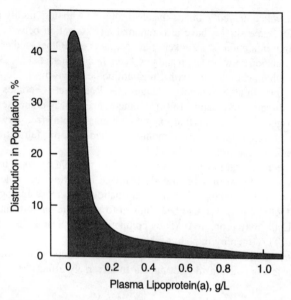

Figure 11.13. Schematic representation of distribution of plasma lipoprotein(a) concentrations in most populations. From Rader DJ, Brewer HB Jr. Lipoprotein(a). Clinical approach to a unique atherogenic lipoprotein. JAMA 1992;267:1109–1112. Reproduced with permission.

Americans than in Caucasians and the distribution is bell-shaped. Elevated Lp(a) levels have been associated with renal failure, poorly controlled insulin-dependent DM, as well as hypothyroidism; levels may normalize following treatment of the underlying disorder.

There have been numerous epidemiologic studies examining the association between Lp(a) levels and CAD event rate. In a prospective, case-control study of middle-aged men, Rosengren and colleagues reported a twofold increase in MI and CAD death among men with the highest Lp(a) levels (greater than 36.5 mg/dL). In the Lipid Research Clinics Primary Prevention Trial of nearly 4,000 middle-aged, hyperlipidemic Caucasian men, Schaefer and associates also found significantly higher levels among cases (23.7 mg/dL) vs controls (19.5 mg/dL). Lp(a) has been shown to be an independent risk factor for early MI (occurring at less than 46 years of age) (see Sandkamp et al.) and for the presence and severity of CAD as assessed by arteriography (see Dahlen). Finally, Hoefler and associates reported that adolescent men with a parental history of MI evidenced an approximate 2.5-fold increase in mean Lp(a) level compared with age-matched subjects without a family history of premature CAD. Some studies have also reported an association between elevated Lp(a) and cerebral infarction (see Zenker et al.; Murai et al.). Other studies have not disclosed an association between Lp(a) and CAD (see Jauhianinen et al.; Ridker et al.).

Immunohistochemical staining with Lp(a) antibodies have disclosed considerable uptake of Lp(a) in atherosclerotic plaques (see Rath et al.). Perhaps the most intriguing data directly implicating Lp(a) in atherogenesis was demonstrated in a study of a transgenic mouse line that expresses human apo(a) (see Lawn et al.). Administration of a high-fat diet for 4 months resulted in aortic fatty streaking in transgenic but not in control mice (Fig. 11.14).

There have been several mechanisms proposed for the role of Lp(a) in accelerating atherosclerosis. Lp(a) may be directly oxidized rendering the molecule susceptible to macrophage uptake and foam cell formation. As a close analog to hepatocyte growth factor, Lp(a) has also been shown to stimulate smooth muscle cell proliferation. Lp(a) may promote CAD by competing with plasminogen for fibrin and endogenous TPA, thereby impeding fibrinolysis.

While *in vitro* studies have shown that Lp(a) inhibits streptokinase-induced fibrinolysis, high levels of Lp(a) do not appear to adversely affect the response to

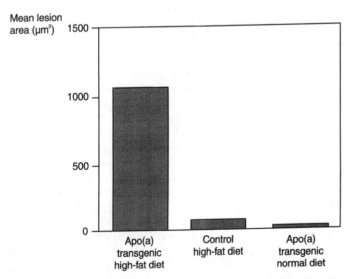

Figure 11.14. Fatty streak lesion areas in apo(a) transgenic mouse aortas. From Wade DP. Lipoprotein(a). Curr Opin Lipidol 1993;4:244–249. Reproduced with permission.

thrombolytic therapy during acute MI. In fact, von Hodenberg and colleagues reported a successful thrombolysis rate of 89% with elevated Lp(a) (greater than or equal to 25 mg/dL) compared to 70% in subjects with normal or lower Lp(a) levels. With regard to revascularization, Lp(a) has been shown to predict saphenous vein graft stenosis following coronary artery bypass grafting (see Hoff et al.) as well as restenosis following PTCA (see Desmarais et al.) (Fig. 11.15).

Conservative management has little impact on Lp(a) levels. For example, a low saturated fat diet produces little if any reduction in Lp(a). Hormonal therapy, however, has been effective in lowering Lp(a). For example, large doses of estrogens (150 μg/day ethinyl estradiol and 80 mg/month polyestradiol phosphate) administered to prostate cancer patients reduced Lp(a) by 50% (see Henriksson et al.). An approximately 15% Lp(a) reduction was reported with conventional post-menopausal estrogen doses (0.625 mg Premarin) (see Sacks et al.). The Lp(a)-lowering mechanism of estrogen is believed to reflect accelerated catabolism of apoB, the primary ligand for LDL-C and presumably, Lp(a). The anabolic steroid stanozolol has also been shown to reduce Lp(a) levels.

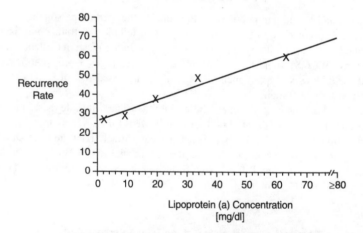

Figure 11.15. Relationship between Lp(a) concentration and recurrence rate. Each data point corresponds to the calculated recurrence rate for each quintile of patients. The median Lp(a) concentration for each quintile was 2, 9, 19, 33, 61, respectively. The curve is a plot of logistic regression model fitted to continuous recurrence rates across the entire patient cohort. With this curve, the recurrence rate for any given value of Lp(a) can be estimated in this or a similar patient population. From Desmarais RL, Sarembock IJ, Ayers CR, Vernon SM, Powers ER, Gimple LW. Elevated serum lipoprotein(a) is a risk factor for clinical recurrence after coronary balloon angioplasty. Circulation 1995;91:1403–1409. Reproduced with permission.

The ability of a variety of other therapies to lower Lp(a) has been evaluated. Lipid lowering medications have produced mixed results. The HMG-CoA reductase inhibitor, lovastatin, was shown to raise Lp(a) in approximately 30% of treated subjects, suggesting stimulation of hepatic synthesis of Lp(a). High-dose (greater than 3 g/d) nicotinic acid appears to be useful as an Lp(a) lowering agent. In combination with neomycin, high-dose nicotinic acid produced a 45% reduction in Lp(a) levels. A more expensive and time consuming procedure, LDL-C apheresis, is also effective in reducing Lp(a) levels. Recently, Gavish and Breslow theorized that a disulfide-bond reducing agent might dissociate apo(a) from Lp(a). Using N-acetylcysteine in two patients with elevated Lp(a), a 70% reduction was obtained; the largest reported to date. Confirmation of these exciting preliminary results may establish an additional indication for N-acetylcysteine.

Measurement of Lp(a) levels may be most reasonable to obtain in subjects with CAD or at high risk who lack traditional risk factors. A trial with nicotinic acid may be useful with elevated levels.

PSYCHOSOCIAL FACTORS

Friedman and Rosenman popularized the concept that certain personality characteristics may predispose to CAD. The notable constellation of traits comprising the so-called Type A personality appears in Table 11.4. In the Western Collaborative Group Study (WCGS), more than 3,100 middle-age men (ages 39–59 years) were followed for 8.5 years. Type A men had a twofold increased risk of CAD events compared with Type B men.

Other studies, however, disputed these findings. The Multiple Risk Factor Intervention Trial (MRFIT) of 3,000 men followed for 9 years, the Aspirin Myocardial Infarction Study, the Beta-Blocker Heart Attack Trial, and the Dutch Heart Study found no association. In fact, the repeat analysis of WCGS after 22 years (see Ragland and Brand) found significantly reduced mortality rates in Type A subjects (Fig. 11.16). Moreover, studies by Case et al., Johnston et al., Shekelle

---

Table 11.4 Characteristics of the Type A Personality

1. Love of competition
2. Need for recognition and advancement
3. Preoccupation with time
4. Goal-oriented obsession
5. Intense and focused concentration
6. Free-floating hostility

From Friedman M, Rosenman RH. Association of specific overt behavior pattern with blood and cardiovascular findings. JAMA 1959; 169:1286–1295.

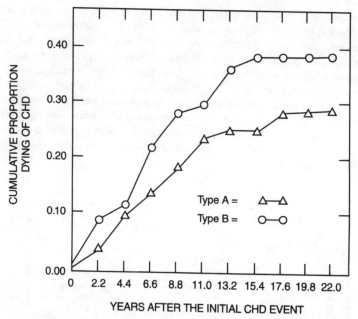

Figure 11.16. Cumulative case fatality rates, according to behavior pattern, in 231 patients with CAD who survived for 24 hours. From Ragland DR, Brand RJ. Type A behavior and mortality from coronary heart disease. N Engl J Med 1988;318:65–69. Reproduced with permission.

et al., and Dimsdale et al., found either no association or an inverse association between Type A and recurrent CAD event rate. These studies suggested Type A subjects may adhere more rigorously to secondary preventive measures.

To correlate specific Type A descriptors with CAD event rate, investigators have exposed hostility and cynicism as prime candidates. Siegler and coworkers observed that hostile behavior occurring during the college years was predictive of an increased tendency toward obesity, hyperlipidemia, and cigarette smoking as subjects approached middle-age. Furthermore, Dembroski and colleagues found that antagonistic hostility (e.g., arrogance, argumentativeness, condescension, and rudeness) was correlated with a 1.5 to 2-fold increased risk of CAD in men younger than 47 years old, even after controlling for other risk factors. In contrast, neuroticism was not shown to predict CAD events (see Costa).

Others have found social isolation to be an important determinant of CAD and total mortality. For example, Hanson and associates noted that CAD rates doubled with reduced social support or isolation. High levels of stress, social isolation, and reduced education were also more likely to result in an adverse outcome among male MI survivors (see Ruberman et al.) (Fig. 11.17). Moreover, in a 10-year prospective study of 150 middle-aged Swedish men, Orth-Gomér and Undén reported that among Type A subjects, there was a significantly higher mortality rate among socially isolated (69%) vs socially integrated (17.3%) men. The stress-related mechanisms of accelerated CAD associated with Type A personality include enhanced catecholamine release leading to elevated heart rate and blood pressure. Endothelial injury may occur owing to increased turbulence and shear stress. Indeed, mental stress has been shown to adversely affect endothelial vasomotor activity (see Specchia et al.). Catecholamines also enhance platelet aggregability and arrhythmogenicity.

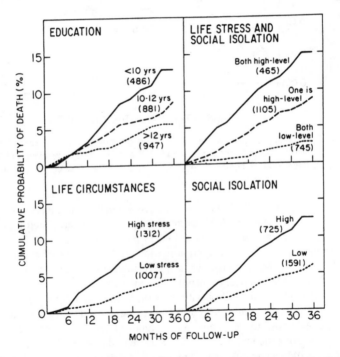

Figure 11.17. Life-table cumulative mortality curves for the health insurance plan-BHAT male survivors of myocardial infarction who completed the psychosocial interview, according to levels of education, life stress (life circumstances), and social isolation. From Ruberman W, Weinblatt E, Goldberg JD, Chaudhary BS. Psychosocial influences on mortality after myocardial infarction. N Engl J Med 1984;311:552–559. Reproduced with permission.

Other biochemical markers affected in stress include apolipoprotein AI and DHEAS. In comparing American and Italian corporate managers, Fava and associates found a more unhealthy psychological and behavioral profile among the Italian managers, characterized by greater hostility and reduced enjoyment in leisure activities. These individuals had lower DHEAS and apolipoprotein levels compared to their American counterparts. With stress reduction, DHEAS levels may be increased (see Littman et al.).

Another important biochemical marker of CAD is cholesterol. While stress often reduces total cholesterol, certain behavioral habits may paradoxically raise cholesterol levels and increase CAD risk. They include enhanced coffee consumption (greater than 5 cups daily) (see LaCroix et al.) and sleep disturbances (see Mattiasson et al.).

Certain occupations are associated with increased rate of CAD. Based on the U.S. Department of Labor Quality of Employment Surveys, a plot of various occupations depicting psychological job demands and decision latitude was generated by Karasek and associates (Fig. 11.18). High job strain positions were defined as high in psychological demand and low in decision making latitude and include firemen, waiters and freight handlers. Such occupations are associated with the highest CAD rates in men based on the U.S. Health Examination Survey (HES) and Health and Nutrition Examination Survey (HANES) (Fig. 11.19). The relative risk of MI in high job strain occupations is nearly fivefold greater than low job stress positions (e.g., watchman, janitor). Occupations characterized by high psychological demands but high decision making latitude (e.g., physicians, public officials) were also at lower risk of CAD. In Sweden, factory and shift work have been associated with up to a threefold increased risk of CAD (see Knutsson et al.). A sevenfold increased risk of MI was reported in men who were always working "against the clock."

The effect of marital status appears to impact on CAD risk. A Finnish study found that divorced men had an approximate twofold increased risk of CAD compared with married men (happily or otherwise). Moreover, Chandra and coworkers reported an approximate 50% higher in-hospital death rate post-MI among unmarried men and women. Increased CAD mortality has also been observed shortly after the death of a male or female spouse (see Jones). In a prospective study conducted in Maryland, Helsing and colleagues found significantly reduced mortality rates among middle-aged widowed males who remarried (Fig. 11.20). Survivorship remained unaffected in widowed females regardless of remarital status.

Interestingly, the educational status of the wife may adversely impact on CAD event rates among married couples (see Haynes et al.). In the Framingham Heart Study, a man who was married to a more educated woman had a higher risk of CAD. This was most prominently displayed in grammar school-educated men where the risk of CAD was 4.4-fold greater (Fig. 11.21). Suarez and Barrett-Connor

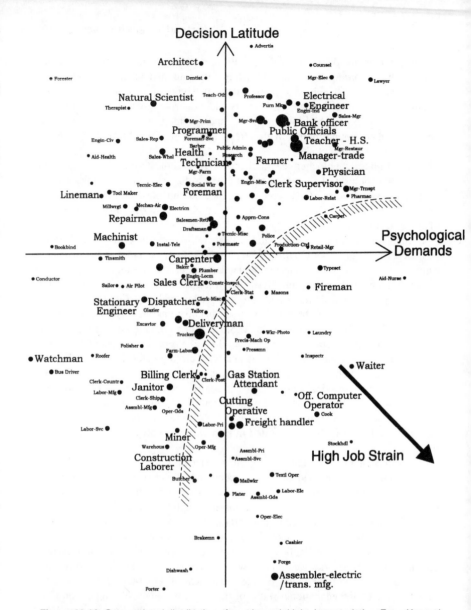

Figure 11.18. Occupational distribution of psychosocial job characteristics. From Karasek RA, Theorell T, Schwartz JE, Schnall PL, Pieper CF, Michela JL. Job characteristics in relation to the prevalence of myocardial infarction in the U.S. Health Examination Survey (HES) and the Health and Nutrition Examination Survey (HANES). Am J Public Health 1988;78:910–918. Reproduced with permission.

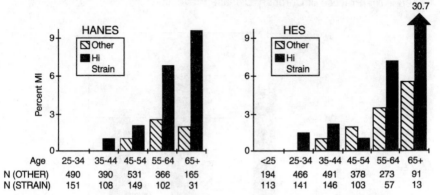

Figure 11.19. Prevalence of myocardial infarction by age and job strain, U.S. HANES and HES, employed males. From Karasek RA, Theorell T, Schwartz JE, Schnall PL, Pieper CF, Michela JL. Job characteristics in relation to the prevalence of myocardial infarction in the U.S. Health Examination Survey (HES) and the Health and Nutrition Examination Survey (HANES). Am J Public Health 1988;78:910–918. Reproduced with permission.

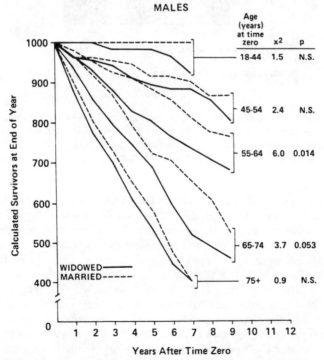

Figure 11.20. Calculated survivorship of widowed and married males by age group and by years after time zero. From Helsing KJ, Szklo M, Comstock GW. Factors associated with mortality after widowhood. Am J Public Health 1981;71:802–809. Reproduced with permission.

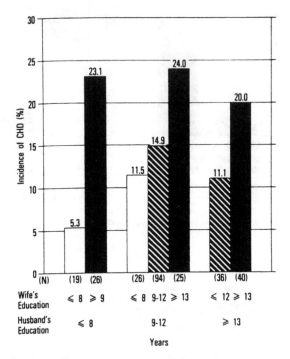

Figure 11.21. Ten-year incidence of CAD among men aged 45–64 years by educational level of husbands and wives. Haynes SG, Eaker ED, Feinleib M. Spouse behavior and coronary heart disease in men: Prospective results from the Framingham Heart Study. Am J Epidemiol 1983;118:1–22. Reproduced with permission.

also observed significantly greater increases in CAD rate among men who lacked a college education but had college educated wives. CAD risk was attenuated when educational status of the spouses was equivalent. While there were no differences in husband's CAD rate based on wife's employment status, occupation was predictive of CAD events. A middle-aged man experienced an approximate fourfold increased incidence of CAD if his wife was a white-collar employee vs clerical, blue-collar or a housewife (Fig. 11.22).Working women with 13+ years of education whose husbands developed CAD were also more likely to have a nonsupportive supervisor and less likely to have been promoted, suggesting that occupational frustration rather than educational level may be a more important contributing factor for the elevated CAD rates observed in husbands. Similarly, men married to angry or hostile women were also at higher risk of CAD.

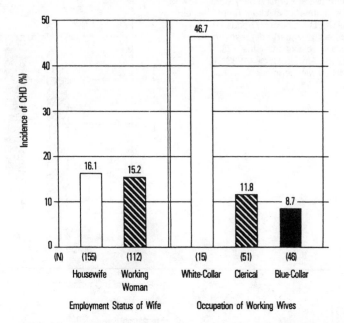

Figure 11.22. Ten-year incidence of CAD among men aged 45–64 years by employment and occupational status of wives. From Haynes SG, Eaker ED, Feinleib M. Spouse behavior and coronary heart disease in men: Prospective results from the Framingham Heart Study. Am J Epidemiol 1983;118:1–22. Reproduced with permission.

Incidence of CAD in men was also related to number of children in the household; three or more children conferred an approximate 2.5-fold increased risk of CAD events in men compared with no children (Fig. 11.23). It is important to note that the Framingham cohort examined middle-aged subjects (ages 45–64 years) in which the incidence of CAD in women was low; therefore no data was available regarding CAD rates in women.

Psychosocial intervention studies designed to reduce CAD event rate have been performed. Friedman and coworkers examined 1,000 male heart attack survivors randomized to either cardiac rehabilitation or behavior modification and found a 45% reduction in subsequent CAD events among subjects in the behavior modification group during the 3-year period. Powell and Thoresen observed reduced CAD deaths only among post-MI Type A patients with preserved left ventricular function who received behavioral counseling (Fig. 11.24). Type A patients with impaired cardiac function, however, did not experience greater benefit from the behavioral counseling program.

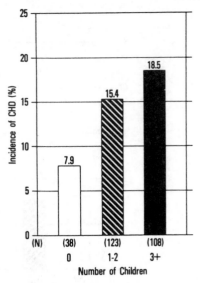

Figure 11.23. Ten-year incidence of coronary heart disease among men aged 45–64 years by number of children. From Haynes SG, Eaker ED, Feinleib M. Spouse behavior and coronary heart disease in men: Prospective results from the Framingham Heart Study. Am J Epidemiol 1983;118:1–22. Reproduced with permission.

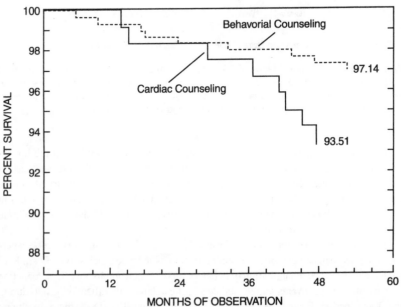

Figure 11.24. Survival in asymptomatic patients with good cardiac function, defined by mild prior acute MI using the Peel index. From Powell LH, Thoresen CE. Effects of type A behavioral counseling and severity of prior acute myocardial infarction on survival. Am J Cardiol 1988;62:1159–1163. Reproduced with permission.

Suggested Readings

Dehydroepiandrosterone Sulfate

Arad Y, Badimon JO, Badimon L, Hembrec W, Ginsberg HN. Dehydroepiandrosterone feeding prevents aortic fatty stream formation and cholesterol accumulation in cholesterol-fed rabbits. Arteriosclerosis 1989; 9:159–166.

Barrett-Connor E, Khaw K-T, Yen SSC. A prospective study of dehydroepiandrosterone sulfate, mortality, and cardiovascular disease. N Engl J Med 1986;315: 1519–1524.

Dworkin CR, Gorman SD, Pashko LL, Christofalo VJ, Schwartz AG. Inhibition of growth of HeLa and WI-38 cells by dehydroepiandrosterone and its reversal by ribo- and deoxyribonucleosides. Life Sci 1986;38:1451–1457.

Eich DM, Nestler JE, Johnson DE, et al. Inhibition of accelerated coronary atherosclerosis with dehydroepiandrosterone in the heterotopic rabbit model of cardiac transplantation. Circulation 1993;87: 261–269.

Gordon GB, Bush DE, Weisman HF. Reduction of atherosclerosis by administration of dehydroepiandrosterone. J Clin Invest 1988;82:712–720.

Haffner SM, Mykkänen L, Valdez RA, Katz MS. Relationship of sex hormones to lipids and lipoproteins in nondiabetic men. J Clin Endocrinol Metab 1993;77:1610–1615.

Haffner SM, Valdez RA, Mykkänen L, Stern MP, Katz MS. Decreased testosterone and dehydroepiandrosterone sulfate concentrations are associated with increased insulin and glucose concentrations in nondiabetic men. Metabolism 1994;43:599–603.

Herrington DM, Gordon GB, Achuff SC, et al. Plasma dehydroepiandrosterone and dehydroepiandrosterone sulfate in patients undergoing diagnostic coronary angiography. J Am Coll Cardiol 1990;16:862–870.

LaCroix AZ, Yano K, Reed DM. Dehydroepiandrosterone sulfate, incidence of myocardial infarction, and extent of atherosclerosis in men. Circulation 1992;86: 1529–1535.

Marmorston J, Lewis JJ, Bernstein JL, et al. Excretion of urinary steroids by men and women with myocardial infarction. Geriatrics 1957; 12:297–300.

Oertel GW, Benes P. The effects of steroids on glucose-6-phosphate dehydrogenase. J Steroid Biochem 1972;3:493–496.

Schwartz A. The effects of dehydroepiandrosterone on the rate of development of cancer and autoimmune processes in laboratory rodents. Basic Life Sci 1985;35:181–191.

Slowinska-Srzednicka J, Zgliczynski S, Ciswicka-Sznajderman M, et al. Decreased plasma dehydroepiandrosterone sulfate and dihydrotestosterone concentrations in young men after myocardial infarction. Atherosclerosis 1989;79:197–203.

Yen TT, Allan JA, Pearson DV, Acton JM, Greenberg MM. Prevention of obesity in Avy/a mice by dehydroepiandrosterone. Lipids 1977;12:409–413.

Fibrinogen

Bolibar I, Kienast J, Thompson SG, Matthias R, Niessner H, Fechtrup C. Relation of fibrinogen to presence and severity of coronary artery disease is independent of other coexisting heart disease. The ECAT Angina Pectoris Study Group. Am Heart J 1993;125:1601–1605.

Fowkes FGR, Lowe GDO, Housley E, Rattray A, Rumley A, Elton RA, MacGregor IR, Dawes J. Cross-linked fibrin degradation products, progression of peripheral arterial disease, and risk of coronary heart disease. Lancet 1993;342:84–86.

Hamsten A, Blombäck M, Wiman B, et al. Haemostatic function in myocardial infarction. Br Heart J 1986;55:58–66.

Joensuu T, Salonen R, Winblad I, Korpela H, Salonen JT. Determinants of femoral and carotid artery atherosclerosis. J Intern Med 1994;236:79–84.

Kannel WB, Wolf PA, Castelli WP, D'Agostino RB. Fibrinogen and risk of cardiovascular disease. The Framingham Study. JAMA 1987;258:1183–1186.

Lowe GDO, Drummond MM, Lorimer AR, et al. Relation between extent of coronary artery disease and blood viscosity. Br Med J 1980;1:673–674.

McDonald L, Edgill M. Coagulability of the blood in ischaemic heart disease. Lancet 1957;2:457–460.

Meade TW, Brozovic M, Chakrabarti RR, et al. Haemostatic function and ischaemic heart disease: Principal results of the Northwick Park Heart Study. Lancet 1986;2:533–537.

Meade TW, Chakrabarti R, Haines AP, North WR, Stirling Y. Characteristics affecting fibrinolytic activity and plasma fibrinogen concentrations. Br Med J 1979;1:153–156.

Nabulsi AA, Folsom AR, White A, et al. Association of hormone-replacement therapy with various cardiovascular risk factors in postmenopausal women. N Engl J Med 1993;328:1069–1075.

Ogston CM, Ogston D. Plasma fibrinogen and plasminogen levels in health and in ischaemic heart disease. J Clin Pathol 1966;19:352–356.

Sanguigni V, Gallu M, Novo S, Strano A. Cholesterol and fibrinogen as predictive factors of progressive carotid atherosclerosis. Int Angiol 1993;12:335–336.

Stone MC, Thorp JM. Plasma fibrinogen—a major coronary risk factor. In: Lenzi S, Descovich GC, eds. Atherosclerosis and cardiovascular disease. Bologna: Editrice Compositori, 1984:3–10.

Wilhelmsen L, Svärdsudd K, Korsan-Bengtsen K, Larsson B, et al. Fibrinogen as a risk factor for stroke and myocardial infarction. N Engl J Med 1984;311:501–505.

Yarnell JWG, Baker IA, Sweetnam PM, et al. Fibrinogen, viscosity, and white blood cell count are major risk factors for ischemic heart disease. The Caerphilly and Speedwell Collaborative Heart Disease Studies. Circulation 1991;83:836–844.

Homocysteine

Boers GHJ, Smals AGH, Trijbels FJM, et al. Heterozygosity for homocystinuria in premature peripheral and cerebral occlusive arterial disease. N Engl J Med 1985;313: 709–715.

Brattström L, Israelsson B, Norrving B, et al. Impaired homocysteine metabolism in early-onset cerebral and peripheral occlusive arterial disease. Effects of pyridoxine and folic acid treatment. Atherosclerosis 1990;81:51–60.

Crouse JR, Toole JF, McKinney WM, et al. Risk factors for extracranial carotid artery atherosclerosis. Stroke 1987;18:990–996.

Genest JJ Jr, McNamara JR, Salem DN, Wilson PWF, Schaefer EJ, Malinow MR. Plasma homocyst(e)ine levels in men with premature coronary artery disease. J Am Coll Cardiol 1990;16:1114–1119.

Kang SS, Wong PWK, Malinow MR. Hyperhomocyst(e)inemia as a risk factor for occlusive vascular disease. Annu Rev Nutr 1992;12:279–298.

Malinow MR, Nieto FJ, Szklo M, Chambless LE, Bond G. Carotid artery intimal-medial wall thickening and plasma homocyst(e)ine in asymptomatic adults: The Atherosclerosis Risk in Communities Study. Circulation 1993;87:1107–13.

Masser PA, Taylor LM Jr, Porter JM. Importance of elevated plasma homocysteine levels as a risk factor for atherosclerosis. Ann Thorac Surg 1994;58: 1240–1246.

McCully KS. Atherosclerosis, serum cholesterol and the homocysteine theory: A study of 194 consecutive autopsies. Am J Med Sci 1990;299:217–221.

McCully KS. Vascular pathology of homocysteinemia: Implications for the pathogenesis of arteriosclerosis. Am J Pathol 1969; 56:111–128.

O'Leary DH, Polak JF, Kronmal RA, et al. Distribution and correlates of sonographically detected carotid artery disease in the Cardiovascular Health Study. Stroke 1992;23:1752–60.

Olszewski AJ, McCully KS. Fish oil decreases serum homocysteine in hyperlipemic men. Coron Artery Dis 1993;4:53–60.

Selhub J, Jacques PF, Bostom AG, et al. Association between plasma homocysteine concentrations and extracranial carotid-artery stenosis. N Engl J Med 1995; 332:286–291.

Stamler JS, Osborne JA, Jaraki O, et al. Adverse vascular effects of homocysteine are modulated by endothelium-derived relaxing factor and related oxides of nitrogen. J Clin Invest 1993;91:308–318.

Stampfer MJ, Malinow RM, Willett WC, et al. A prospective study of plasma homocyst(e)ine and risk of myocardial infarction in US physicians. JAMA 1992;268: 877–881.

Taylor LM Jr, Porter JM. Elevated plasma homocysteine as a risk factor for atherosclerosis. Semin Vasc Surg 1993;36–45.

Tsai J-C, Perrella MA, Yoshizumi M, et al. Promotion of vascular smooth muscle cell growth by homocysteine: A link to atherosclerosis. Proc Natl Acad Sci USA 1994; 91:6369–6373.

Ubbink JB, Vermaak WJH, van der Merwe A, Becker PJ. Vitamin B-12, vitamin B-6, and folate nutritional status in men with hyperhomocysteinemia. Am J Clin Nutr 1993;57:47–53.

Ueland PM, Refsum H. Plasma homocysteine, a risk factor for vascular disease: Plasma levels in health, disease, and drug therapy. J Lab Clin Med 1989;114:473–501.

Iron

Ascherio A, Willett WC, Rimm EB, Giovannucci EL, Stampfer MJ. Dietary iron intake and risk of coronary disease among men. Circulation 1994;89: 969–974.

Magnusson MK, Sigfusson N, Sigvaldason H, Johannesson GM, Magnusson S, Thorgeirsson G. Low iron-binding capacity as a risk factor for myocardial infarction. Circulation 1994;89:102–108.

Miller M, Hutchins GM. Hemochromatosis, multiorgan hemosiderosis, and coronary artery disease. JAMA 1994;272:231–233.

Salonen JT, Nyyssönen K, Korpela H, Tuomilehto J, Seppänen R, Salonen R. High stored iron levels are associated with excess risk of myocardial infarction in Eastern Finnish men. Circulation 1992; 86:803–811.

Sempos CT, Looker AC, Gillum RF, Makuc DM. Body iron stores and the risk of coronary heart disease. N Engl J Med 1994;330:1119–1124.

Steinberg D, Parthasarathy S, Carew TE, Khoo JC, Witztum JL. Modifications of low-density lipoprotein that increase its atherogenicity. N Engl J Med 1989;320:915–924.

Sullivan JL. Stored iron and ischemic heart disease. Empirical support for a new paradigm. Circulation 1992;86:1036–1037.

Sullivan JL. Iron and the sex difference in heart disease risk. Lancet 1981; 1: 1293–1294.

Lipoprotein(a)

Dahlen GH, Guyton JR, Attar M, Farmer JA, Kautz JA, Gotto AM Jr. Association of levels of lipoprotein Lp(a), plasma lipids, and other lipoproteins with coronary artery disease documented by angiography. Circulation 1986;74:758–765.

Desmarais RL, Sarembock IJ, Ayers CR, Vernon SM, Powers ER, Gimple LW. Elevated serum lipoprotein(a) is a risk factor for clinical recurrence after coronary balloon angioplasty. Circulation 1995;91: 1403–1409.

Gavish D, Breslow JL. Lipoprotein(a) reduction by N-acetylcysteine. Lancet 1991; 337:203–204.

Guraker A, Hoeg JM, Kostner G, Papadopoulos NM, Brewer HB. Levels of lipoprotein Lp(a) decline with neomycin and niacin treatment. Atherosclerosis 1985;57:293–301.

Guyton JR, Dahlen GH, Patsch W, Kautz JA, Gotto AM Jr. Relationship of plasma lipoprotein Lp(a) levels to race and to apolipoprotein B. Arteriosclerosis 1985; 5:265–272.

Henriksson P, Angelin B, Berglund L. Hormonal regulation of serum Lp(a) levels. Opposite effects after estrogen treatment and orchidectomy in males with prostatic carcinoma. J Clin Invest 1992; 89:1166–1171.

Hoefler G, Harnoncourt F, Paschke E, Mirtl W, Pfeiffer KH, Kostner GM. Lipoprotein(a): A risk factor for myocardial infarction. Arteriosclerosis 1988;8:398–401.

Hoff HF, Beck GJ, Skibinski CI, et al. Serum Lp(a) level as a predictor of vein graft stenosis after coronary artery bypass surgery in patients. Circulation 1988; 77:1238–1244.

Jauhiainen M, Koskinen P, Ehnholm C, et al. Lipoprotein(a) and coronary heart disease risk: A nested case-control study of the Helsinki Heart Study participants. Atherosclerosis 1991;89:59–67.

Karadi I, Kostner GM, Gries A, Nimpf J, Romics L, Malle E. Lipoprotein(a) and plasminogen are immunochemically related. Biochem Biophys Acta 1988; 960:91–97.

Kostner GM, Gavish D, Leopold B, Bolzano K, Weintraub MS, Breslow JL. HMG CoA reductase inhibitors lower LDL cholesterol without reducing Lp(a) levels. Circulation 1989;80:1313–1319.

Lawn RM, Wade DP, Hammer RE, Chiesa G, Verstuyft JG, Rubin EM. Atherogenesis in transgenic mice expressing human apolipoprotein(a). Nature 1992;360:670–672.

Murai A, Miyahara T, Fujimoto N, Matsuda M, Kameyama M. Lp(a) lipoprotein as a risk factor for coronary heart disease and cerebral infarction. Atherosclerosis 1986; 59:199–204.

Ramirez LC, Arauz-Pacheco C, Lackner C, Albright G, Adams BV, Raskin P. Lipoprotein (a) levels in diabetes mellitus: Relationship to metabolic control. Ann Intern Med 1992;117:42–47.

Rader DJ, Brewer HB Jr. Lipoprotein(a). Clinical approach to a unique atherogenic lipoprotein. JAMA 1992;267:1109–1112.

Rath M, Niendorf A, Reblin T, Dietel M, Krebber HJ, Beisiegel U. Detection and quantification of lipoprotein(a) in the arterial wall of 107 coronary bypass patients. Arteriosclerosis 1989;9:579–592.

Ridker PM, Hennekens CH, Stampfer MJ. A prospective study of lipoprotein(a) and the risk of myocardial infarction. JAMA 1993;270:2195–2199.

Rosengren A, Wilhelmsen L, Eriksson E, Risberg B, Wedel H. Lipoprotein(a) and coronary heart disease: A prospective case-control study in a general population of middle aged men. Br Med J 1990;301: 1248–1251.

Sacks FM, McPherson R, Walsh BW. Effect of postmenopausal estrogen replacement on plasma Lp(a) lipoprotein concentrations. Arch Intern Med 1994;154:1106–1110.

Sandkamp M, Funke H, Schuke H, Köhler E, Assmunn G. Lipoprotein(a) is an independent risk factor for myocardial infarction at a young age. Clin Chemistry 1990;36: 20–23.

Scanu AM. Lipoprotein(a). A genetic risk factor for premature coronary heart disease. JAMA 1992;267:3326–3329.

Scanu AM, Fless GM. Lipoprotein(a). Heterogeneity and biological relevance. J Clin Invest 1990;85:1709–1715.

Schaefer EJ, Lamon-Fava S, Jenner JL, McNamara JR, Ordovas JM, Davis CE, et al. Lipoprotein(a) levels and risk of coronary heart disease in men. The Lipid Research Clinics Coronary Primary Prevention Trial. JAMA 1994;271: 999–1003.

Seed M, Hoppichler F, Reaveley D, McCarthy S, Thompson GR, Boerwinkle E. Relation of serum lipoprotein(a) concentration and apolipoprotein(a) phenotype to coronary heart disease in patients with familial hypercholesterolemia. N Engl J Med 1990;332:1491–1499.

Smith EB, Cochran S. Factors influencing the accumulation in fibrous plaques of lipid derived from low density lipoprotein II: Preferential immobilization of lipoprotein (a). Atherosclerosis 1990;84:173–181.

Utermann G. The mysteries of lipoprotein(a). Science 1989;246:904–910.

von Hodenberg E, Kreuzer J, Hautmann M, Nordt T, Kübler, Bode C. Effects of lipoprotein (a) on success rate of thrombolytic therapy in acute myocardial infarction. Am J Cardiol 1991;67:1349–1353.

Wade DP. Lipoprotein (a). Curr Opin Lipidol 1993;4:244–249.

Zenker G, Költringer P, Boné G, Niederkorn K, Pfeiffer K, Jürgens G. Lipoprotein(a) as a strong indicator for cerebrovascular disease. Stroke 1986;17:942–945.

Psychosocial Factors

Case RB, Heller SS, Case NB, Moss AJ. Multicenter Post-Infarction Research Group. Type A behavior and survival after acute myocardial infarction. N Engl J Med 1985;312:737–741.

Chandra V, Szklo M, Goldberg R, Tonascia J. The impact of marital status on survival after an acute myocardial infarction: A population-based study. Am J Epidemiol 1983;117:320–325.

Costa PT Jr. Influence of the normal personality dimension of neuroticism on chest pain symptoms and coronary artery disease. Am J Cardiol 1987;60:20J–26J.

Dembroski TM, MacDougall JM, Costa PT Jr, Grandits GA. Components of hostility as predictors of sudden death and myocardial infarction in the multiple risk factor intervention trial. Psychosom Med 1989; 51:514–522.

Dembroski TM, MacDougall JM, Williams RB, Haney TL, Blumenthal JA. Components of Type A, hostility, and anger-in: Relationship to angiographic findings. Psychosom Med 1985;47: 219–233.

Dimsdale JE, Gilbert J, Hutter AM Jr, Hackett TP, Block PC. Predicting cardiac morbidity based on risk factors and coronary angiographic findings. Am J Cardiol 1981;47:73–76.

Fava M, Littman A, Lamon-Fava S, Milani R, Shera D, MacLaughlin R, et al. Psychological, behavioral and biochemical risk factors for coronary artery disease among American and Italian male corporate managers. Am J Cardiol 1992;70: 1412–1416.

Friedman M, Rosenman RH. Association of specific overt behavior pattern with blood and cardiovascular findings. JAMA 1959;169:1286–1295.

Friedman M, Thoresen CE, Gill JJ, Ulmer D, Powell LH, Price VA. Alteration of type A behavior and its effect on cardiac recurrences in post myocardial infarction patients: Summary results of the recurrent coronary prevention project. Am Heart J 1986;112:653–665.

Hanson BS, Isacsson SO, Janzon L, Lindell SE. Social network and social support influence mortality in elderly men. The prospective population of "men born in

1914" Malmo, Sweden. Am J Epidemiol 1989;130:100–111.

Haynes SG, Eaker ED, Feinleib M. Spouse behavior and coronary heart disease in men: Prospective results from the Framingham Heart Study. Am J Epidemiol 1983;118:1–22.

Haynes SG, Levine S, Scotch N, Feinleib M, Kannel WB. The relationship of psychosocial factors to coronary heart disease in the Framingham Study. Am J Epidemiol 1978;107:362–383.

Helsing KJ, Szklo M, Comstock GW. Factors associated with mortality after widowhood. Am J Public Health 1981;71: 802–809.

Howard JH, Rechnitzer PA, Cunningham DA, Wong D, Brown H. Personality. Type A behavior, and the effects of β-blockade. J Cardiovasc Pharmacol 1991;18:267–277.

Johnston DW, Cook DG, Shaper AG. Type A behaviour and ischaemic heart disease in middle aged British men. Br Med J 1987;295:86–89.

Jones DR. Heart disease mortality following widowhood: Some results from the OPCS Longitudinal Study. J Psychosom Res 1987;31:325–333.

Karasek RA, Theorell T, Schwartz JE, Schnall PL, Pieper CF, Michela JL. Job characteristics in relation to the prevalence of myocardial infarction in the US Health Examination Survey (HES) and the Health and Nutrition Examination Survey (HANES). Am J Public Health 1988; 78:910–918.

Knutsson A, Akerstedt T, Jonsson BG, Orth-Gomer K. Increased risk of ischaemic heart disease in shift workers. Lancet 1986;2:89–92.

LaCroix AZ, Mead LA, Liang K-Y, Thomas CB, Pearson TA. Coffee consumption and the incidence of coronary heart disease. N Engl J Med 1986;315:977–982.

Littman AB, Fava M, Halperin P, et al. Physiologic benefits of a stress reduction program for healthy middle-aged army officers. J Psychosom Res 1993;37: 345–354.

Matthews KA, Haynes SG. Type A behavior pattern and coronary disease risk. Update and critical evaluation. J Epidemiol 1986;123:923–960.

Mattiasson I, Lindgärde F, Nilsson JA, Theorell T. Threat of unemployment and cardiovascular risk factors: Longitudinal study of quality of sleep and serum cholesterol concentrations in men threatened with redundancy. Br Med J 1990; 301:461–466.

Orth-Gomér K, Undén A-L. Type A behavior, social support, and coronary risk: Interaction and significance for mortality in cardiac patients. Psychosom Med 1990;52:59–72.

Powell LH, Thoresen CE. Effects of type A behavioral counseling and severity of prior acute myocardial infarction on survival. Am J Cardiol 1988;62:1159–1163.

Ragland DR, Brand RJ. Type A behavior and mortality from coronary heart disease. N Engl J Med 1988;318:65–69.

Rosenman RH, Brand RJ, Sholtz RI, Friedman M. Multivariate prediction of coronary heart disease during 8.5 year follow-up in the Western Collaborative Group Study. Am J Cardiol 1976;37:903–910.

Ruberman W, Weinblatt E, Goldberg JD, Chaudhary BS. Psychosocial influences on mortality after myocardial infarction. N Engl J Med 1984;311:552–559.

Shekelle RB, Gale M, Norusis M. Type A score (Jenkins Activity Survey) and risk of recurrent coronary heart disease in the Aspirin Myocardial Infarction Study. Am J Cardiol 1985;56:221–225.

Shekelle RB, Hulley SB, Neaton JD, et al. The MRFIT Behavior Pattern Study. II. Type A behavior and incidence of coronary heart disease. Am J Epidemiol 1985;122: 559–570.

Shekelle RB, Vernon SW, Ostfield AM. Personality and coronary heart disease. Psychosom Med 1991;53:176–184.

Siegel WC, Hlatky MA, Mark DB, Barefoot JC, Harrell FE Jr, Pryor DB. Effect of Type A behavior on exercise test outcome in coronary artery disease. Am J Cardiol 1990;66:179–182.

Siegler IC, Peterson BL, Barefoot JC, Williams RB. Hostility during late adolescence predicts coronary risk factors at midlife. Am J Epidemiol 1992;136:146–154.

Specchia G, Falcone C, Traversi E, et al. Mental stress as a provocative test in patients with various clinical syndromes of coronary heart disease. Circulation 1991; 83(4 suppl):II108–114.

Suarez L, Barrett-Connor E. Is an educated wife hazardous to your health? Am J Epidemiol 1984;119:244–249.

12/ Nontraditional Therapies: Alcohol, Antioxidants, Chelation Therapy, Fish Oils, Garlic, and Onions

ALCOHOL CONSUMPTION

As discussed in previous chapters, moderate alcohol consumption (1 oz alcohol=24 oz beer, 8 oz table wine or 2 shots of 80 proof spirits) is cardioprotective (see also Chapter 5). The flagship mechanism appears to be significant elevation in HDL-C and its subfractions (see Gaziano et al.). Other important mechanisms include enhancement of fibrinolysis by stimulating endogenous production of tissue-type plasminogen activator (t-PA) (Fig. 12.1), inhibition of platelet aggregation (see Renaud et al.), and reduction in fibrinogen.

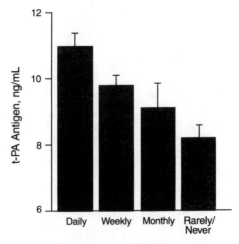

Reported Alcohol Use

Figure 12.1. Mean plasma concentration of endogenous tissue-type plasminogen activator (t-PA) antigen among daily, weekly, monthly, and rarely-or-never consumers of alcohol (P trend=0.0002). Error bars represent SEM. From Ridker PM, Vaughan DE, Stampfer MJ, Glynn RJ, Hennekens CH. Association of moderate alcohol consumption and plasma concentration of endogenous tissue-type plasminogen activator. JAMA 1994;272:929–933. Reproduced with permission.

Moderate drinking may also reduce the risk of non-insulin-dependent diabetes mellitus (NIDDM) as recently observed in a study of elderly subjects who consumed up to 1 oz of alcohol daily (see Gurwitz et al.).

What compounds contained in alcohol are responsible for the cardioprotective effect? Renaud and De Lorgeril reported findings from the International World Health Organization Monitoring Trends and Determinants in Cardiovascular Disease (WHO MONICA) Project which investigated cardiovascular mortality rates in various countries. Despite the high intake of saturated fat, mortality rates from ischemic heart disease in France were among the lowest of the 17 participating countries (Fig. 12.2). This "French" paradox (also applicable for Switzerland) was reportedly due to a high consumption of red wine. Moderate daily alcohol consumption translated into a 40% reduction in CAD events. It has been proposed that red wine is especially cardioprotective because nonalcoholic compounds (tannins) present in red wine contain resveratrol and polyphenols, members of the flavonoid

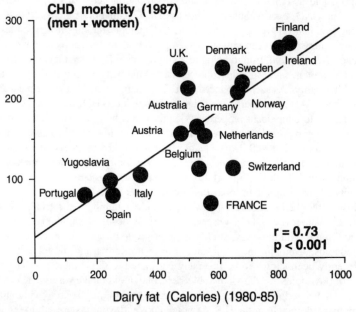

Figure 12.2. Relation between mean age-standardized death rate from CHD for men and women and consumption of dairy fat in countries reporting wine consumption. From Renaud S, De Lorgeril M. Wine, alcohol, platelets, and the French paradox for coronary heart disease. Lancet 1992;339:1523–1526. Reproduced with permission.

group of antioxidants. Indeed, Frankel and associates showed that phenolic compounds present in red wine were more potent antioxidants than α-tocopherol (vitamin E). Moreover, Ruf and colleagues found that tannins prevented the rebound effect on platelet aggregation commonly observed following alcohol withdrawal.

In a large prospective cohort study, Klatsky and associates found an approximate 40% reduction in mortality from cardiovascular causes among moderate consumers of wine (red and white wine were not differentiated) compared with beer. In contrast, heavy alcohol consumption of any kind (more than six drinks daily) is harmful, resulting in a twofold increased risk of supraventricular arrhythmias. Other complications include gastritis and hypertension, as well as the most feared sequalae, cardiomyopathy (8–10 oz daily for 10 years), hemorrhagic stroke, and cirrhosis.

ANTIOXIDANTS

The oxidative modification of LDL-C is a critical step in atherosclerosis (see Chapter 2). Lipid soluble antioxidants such as ß-carotene (vitamin A) and α-tocopherol are avidly incorporated into LDL-C, thereby preventing lipid peroxidation. Regnstrom and associates reported a direct correlation between LDL-C oxidative capacity and CAD severity. Susceptibility to LDL-C oxidation is increased in diabetics owing to enhanced glycosylation of LDL-C. Cigarette smoking also promotes oxidation by generating oxygen radicals which prevent dehydroascorbate, the oxidized product of ascorbic acid, from binding to apolipoprotein B. Plasma levels of ascorbic acid and ß-carotene are also reduced in smokers. Finally, HDL-C may directly inhibit LDL-C oxidation. As such, enhanced LDL-C oxidation may be another mechanism for the higher CAD rate observed in subjects with reduced HDL-C.

In addition to antioxidant properties, vitamin E has been shown to affect platelet adhesion. Steiner reported reductions in platelet adhesion in subjects receiving vitamin E supplementation (200–400 IU/d). The mechanism invoked by α-tocopherol involves changes in the cytoskeletal structure and reduced development of platelet pseudopodia.

Countries with high CAD mortality rates, such as Great Britain and Scotland, have reduced consumption of foods that are nutritionally rich sources of antioxidant vitamins (Table 12.1). As the only water soluble vitamin of the triad, maximal Vitamin C tissue levels may be observed with daily doses of 250–500 mg.

In addition to vitamins A, C, and E, another group of antioxidant compounds is the flavonoids. Although these substances have no known nutritional value, they have recently been shown to be inversely correlated to CAD mortality. The main sources of flavonoids are shown in Table 12.2. Flavonoid intake varies considerably between countries. For example, in Japan, tea is the primary source, while apples and onions predominate in the U.S. As noted above, flavonoids present in red wine have also been theorized to partially account for the "French Paradox."

Observational studies have also documented the cardioprotective effect of antioxidant vitamins. In the Nurses' Health Study, there was a 34% reduction in

Table 12.1 Nutritionally Rich Sources of Beta-Carotene, Vitamin C, and Vitamin E (α-Tocopherol)

Food Source	Serving Size	Beta-Carotene (mg)
Carrot juice	1 cup	24.2
Gazpacho	1 cup	11.7
Sweet potato	1 med	10.0
Apricots, dried	10 halves	6.2
Chicory, raw	1 cup	6.2
Carrot, raw	1 med	5.7
Spinach	½ cup	4.9
Cantaloupe	½	4.8
Turnip greens	½ cup	3.9
Pumpkin	½ cup	3.7

RDA is 3 mg (5,000 IU Vitamin A).

Food Source	Serving Size	Vitamin C (mg)
Orange juice	1 cup	124
Papaya	1	188
Cantaloupe	½	113
Broccoli, cooked	1 cup	98
Brussel sprouts	1 cup	97
Green peppers	1	95
Grapefruit juice	1 cup	94
Strawberries	1 cup	85
Orange	1 med	75
Oysters, raw	1 cup	72

RDA is 60 mg.

Food Source	Serving Size	α-Tocopherol (mg)	C	Fat (g)
Wheat germ oil	1 tbsp	20.3	120	13.6
Sunflower seeds	1 oz	14.2	120	13.6
Mayonnaise, Hellman	1 tbsp	11.0	99	11.0
Margarine, Mazola	1 tbsp	8.0	100	10.0
Almonds, dried	24 nuts	6.7	180	16.2
Hazelnuts	20 nuts	6.7	194	19
Sunflower oil	1 tbsp	6.3	120	13.6
Sweet potato, raw	1 med	5.9	141	0.5
Almond oil	1 tbsp	5.3	120	13.6
Cottonseed oil	1 tbsp	4.8	120	13.6

RDA is 8-10 mg (30 IU Vitamin E).
α-Tocopherol is the biologically active form of Vitamin E.
C = calories.

Table 12.2. Flavonoid Levels of Selected Foods*

Flavonoid Level	Foods
Low (<10 mg/kg or <10 mg/L)	Cabbage, carrot, mushroom, pea, spinach, peach, white wine, coffee, orange juice
Medium (<50 mg/kg or <50 mg/L)	Lettuce, tomato, red pepper, broad bean, strawberry, apple, grape, red wine, tea, tomato juice
High (>50 mg/kg)	Onion, kale, French bean, broccoli, endive, celery, cranberry

*Sum of quercetin, kaempferol, myricetin, luteolin, and apigenin.
From Hertog MGL, Kromhout D, Aravanis C, et al. Flavonoid intake and long-term risk of coronary heart disease and cancer in the seven countries study. Arch Intern Med 1995;155:381–386. Reproduced with permission.

CAD event rate in women receiving vitamin E supplements and a 22% reduction among the highest consumers of ß-carotene (see Stampfer et al.). In the Health Professionals Follow-up Study of nearly 40,000 men, 100 IU of vitamin E daily was associated with an approximate 40% reduction of CAD events (see Rimm et al.). A subgroup with pre-existing CAD in the Physicians' Health Study evidenced a 50% reduction in major events (inclusive of nonfatal and fatal MI as well as coronary revascularization) associated with alternate day doses (50 mg) of ß-carotene (see Gaziano).

While these studies demonstrated a powerful association between antioxidant use and CAD event rate, a recent Finnish study of nearly 30,000 men found no differences in CAD mortality rates among subjects receiving α-tocopherol, ß-carotene, or both. However, the Finnish study employed lower doses of α-tocopherol (50 mg) than that used in the Health Professionals Follow-up Study. Further studies underway to resolve this discrepancy include The Physicians' Health Study (50 mg of ß-carotene on alternate days), The Women's Health Study (ß-carotene, vitamin E, and aspirin in primary prevention), and the Women's Antioxidant Cardiovascular Disease Study (20 mg ß-carotene, 400 IU vitamin E, and 1 gram vitamin C for secondary prevention).

CHELATION THERAPY

It is believed that nearly one-half million CAD subjects will undergo ethylenediamine tetraacetic acid (EDTA) chelation therapy. Because LDL-C oxidation is accentuated in the presence of metal ions (e.g., copper and iron), it has been proposed that EDTA chelation of these ions might interrupt the oxidative process. Indeed, *in vitro* studies have demonstrated enhanced peroxidation with copper sulfate incubation with LDL-C and prevention of further oxidation following administration of EDTA. Moreover, EDTA chelation also binds calcium and may aid in removing excess deposits from atherosclerotic plaques.

In review of published literature addressing the use of EDTA chelation therapy for CAD, Grier and Meyers reported that most studies were either case reports or noncontrolled trials. Furthermore, these studies were inherently biased because subjective measures were used to assess outcome. In the only prospective, double-blind, placebo-controlled study, Guldager and colleagues evaluated 153 patients with claudication. During a 5-9 week period, subjects received a total of 20 infusions of either sodium EDTA (3 g) or sodium chloride. Walking distance, systemic ankle blood pressure index, and symptoms were assessed post–treatment and during follow-up at 3 and 6 months. The EDTA-chelation treated group did not demonstrate improvement in claudication symptoms compared to the placebo group.

In addition to the lack of proven efficacy, side effects of chelation therapy include phlebitis at the infusion site, hypotension, hypocalcemia with tetany, and cardiac arrhythmias. A specific and more innocuous protocol for EDTA infusion has been recommended by the American College of Advancement in Medicine (see Cranton).

Until randomized, double-blind, placebo-controlled trials demonstrate reduction in CAD event rate, there is no evidence to support the use of EDTA chelation for the treatment of CAD atherosclerosis.

FISH AND FISH OILS

The astute observation of an increased bleeding tendency and reduced CAD rate associated with ω-3 fatty acids intake in Greenland Eskimos launched a series of formidable investigations (see von Schacky). The two main sources of ω-3 fatty acids are eicosapentanoic acid (EPA) and docosahexanoic acid (DHA) (Fig. 12.3).

In a 20-year observational study from Zutphen, the Netherlands, a 50% reduction in cardiovascular mortality was found in middle-aged men who consumed 30g of fish daily compared with non-fish-eaters. Similarly, the Western Electric Study (Chicago) demonstrated a strong and graded inverse relationship between fish consumption and CAD death (Table 12.3). Interestingly, in the Zutphen study, the consumption of arctic mammals and fish containing high amounts of ω-3 fatty acids was low, suggesting that there were additional cardioprotective factors in fish. Other studies have failed to show a beneficial effect of fish oil supplementation on CAD event rate (see Curb and Reed, Lapidus et al., Guallar et al.).

As selenium was shown to be inversely associated with MI and cardiovascular death, Kromhout and coworkers speculated that this trace element contributes to cardioprotection by prolonging bleeding time and increasing production of prostacyclin.

Perhaps the most influential secondary prevention study of fish consumption was the 2 year prospective Diet and Reinfarction Trial (DART). More than 2,000 MI survivors were randomized to either fatty fish (2–3 times weekly), a low satu-

Common Name	Abbreviation	Systematic Name	Source	Omega Bond	Structure
A. Saturated Fatty Acids					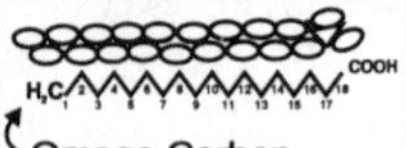
Stearic	18:0	n-Octadecanoic	Animal Fat	Sat	Omega Carbon
Palmitic	16:0	n-Hexadecanoic	Animal Fat	Sat	
B. Unsaturated Fatty Acids					
Oleic	18:1	*cis*-9-Octadecanoic	Vegetable Oil	9	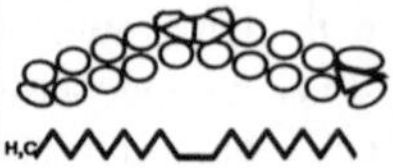
Linoleic	18:2	*cis, cis*, 9,12 - Octadecadienoic	Safflower Oil	6	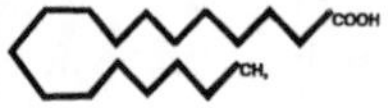
Linolenic	18:3	all *cis*, 9,12,15 - Octadecatrienoic	Linseed Oil	3	
Eicosapentanoic	20:5	all *cis*-5,8,11,14,17 - Eicosapentanoic	Fish Oil	3	
Docosahexanoic	22:6	all *cis*-4,7,10,13,16,19- Docosahexanoic	Fish Oil	3	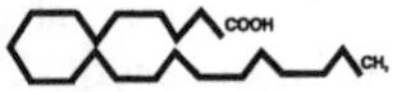
Arachidonic	20:4	all *cis*-5,8,11,14 - Eicosatetraenoic	Synthesized Endogenously	6	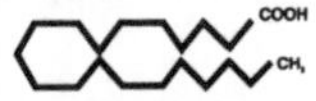

Figure 12.3. Nomenclature of fatty acids. Fatty acids are named by either their source, abbreviation (number of carbon atoms:number of double bonds), systemic name (chemical structure including position of double bonds), or position of last double bond. ω Bond number indicates carbon-carbon double bond closest to methyl end (ω-carbon) of fatty acid; i.e., ω-3 indicates double bond between 3rd and 4th ω-carbon atoms. Representative structures of fatty acids are shown in last column. From Malasanos TH, Stacpoole PW. Biological effects of ω-3 fatty acids in diabetes mellitus. Diabetes Care 1991;14: 1160–1179. Reproduced with permission.

rated fat diet, or a high-fiber diet. Although reinfarction rate was not affected, subjects assigned to fish consumption experienced a 29% reduction in all-cause mortality. Adipose tissue biopsies and segments of coronary arteries from 40 consecutive autopsied patients demonstrated an inverse association between CAD severity and adipose tissue concentration of the ω-3 fatty acid, DHA (see Burr et al.). Fish consumption and risk of stroke was investigated in the Zutphen study, where consumption of at least 20 grams daily coincided with reduced risk of stroke and improved survival (Fig. 12.4).

There have been many randomized controlled trials assessing the efficacy of fish oil on restenosis rates following coronary angioplasty. In a review by Kristensen

Table 12.3. Twenty-five-Year Risk of Death, by Amount of Fish Consumed, among Middle-Aged Men Who Were Free of Coronary Heart Disease at Entry

Fish Consumption	No. of Men at Risk	Coronary Heart Disease		Other CVR Diseases*		Malignant Neoplasms		Other Causes		Total Deaths	
		no.	%	no.	%	no.	%	no.	%	no.	%
g/day											
0	205	42	20.5	15	7.3	13	6.3	14	6.8	84	41.0
1–17	686	128	18.7	39	5.7	72	10.5	25	3.6	264	38.5
18–34	779	121	15.5	31	4.0	78	10.0	38	4.9	268	34.4
>35	261	34	13.0	16	6.1	27	10.3	14	5.4	91	34.9
Total	1931	325	16.8	101	5.2	190	9.8	91	4.7	707	36.6
P value for trend		0.008		0.264		0.318		0.965		0.051	

*CVR denotes cardiovascular-renal.
From Shekelle RB, Missell LV, Paul O, Shryock AM, Stamler J. Fish consumption and mortality from coronary heart disease. N Engl J Med 1985;313:820. Reproduced with permission.

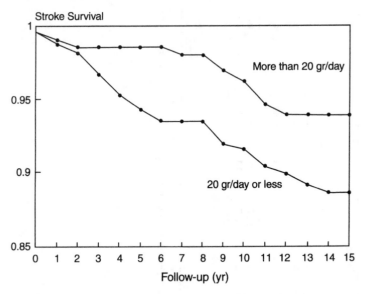

Figure 12.4. Fifteen-year stroke incidence by categories of fish consumption in 1970 in 552 men aged 50 to 69 years. From Keli SO, Feskens EJM, Kromhout D. Fish consumption and risk of stroke. The Zutphen Study. Stroke 1994;25:328–332. Reproduced with permission.

and associates, restenosis rates were favorably affected in five of eight trials, although the number of patients in each study was small (Table 12.4). In the largest randomized study to date, however, Leaf and colleagues failed to demonstrate an effect of fish-oil supplementation (8 grams of ω-3 fatty acids/day) on coronary restenosis rates.

Several beneficial effects result from fish oils. In addition to reducing hepatic production of VLDL-C (see Chapter 6) and plasma homocysteine levels (see Chapter 11), fish oils also impair leukocyte adhesion to the endothelium and monocyte chemotaxis (see Chapter 2). Moreover, the ω-3 fatty acids decrease synthesis of interleukin-1, oxygen-free radicals, TNF, PDGF, platelet-activating factor, and fibrinogen. In rats, fish-oil supplementation reduced arrhythmias and increased the threshold for ventricular fibrillation during myocardial ischemia. In a canine model, fish oils reduced the size of an MI and enhanced the thrombolytic effect of TPA.

A very important effect of fish oils is vasodilation owing to PGI_2 and EDRF-NO activation. In heart transplant recipients receiving dietary supplementation with ω-3 fatty acids, Fleischhauer and colleagues observed a normal vasodilatory response to intracoronary acetylcholine (Fig. 12.5). In contrast, control heart transplant

Table 12.4. Randomised Controlled Trials on the Effect of Fish Oil on the Rate of Restenosis After Percutaneous Coronary Angioplasty (PTCA)

Study	No of restenoses Fish oil (%)	No of cases Control (%)	Main result	n-3 PUFA/day	Treatment started before PTCA? (days)
Slack et al.	8/50 (16)	21/63 (33)	+	2·7	No
Dehmer et al.	8/43 (19)	18/39 (46)	+	5·4	Yes (7)
Grigg et al.	15/54 (28)	19/60 (32)	0	3·0	No
Milner et al.	21/95 (22)	35/99 (35)	+	4·5	No
Reis et al.	44/124 (35)	15/62 (24)	0	6·0	Yes (1–7)
Nye et al.	5/36 (14)	18/71 (25)	+	3·6	No
Bairati et al.	18/59 (31)	29/60 (48)	+	4·5	Yes (21)
Kaul et al.	19/58 (33)	13/49 (27)	0	3·0	Yes (1–7)
Total	138/519 (27%)	168/503 (33%)			

PUFA, polyunsaturated fatty acids. + = statistically significant reduction in restenosis rate in the fish oil group compared with the control group. 0 = no statistically significant difference between the groups.
From Kristensen SD, De Caterina R, Schmidt EB, Endres S. Br Heart J 1993;70:212–214. Reproduced with permission.

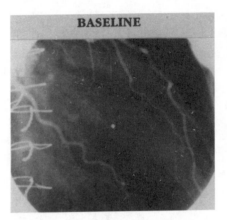 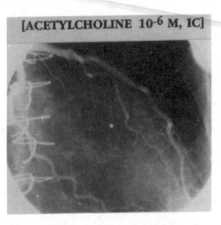

BASELINE   [ACETYLCHOLINE 10^{-6} M, IC]

Figure 12.5. Example of acetylcholine-mediated vasodilation in a 27-year-old woman 2 years after heart transplantation. Baseline angiogram demonstrates left anterior descending coronary artery before infusion of acetylcholine. At an estimated intracoronary concentration of 10^{-6} mol/L (infused concentration of 10^{-4} mol/L) there was a 34% increase in diameter of the artery versus baseline measurements. From Fleischhauer FJ, Yan W, Fischell TA. Fish oil improves endothelium-dependent coronary vasodilation in heart transplant recipients. J Am Coll Cardiol 1993;21:982–989. Reproduced with permission.

patients demonstrated vasoconstrictor responses, suggesting that fish oils improve endothelial-dependent vasomotor function. The vasodilatory effect may also account for the reduction in blood pressure observed in hypertensive (Fig. 12.6) and normotensive subjects receiving fish oil supplements.

The effect of fish-oil therapy in diabetic subjects has also been explored. In contrast to IDDM where glycemic control is often unaffected, fish oils (greater than 4 gm daily) impair glucose tolerance in NIDDM by increasing hepatic glucose production and inhibiting insulin secretion. The increased caloric burden of fish-oil supplementation (see Chapter 6) is also associated with worsening glucose tolerance.

The effect of ω-3 fatty acids on atherosclerotic progression and regression has not been systematically investigated. As fish consumption may reduce CAD risk, two to three servings weekly is heartily recommended. Until compelling data dictate otherwise, fish-oil supplementation is advocated primarily in patients with hypertriglyceridemia.

GARLIC AND ONIONS

Diverse indications for garlic have evolved over the centuries. Aristotle recommended it for the treatment of rabies, Hippocrates for pneumonia, and Mohammed for scorpion stings. The active ingredients contained within garlic and onions are sulfur-derived compounds (e.g., diallyldisulfide and allyl propyldisulfide). The concentration of the oil derived from these compounds is 10-fold greater in garlic than in onions. When a garlic clove is compressed, the enzyme allinase converts odorless alliin to the biologically active odoriferous compound, allicin.

Both garlic and onions reduce the postprandial response to a fat load, enhance fibrinolytic activity, and reduce platelet adhesiveness and aggregability. In a recent double-blind, placebo-controlled study, Kiesewetter and colleagues administered 800 mg of garlic powder (4 coated tablets containing 200 mg) over a 4 week period and observed an approximate 60% reduction in spontaneous platelet aggregation.

The effect of garlic on blood pressure has also been assessed. In a meta-analysis of 415 subjects encompassing seven separate trials, there were significant reductions in systolic blood pressure in three and diastolic blood pressure in four studies, suggesting that garlic may possess antihypertensive properties.

Garlic has also been touted as a cholesterol-lowering agent. A meta-analysis by Warshafsky and associates (Fig. 12.7), involving 325 subjects, demonstrated mean reductions in cholesterol of 23 mg/dL in garlic-treated individuals who had TC lev-

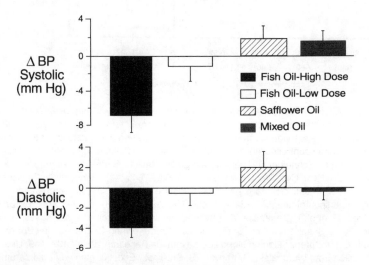

Figure 12.6. Demonstration of dose-dependent antihypertensive effects of fish oils. Subjects were given high-dose (15 g/day) or low-dose (3 g/day) ω-3 fatty acids, ω-6 fatty acids as safflower oil (50 mL/day), or mixed oils to mimic average American diet. From Knapp HR, FitzGerald GA. The antihypertensive effects of fish oil: A controlled study of polyunsaturated fatty acid supplements in essential hypertension. N Engl J Med 1989;320:1037–1043. Reproduced with permission.

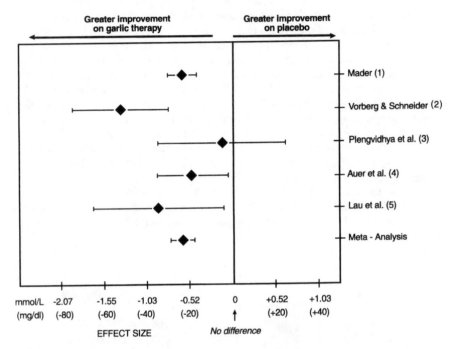

Figure 12.7. Effect sizes with 95% confidence intervals for mean improvement during garlic therapy compared with placebo. (1) Mader FH. Treatment of hyperlipidaemia with garlic-powder tablets. Evidence from the German Association of General Practitioners' multicentric placebo-controlled double-blind study. Arzneimittelforschung 1990;40:1111–1116. (2) Vorberg G, Schneider B. Therapy with garlic: Results of a placebo-controlled, double-blind study. Br J Clin Pract Sym Suppl 1990;69:7–11. (3) Plengvidhya C, Sitprija S, Chinayon S, Pasatrat S, Tankeyoon M. Effects of spray dried garlic preparation on primary hyperlipoproteinemia. J Med Assoc Thai 1988;71:248–252. (4) Auer W, Eiber A, Hertkorn E, et al. Hypertension and hyperlipidemia: Garlic helps in mild cases. Br J Clin Pract Symp Suppl 1990;69:3–6. (5) Lau BH, Lam F, Wang-Cheng R. Effect of an odor modified garlic preparation on blood lipids. Nutrition Research 1987;7:139–149. Used with permission from Warshafsky S, Kamer RS, Sivak SL. Effect of garlic on total serum cholesterol. A meta-analysis. Ann Intern Med 1993;119:599–605.

els exceeding 200 mg/dL. The duration of the studies varied from 8–24 weeks; however, a minimum of 12 weeks was required to detect significant changes in TC levels. The garlic preparations ranged from Kwai powder tablets (600–800 mg/day) to spray-dried garlic powder (700 mg/day) and Kyolic aqueous extract (4 mL or 1 g/day). Kwai powder tablets totaling 600 mg are equivalent to 1.8 g of fresh garlic or slightly more than ½ clove of garlic (1 clove=3 g fresh garlic). Thus, the equivalent of ½ to 1 clove of fresh garlic daily (Kwai tablets, 600–800 mg) reduces TC nearly 10%. In their meta-analysis, Silagy and Neil reported 13% reductions in TG levels in addition to TC. There were no changes attributable to HDL-C with garlic use. The proposed mechanisms for these effects are reduction in hepatic cholesterol and TG synthesis as demonstrated *in vitro* by Yeh and Yeh.

Onions are also a major source of flavonoids (see above). In the Zutphen Elderly Study, onions were the second most common source of flavonoids after tea. As a dietary antioxidant, onion consumption was correlated with reduced CAD mortality. Garlic also appears to possess antioxidant properties. Phelps and Harris reported that 600 mg of Kwai tablets administered for 2 weeks reduced susceptibility to lipoprotein oxidation without lowering cholesterol levels. Further study is needed to confirm these findings as well as define the specific compounds responsible for these important effects.

Suggested Readings

Alcohol

Frankel EN, Kanner J, German JB, Parks E, Kinsella JE. Inhibition of oxidation of human low-density lipoprotein by phenolic substances in red wine. Lancet 1993;341:454–57.

Gaziano JM, Buring JE, Breslow JL, Goldhaber SZ, et al. Moderate alcohol intake, increased levels of high-density lipoprotein and its subfractions, and decreased risk of myocardial infarction. N Engl J Med 1993;329:1829–34.

Gurwitz JH, Field TS, Glynn RJ, et al. Risk factors for non-insulin-dependent diabetes mellitus requiring treatment in the elderly. J Am Geriatr Soc 1994;42:1235–1240.

Klatsky AL, Armstrong MA. Alcoholic beverage choice and risk of coronary artery disease mortality: Do red wine drinkers fare best? Am J Cardiol 1993;71:467–469.

Klatsky AL, Armstrong MA, Friedman GD. Alcohol and mortality. Annals Intern Med 1992;117:646–654.

Renaud SC, Beswick AD, Fehily AM, Sharp DS, Elwood PC. Alcohol and platelet aggregation: The Caerphilly Prospective Heart Disease Study. Am J Clin Nutr 1992;55:1012–1017.

Renaud S, De Lorgeril M. Wine, alcohol, platelets, and the French paradox for coronary heart disease. Lancet 1992;339:1523–26.

Ridker PM, Vaughan DE, Stampfer MJ, Glynn RJ, Hennekens CH. Association of moderate alcohol consumption and plasma concentration of endogenous tissue-type plasminogen activator. JAMA 1994;272:929–933.

Ruf JC, Berger JL, Renaud S. Platelet rebound effect of alcohol withdrawal and wine drinking in rats. Relation to tannins and lipid peroxidation. Arterioscler Thromb Vasc Biol 1995;1:140–144.

Suh I, Shaten J, Cutler JA, Kuller LH for the Multiple Risk Factor Intervention Trial Research Group. Alcohol use and mortality from coronary heart disease: The role of high-density lipoprotein cholesterol. Ann Intern Med 1992;116:881–887.

Taskinen MR, Nikkila EA, Valimaki M, et al. Alcohol-induced changes in serum lipoproteins and in their metabolism. Am Heart J 1987;113(2 Pt 2):458–464.

Taskinen MR, Valimaki M, Nikkila EA, Kuusi T, Ehnholm C, Ylikahri R. High density lipoprotein subfractions and postheparin plasma lipases in alcoholic men before and after ethanol withdrawal. Metabolism 1982;31:1168–1174.

Antioxidants

Alpha Tocopherol, Beta Carotene Cancer Prevention Study Group. The effect of vitamin E and beta carotene on the incidence of lung cancer and other cancers in male smokers. N Engl J Med 1994;330:1029–1035.

Gaziano JM. Antioxidant vitamins and coronary artery disease risk. Am J Med 1994;97:3A–18S—3A–21S.

Hertog MGL, Kromhout D, Aravanis C, et al. Flavonoid intake and long-term risk of coronary heart disease and cancer in the seven countries study. Arch Intern Med 1995;155:381–386.

Hoffman RM, Garewal HS. Antioxidants and the prevention of coronary heart disease. Arch Intern Med 1995;155:241–246.

National Research Council. Fat-soluble vitamins: Vitamin A. In: Recommended Dietary Allowances, 10th Edition. Washington, DC: National Academy Press, 1989:78–92.

National Research Council. Fat-soluble vitamins: Vitamin E. In: Recommended Dietary Allowances, 10th Edition. Washington, DC: National Academy Press, 1989:99–107.

National Research Council. Water-soluble vitamins: Vitamin C: In: Recommended Dietary Allowances, 10th Edition. Washington, DC: National Academy Press, 1989:115–124.

Parthasarathy S, Barnett J, Fong LG. High density lipoprotein inhibits the oxidative modification of low density lipoprotein. Biochem Biophys Acta 1990;1044:275–283.

Pennington JAT. Supplementary Tables: Vitamin E as alpha-tocopherol (mg). In: Bowes & Church's Food Values of Portions Commonly Used, 16th Edition. Philadelphia: J.B. Lippincott Company, 1994:418–420.

Pennington JAT, Church HN. Supplementary Tables: Vitamin E as alpha-tocopherol (mg). In: Bowes & Church's Food Values of Portions Commonly Used, 14th Edition. Philadelphia: J.B. Lippincott Company, 1985:219–222.

Regnstrom J, Nilsson J, Tornvall P, Landou C, Hamsten A. Susceptibility to LDL oxidation and coronary atherosclerosis in man. Lancet 1992;339:1183–1186.

Rimm EB, Stampfer MJ, Ascherio A, Giovannucci E, Colditz GA, Willett WC. Vitamin E consumption and the risk of coronary heart disease in men. N Engl J Med 1993;328:1450–1456.

Scheffler E, Huber L, Fruhbis J, Schulz I, Ziegler R, Dresel HA. Alteration of plasma low density lipoprotein from smokers. Atherosclerosis 1990;82:261–265.

Stampfer MJ, Hennekens CH, Manson JE, Colditz GA, Rosner B, Willett WC. Vitamin E consumption and the risk of coronary disease in women. N Engl J Med 1993;328:1444–1449.

Steiner M. Vitamin E: More than an antioxidant. Clin Cardiol 1993;16(4 Suppl 1):I16–I18.

Whitney EN, Cataldo CB, Rolfes SR. The fat-soluble vitamins: Vitamin A in foods. In:

Understanding Normal and Clinical Nutrition, 2nd Edition. St. Paul, MN: West Publishing Company, 1987:353.

Whitney EN, Cataldo CB, Rolfes SR. The water-soluble vitamins: Vitamin C. In: Understanding Normal and Clinical Nutrition, 2nd Edition. St. Paul, MN: West Publishing Company, 1987:321.

Yokode M, Kita T, Arai H, Kawai C, Narumiya S, Fujiwara M. Cholesterol ester accumulation in macrophages incubated with low density lipoprotein pretreated with cigarette smoke extract. Proc Natl Acad Sci USA 1988;85:2344–2348.

Chelation

Cranton EM. Protocol of the American College of Advancement in Medicine for the safe and effective administration of EDTA chelation therapy. In: A textbook on EDTA chelation therapy. New York: Human Sciences Press, 1989:269–306.

Grier MT, Meyers DG. So much writing, so little science: A review of 37 years of literature on edetate sodium chelation therapy. Ann Pharmacother 1993;27:1504–1509.

Guldager B, Jelnes R, Jørgensen SJ, et al. EDTA treatment of intermittent claudication—a double-blind, placebo-controlled study. J Intern Med 1992;231:261–267.

Olszewer E, Carter JP. EDTA chelation therapy in chronic degenerative disease. Med Hypotheses 1988;27:41–49.

Parthasarathy S, Steinberg D. Cell-induced oxidation of LDL. Curr Opin Lipidol 1992;3:313–317.

Fish Oils

Braden GA, Knapp HR, Fitzgerald DJ, Fitz-Gerald GA. Dietary fish oil accelerates the response to coronary thrombolysis with tissue-type plasminogen activator. Circulation 1990;82:1788–187.

Burr ML. Fish food, fish oil and cardiovascular disease. Clin and Exper Hypertens [A] 1992;14(1–2):181–192.

Burr ML, Gilbert JF, Holliday RM, et al. Effects of changes in fat, fish, and fibre intakes on death and myocardial reinfarction: Diet and Reinfarction Trial (DART). Lancet 1989;2:757–761.

Curb JD, Reed DW. Fish consumption and mortality from coronary heart disease [letter]. N Engl J Med 1985;313:821–822.

Fleischhauer FJ, Yan W, Fischell TA. Fish oil improves endothelium-dependent coronary vasodilation in heart transplant recipients. J Am Coll Cardiol 1993;21:982–989.

Guallar E, Hennekens CH, Sacks FM, Willett WC, Stampfer MJ. A prospective study of plasma fish oil levels and incidence of myocardial infarction in U.S. male physicians. J Am Coll Cardiol 1995;25:387–394.

Israel DH, Gorlin R. Fish oils in the prevention of atherosclerosis. J Am Coll Cardiol 1992;19:174–185.

Keli SO, Feskens EJM, Kromhout D. Fish consumption and risk of stroke. The Zutphen Study. Stroke 1994;25:328–332.

Knapp HR, Reilly IAG, Alessandrini P, FitzGerald GA. In vivo indexes of platelet and vascular function during fish-oil administration in patients with atherosclerosis. N Engl J Med 1986;314:937–942.

Kristensen SD, De Caterina R, Schmidt EB, Endres S. Fish oil and ischaemic heart disease. Br Heart J 1993;70:212–214.

Kromhout D, Bosschieter EB, Coulander C. The inverse relation between fish consumption and 20-year mortality from coronary heart disease. N Engl J Med 1985;312:1205–1209.

Lapidus L, Andersson H, Bengtsson C, Bosaeus I. Dietary habits in relation to incidence of cardiovascular disease and death in women: A 12-year follow-up of participants in the population study of women in Gothenburg, Sweden. Am J Clin Nutr 1986;44:444–448.

Leaf A. Cardiovascular effects of fish oils. Beyond the platelet. Circulation 1990;82: 624–628.

Leaf A, Jorgensen MB, Jacobs AK, et al. Do fish oils prevent restenosis after coronary angioplasty? Circulation 1994;90:2248–2257.

Malasanos TH, Stacpoole PW. Biological effects of ω-3 fatty acids in diabetes mellitus. Diabetes Care 1991;14:1160–1179.

Olszewski AJ, McCully KS. Fish oil decreases serum homocysteine in hyperlipemic men. Coron Artery Dis 1993;4:53–60.

Seidelin KN, Myrup B, Fischer-Hansen B. n-3 fatty acids in adipose tissue and coronary artery disease are inversely related. Am J Clin Nutr 1992;55:1117–1119.

Shekelle RB, Missell LV, Paul O, Shryock AM, Stamler J. Fish consumption and mortality from coronary heart disease. N Engl J Med 1985;313:820.

Shekelle RB, Shryock AM, Paul O, et al. Diet, serum cholesterol, and death from coronary heart disease: The Western Electric Study. N Engl J Med 1981;304:65–70.

von Schacky C. Prophylaxis of atherosclerosis with marine omega-3 fatty acids. Ann Int Med 1987;107:890–899.

Garlic and Onion

Bordia A, Bansal HC, Arora SK, Singh SV. Effect of the essential oils of garlic and onion on alimentary hyperlipemia. Atherosclerosis 1975;21:15–19.

Gupta MK, Mittal SR, Mathur AK, Bhan AK. Garlic—the other side of the coin [letter]. Int J Cardiol 1993;38:333.

Hertog MG, Feskens EJ, Hollman PC, Katan MB, Kromhout D. Dietary antioxidant flavonoids and risk of coronary heart disease: The Zutphen Elderly Study. Lancet 1993;342:1007–1011.

Jain AK, Vargas R, Gotzkowsky S, McMahon FG. Can garlic reduce levels of serum lipids? A controlled clinical study. Am J Med 1993;94:632–635.

Kamer RS, Warshafsky S, Sivak SL. A response to "Does Eating Garlic Lower Cholesterol?" Ann Intern Med 1994;120: 969–970.

Kiesewetter H, Jung F, Pindur G, Jung EM, Mrowietz C, Wenzel E. Effect of garlic on thrombocyte aggregation, microcirculation, and other risk factors. Int J Clin Pharmacol Ther Toxicol 1991;29:151–155.

Phelps S, Harris WS. Garlic supplementation and lipoprotein oxidation susceptibility. Lipids 1993;28:475–477.

Rietz B, Isensee H, Strobach H, Makdessi S, Jacob R. Cardioprotective actions of wild garlic (Allium ursinum) in ischemia and reperfusion. Mol Cell Biochem 1993;119: 143–150.

Silagy C, Neil A. Garlic as a lipid lowering agent—a meta-analysis. J R Coll Physicians Lond 1994;28:39–45.

Silagy CA, Neil HAW. A meta-analysis of the effect of garlic on blood pressure. J Hyper 1994;12:463–468.

Warshafsky S, Kamer RS, Sivak SL. Effect of garlic on total serum cholesterol. A meta-analysis. Ann Intern Med 1993;119: 599–605.

Yeh YY, Yeh SM. Garlic reduces plasma lipids by inhibiting hepatic cholesterol and triacylglycerol synthesis. Lipids 1994;29:189–193.

13/ Women and Heart Disease

Cardiovascular disease remains the number one killer in the U.S., causing more deaths in women than in men (Table 13.1). Based on the Framingham Heart Study, the initial manifestations of CAD occur on average, one decade later in women and accelerate after menopause. By the latter part of the eighth decade, the percentage of CAD deaths rival their male counterparts (Fig. 13.1). While reduction in CAD death rates have been observed for both sexes (see Chapter 1), the percent change events lag in women (Table 13.2). Among cardiovascular deaths in women, nearly 250,000 result from MI and 90,000 from stroke. In contrast, the two most common causes of cancer in women, lung and breast, account for 56,000 and 46,000 yearly deaths, respectively. A comparison between CAD and breast cancer deaths (Figure 13.2) illustrates that although death rates from breast cancer are approximately one-fifth that of CAD, deaths from breast cancer occur more commonly in pre-menopausal women. This section will elaborate upon cardiovascular risk factors and the diagnosis and treatment of CAD. We will also explore inherent biases which may affect initiation of appropriate management strategies in women.

CARDIOVASCULAR RISK FACTORS IN WOMEN

Women are afflicted with the same cardiovascular risk factors as men (Table 13.3). The prevalence of risk factors are particularly high in women over age 55 years. Approximately 50% of women in this age group are overweight and have elevated cholesterol and blood pressure.

Table 13.1 Cardiovascular Morbidity and Mortality in United States 1988 to 1990

	Women	Men
Deaths	478,000	453,000
Hospitalizations	2.5 million	2.7 million
Physician's office visits	32 million	25 million
Prevalence		
Hypertension	30 million	32 million
Heart Disease	9.6 million	8.0 million
Population	127 million	121 million

From Higgins M, Thom T. Cardiovascular disease in women as a public health problem. In: Wenger NK, Speroff L, Packard B, eds. Cardiovascular health and disease in women. Greenwich: Le Jacq Communications, Inc., 1993:15–19. Reproduced with permission.

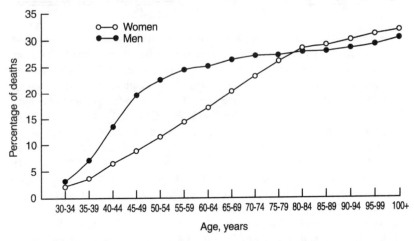

Figure 13.1. Percentage of male deaths due to ischemic heart disease during 1988, relative to total number of male deaths during that same year, compared with percentage of female deaths due to ischemic heart disease, relative to total number of female deaths. From Holm K, Penckofer S. Cardiovascular risk factors in women. J Myocard Ischemia 1992;4:25–46. Reproduced with permission.

Table 13.2. Percent Change in Cardiovascular Disease Death Rates in US Men and Women 1983 to 1988

	Men	Women
Total cardiovascular disease	−14	−10
Coronary heart disease	−20	−16
Stroke	−14	−13
Other cardiovascular disease	+ 1	+ 2

From Higgins M, Thom T. Cardiovascular disease in women as a public health problem. In: Wenger NK, Speroff L, Packard B, eds. Cardiovascular health and disease in women. Greenwich: Le Jacq Communications, Inc., 1993:15–19. Reproduced with permission.

Cholesterol

A comparison between lipoprotein levels at various ages in men and women is illustrated in Figure 13.3. While HDL-C levels remain fairly constant, small increases in VLDL-C and more substantial elevations in LDL-C coincide with the aging process in women. Total cholesterol levels exceeding 260 mg/dL yield an approximate threefold increased risk of CAD in women compared with desirable levels (less than 200 mg/dL). Studies from Framingham have demonstrated an age-

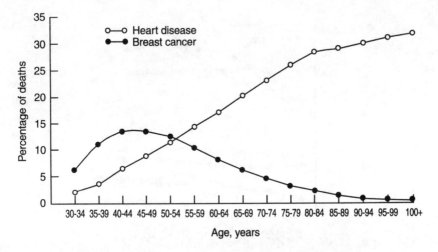

Figure 13.2. Percentage of deaths due to breast cancer or heart disease in US women during 1988, relative to total number of female deaths during the same year. From Holm K, Penckofer S. Cardiovascular risk factors in women. J Myocard Ischemia 1992;4:25–46. Reproduced with permission.

Table 13.3. Prevalence of Cardiovascular Disease Risk

Factors NHANES II, Ages 20 to 74 Years[1]		
Risk Factor	Men (%)	Women (%)
High serum cholesterol[2]	26	29
Hypertension[3]	45	36
Cigarette smoking (1990)	28	23
Overweight[4]	25	27
Diabetes mellitus[5]	6	7

[1] Age-adjusted
[2] ≥ 240 mg/dL
[3] $\geq 140/90$ mm Hg or on medication
[4] Body mass index ≥ 27.8 kg/m^2 for women
[5] Diagnosed and undiagnosed (glucose tolerance test positive)
From Higgins M, Thom T. Cardiovascular disease in women as a public health problem. In: Wenger NK, Speroff L, Packard B, eds. Cardiovascular health and disease in women. Greenwich: Le Jacq Communications, Inc., 1993:15–19. Reproduced with permission.

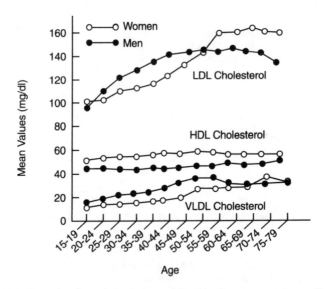

Figure 13.3. Age-related trends in cholesterol fractions in women and men: Framingham Heart Study. From Kannel WB. Nutrition and the occurrence and prevention of cardiovascular disease in the elderly. Nutr Rev 1988;46:68–78.

independent association between TC and CAD; for each 1% increase in TC there is a 2% increase in CAD rate. HDL-C inversely predicts CAD in women, and the total cholesterol:HDL-C ratio may be a better predictor of CAD than TC alone. Women with elevated LDL-C appear to be at reduced CAD risk if accompanied by high HDL-C and favorable total cholesterol:HDL-C ratio (less than 4:1).

Cigarette Smoking

There are currently 22 million female cigarette smokers in the U.S. Although the smoking rate continues to decrease (see also Chapter 9), it has been projected that by the next millennium, there will be more women who smoke (23%) than men (20%). In addition to the known adverse consequences of smoking such as reduced HDL-C, elevated fibrinogen, and enhanced platelet aggregability, cigarette smoking has also been associated with reduced levels of cardioprotective estrogen and increased adrenal androgens. Importantly, while the relative risk of MI is nearly four times greater among women smokers than nonsmokers, this risk is markedly attenuated within 1 to 2 years of smoking cessation.

Smoking also increases the risk of stroke (thromboembolic and subarachnoid hemorrhage) in women. In the Nurses' Health Study, Colditz and coworkers reported data that, compared to nonsmokers, CVA events were two-fold greater in moderate smokers (up to 14 cigarettes daily) and nearly four-fold greater in heavy smokers (25 cigarettes or more per day). These results were not materially affected after adjustment for other risk factors or hormone replacement therapy.

Diabetes Mellitus

Diabetes mellitus is an especially important risk factor in women (see also Chapter 8). The cardiovascular protection afforded women is lost with DM and the risk of cardiovascular death is enhanced threefold. These effects are particularly noteworthy in younger women (aged 35–64 years) (Fig. 13.4). In the U.S. there are approximately 2.7 million Caucasian and 0.7 million African-American women with DM. Diabetic women often have other risk factors, including hypertension, dyslipidemia, and central adiposity.

Hypertension

As reviewed in Chapter 7, CAD rates increase with BP elevation. In women, for each 10-mm Hg rise in blood pressure, there is a 20–30% increase in cardiovascular event rate. Overall, hypertensive women bear a 3.5-fold increased risk of CAD and a nearly 3-fold increased risk of CVA. The latter finding is particularly noteworthy because strokes are the third leading cause of death in the United States and are more common in women (90,000/year) than in men (60,000/year). As reviewed

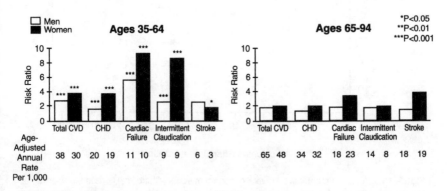

Figure 13.4. Risk ratios of cardiovascular disease events in diabetic women and men; Framingham Heart Study 30-year follow-up. From Copyright © Wilson PWF, Kannel WB. In: Ruderman N, et al., eds. Hyperglycemia, diabetes, and vascular disease. New York: Oxford University Press, 1992:22–29. Reproduced with permission.

above, rigorous control of blood pressure has produced favorable reductions in cardiovascular event and death rate.

Menopause

The prevalence of CAD risk factors increases with age, with a tendency for elevations in blood pressure, glucose, LDL-C, TG, and fibrinogen levels. Although an uncommon occurrence, natural menopause before age 35 years (without estrogen replacement) triples the risk of subsequent cardiovascular events. As well, the absence of hormone-replacement therapy (HRT) increases the mortality rate in post-menopausal women with CAD (see Fig. 10.3). Without angiographic CAD, however, HRT did not impact on survival rates (Fig. 13.5).

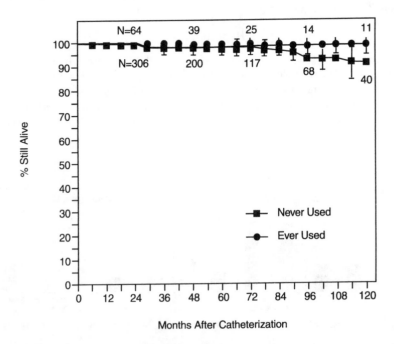

Figure 13.5. Ten-year cumulative survival of control patients with normal coronary angiograms. Number of patients being followed indicated by numbers on survival curves. Actuarial methods used to calculate survival. From Sullivan JM, Vander Zwaag R, Hughes JP, Maddock V, Kroetz FW, Ramanathan KB, Mirvis DM. Estrogen replacement and coronary artery disease. Effect on survival in postmenopausal women. Arch Intern Med 1990;150:2557–2562. Reproduced with permission. Copyright © 1990, American Medical Association.

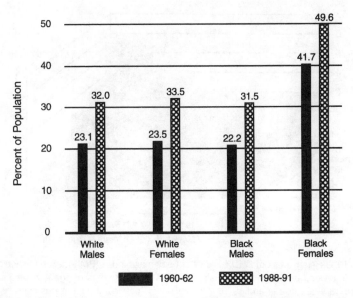

Figure 13.6. Overweight (approximately 20% or more above desirable weight) trends by sex and race, adults age 20 and over. Reproduced with permission. Heart and Stroke Facts: 1995 Statistical Supplement. Copyright © 1994, American Heart Association.

To prospectively evaluate initial CAD event rate, the Nurses' Health Study compared women (aged 30 and 55 yrs) who had natural or surgical menopause. No increased risk in CAD was observed with either natural or surgical menopause and removal of one ovary only during a 6-yr follow-up period. Bilateral oophorectomy, however, conferred a two-fold increased risk of CAD events; this risk was mitigated with HRT.

Obesity

The prevalence of obesity (greater than 20% above ideal body weight) has increased during the past 20 years (Fig. 13.6). Especially noteworthy is the high prevalence of obesity among African-American women. In a 14-year follow-up among women in the Nurses' Health Study, body mass index was positively correlated with CAD risk. Subjects gaining the most weight posed the highest risk of CAD (Fig. 13.7). Perhaps an even greater predictor is the waist/hip circumference; a ratio of >0.8 enhances CAD risk. In a study by Folsom and associates, for each 6 inch increment in waist in a woman with a 40-inch hip size, there was a corresponding 60% increase in overall mortality.

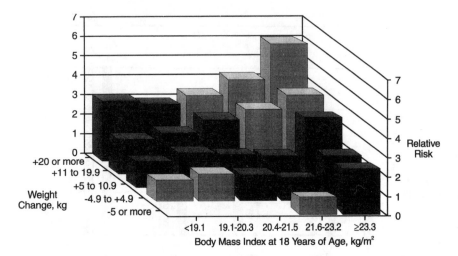

Figure 13.7. Relative risk of CHD by level of body mass index (BMI) (defined as weight in kilograms divided by the square of height in meters) at 18 years of age and weight gain between 18 years of age and 1976. Plus signs indicate weight gain; minus signs, weight loss. Women with a BMI of less than 19.1 kg/m² at 18 years of age and with stable weight were the reference category. From Willett WC, Manson JE, Stampfer MJ, et al. Weight, weight change, and coronary heart disease in women. Risk within the 'normal' weight range. JAMA 1995;273:461–465. Reproduced with permission. Copyright © 1995, American Medical Association.

Triglycerides

In contrast to men, TG appears to be a better predictor of CAD in women. In the Lipid Research Clinics' Follow-up Study, plasma TG was an independent predictor of CAD mortality (see Bass et al.). The risk of death was highest with TG greater than 4.5 mmol/L (400 mg/dL) associated with HDL-C less than 1.3 mmol/L (50 mg/dL) (Fig. 13.8). Similarly, elevated CAD rates were found in the Framingham Heart Study among women with elevated TG and low HDL-C (see Castelli).

DIAGNOSIS OF CAD IN WOMEN

Presentation of angina pectoris is different between the sexes. In the Framingham Heart Study, women were twice as likely as men to present with angina. However, the long-term prognosis was more favorable in women; 25% of men compared with 14% of women suffered an MI within 5 years.

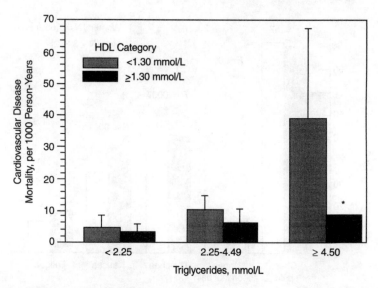

Figure 13.8. Age-adjusted cardiovascular disease mortality rates (with upper 95% confidence intervals) by triglyceride and HDL levels in women aged 50 to 69 years. Asterisk indicates upper confidence interval is undefined for triglyceride levels greater than or equal to 399 mmol/L and HDL levels greater than or equal to 4.5 mmol/L. From Bass KM, Newschaffer CJ, Klag MJ, Bush TL. Plasma lipoprotein levels as predictors of cardiovascular death in women. Arch Intern Med 1993;153:2209–2216. Reproduced with permission. Copyright © 1993, American Medical Association.

The relative lack of adverse consequences in women with angina appears to have contributed to the altered perception of CAD risk between the sexes. Accordingly, women were often excluded from primary and secondary CAD prevention trials. In studies where women were included, such as the Coronary Artery Surgery Study (CASS), nearly three times as many women referred for diagnostic coronary arteriography had minimal or no lesions compared with men. These data suggested that anginal symptoms were different between men and women, inasmuch as the chest pain described by women was not necessarily synonymous with angina pectoris.

The Myocardial Infarction Triage and Intervention (MITI) Project evaluated gender-related clinical presentations of chest pain. In comparing symptoms associated with MI, women were more likely to present with upper abdominal pain, dyspnea, nausea and fatigue than were men (Fig. 13.9). That women present with more atypical symptoms reduced the probability that significant CAD would be deduced.

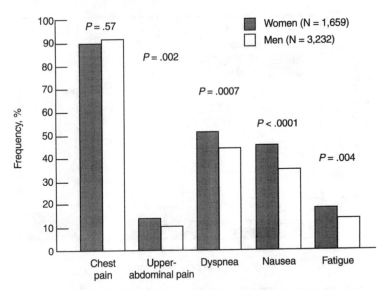

Figure 13.9. Frequency of symptoms in women and men with acute MI in the Myocardial Infarction Triage and Intervention Project registry. P values are adjusted for age. From Maynard C, Weaver WD. Treatment of women with acute MI: New findings from the MITI registry. J Myocard Ischemia 1992;4:27–37. Reproduced with permission.

Accordingly, disease progression would ultimately manifest in higher surgical complication rates. Moreover, women are more likely to reinfarct or die following an MI. Among nearly 6,000 MI patients, Greenland and associates reported higher in-hospital mortality rates in women (23%) than in men (16%). After 1 year of follow-up, the cumulative death rates remained elevated in women (32%) compared with men (23%). In the Framingham Heart Study, women had a threefold greater incidence of reinfarction within the first year. In the Multicenter Investigation of Limitation of Infarct Size (MILIS) study, the death rate in women (36%) remained significantly greater than in men (21%) at 4 years.

Inherent differences in non-invasive cardiac test interpretations may further complicate an accurate diagnosis of CAD in women. Electrocardiographic stress testing is associated with a higher false-positive rate in women (54%) than in men (12%) (see Weiner et al.), owing to a higher prevalence of ST-T wave abnormalities. The sensitivity of the test is also lower in women because of their reduced prevalence of left main and three-vessel disease. A negative exercise stress test, however, is helpful in ruling out critical CAD.

Thallium-201 scintigraphy has a high sensitivity (75%) which is increased with multivessel disease. However, breast tissue induced attenuation of radioactivity may mimic an anterior wall defect and cause a false-positive test in up to 30% of patients. Exercise radionuclide ventriculography, another important non-invasive test in men, is less sensitive in women as the expected rise in the left ventricular ejection fraction is attenuated during exercise (see Higginbotham et al.). Rather, a large increase in end-diastolic volume has been observed. Exercise echocardiography appears to be a promising diagnostic test in women. Preliminary studies have reported both high sensitivity and specificity (greater than 85%).

In regard to thrombolytic therapy, women are more likely to present beyond 6 hours of chest pain onset, thereby reducing the efficacy of these agents. As the onset of CAD is delayed in women (see above), the initial MI may present an age (e.g., older than 75 years) generally deemed ineligible for thrombolytic therapy. The Second International Study of Infarct Survival (ISIS-2) recently demonstrated, however, that octogenarian patients treated with thrombolytic therapy experienced reduced cardiovascular mortality rates. In women receiving thrombolytic therapy, there are no differences in the rate of infarct-vessel patency or recovery of left ventricular function compared to men. However, women experienced higher in-hospital and 6 month mortality rates. The increased morbidity in women is associated with greater age at presentation and increased risk of intracerebral hemorrhage.

Women are less likely to receive invasive diagnostic procedures (e.g., coronary arteriography). Steingart et al. found that only 15.4% of women had coronary arteriography performed, compared with 27.3% of men despite greater functional limitations imposed by worsening anginal symptoms. Ayanian and Epstein corroborated reduced diagnostic testing in women presenting with anginal symptoms or MI.

The relative paucity of procedures in women appears to reflect either a perceived underestimation of CAD severity or the disappointingly high complication rate following PTCA or coronary artery bypass graft (CABG) surgery. Increased complications during PTCA were reported by the National Heart, Lung, and Blood Institute PTCA registry through the mid-1980s. Recently, Kelsey and colleagues reported that women had a higher initial complication and hospital mortality (3% vs 0.3%) rate, reflecting older age and an overall poorer cardiovascular risk profile. Survival rates at 4 years, however, were similar between the sexes, suggesting that with suitable anatomy, PTCA should not be restricted in women.

In regard to CABG, referred women are older and more likely to have unstable angina, CHF, and DM; all portend a less favorable outcome. Seemingly as a consequence of more advanced presentation, women are also more likely to have urgent or emergent CABG performed. Khan and coworkers reported that among patients referred for CABG, women were older on average and suffered a higher in-hospital mortality rate than men (4.6 vs 2.6%). In the CASS study, operative mortality was more than twice as great in women (4.5%) than men (1.9%). A review of the Cleveland Clinic Foundation's experience of nearly 8,000 patients undergoing CABG revealed that while left ventricular function was not different between the sexes, significantly more women evidenced New York Heart Association Class IV impairment (Fig. 13.10). Operative mortality was also higher in women (3.8%) than in men (1.8%) at all age ranges (Fig. 13.11).

It had been hypothesized that the smaller size of coronary vessels corresponding to a reduced body size was an important factor that contributed to higher mortality rates in women. However, when comparing operative mortality between small men and women (body surface area less than 1.75 M^2), the rates remained higher in women (Fig. 13.12). Interestingly, patency rates of saphenous vein grafts and internal mammary arteries were not different at 5 years of follow-up. Moreover, there were no differences in 15-year survival rates between men and women. Perhaps most important was the disappearance of the gender difference when factors such as age and surgical priority were accounted for. Thus, earlier detection of CAD through risk factor assessment and accurate diagnostic testing appears to be paramount in reducing the associated higher morbidity and surgical mortality rates observed in women.

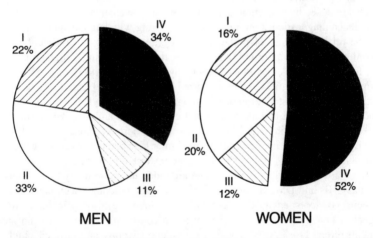

Figure 13.10. Distribution of patients by New York Heart Association functional class prior to CABG. From Cosgrove DM. Coronary artery surgery in women. Cardiovascular Reviews and Reports Sept 1994;54–59. Reproduced with permission.

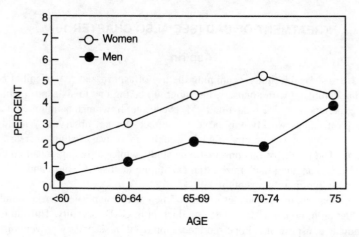

Figure 13.11. Operative mortality by sex and age among patients undergoing CABG. From Cosgrove DM. Coronary artery surgery in women. Cardiovascular Reviews and Reports Sept 1994:54–59. Reproduced with permission.

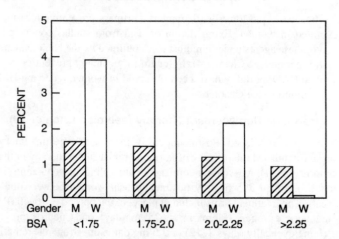

Figure 13.12. Operative mortality by sex and body surface area (BSA) among patients undergoing CABG. From Cosgrove DM. Coronary artery surgery in women. Cardiovascular Reviews and Reports Sept 1994:54–59. Reproduced with permission.

TREATMENT OF CAD (SEE ALSO CHAPTER 10)

Aspirin

The Nurses' Health Study, examining the use of aspirin and risk of initial MI, found that compared with nonusers, the subgroup taking one to six aspirin tablets weekly experienced a 32% reduction in MI event rate. In women taking more than seven aspirin tablets weekly, this protective effect was not observed. With high aspirin consumption (15 or more tablets weekly) there was a slight increase in stroke rate. The results of this observational study, while intriguing, await confirmation from an ongoing randomized trial examining the use of aspirin and antioxidant therapy in primary prevention.

A meta-analysis of antiplatelet use in women with established CAD found a 32% reduction in nonfatal MI and 15% reduction in CAD mortality. Thus, unless contraindicated, aspirin should be routinely employed in secondary prevention. A daily dose of 325 mg has been the most commonly used although doses as low as 40 mg (½ baby aspirin) inhibit platelet thromboxane production.

Lipid-Lowering Medications

The efficacy of lipid-lowering therapy as a primary preventive measure has not been explored in women. Extrapolation of data from studies conducted in men would favor these agents under circumstances outlined by the National Cholesterol Education Program (see Chapter 4). In regard to secondary prevention, significant reductions in CAD mortality have been observed in women receiving HMG-CoA reductase inhibitors (see Chapter 4).

Hormone Replacement Therapy (see also Chapter 10)

The recently published Postmenopausal Estrogen/Progestin Interventions (PEPI) trial established the efficacy of hormone replacement therapy in the primary prevention of CAD. A 3-year randomized, double-blind, placebo-controlled multicenter trial enrolled 875 healthy postmenopausal women between the ages of 45–64 years. The treatment arms included placebo, unopposed estrogen (Premarin, 0.625 mg/day), estrogen (Premarin 0.625 mg/day) and medroxyprogesterone acetate 10 mg cyclically (days 1–12) or 2.5 mg daily, or estrogen (Premarin 0.625 mg/day) plus micronized progesterone 200 mg cyclically (days 1–12). The use of daily progesterone eliminates uterine bleeding.

Endometrial hyperplasia occurred commonly with unopposed estrogen use but did not occur with combination therapy. In women receiving unopposed estrogens, there was an overall 25% reduction in CAD event rate associated with prominent increases in HDL-C. Reduction in TC was evident with combination of estrogen and medroxyprogesterone acetate (Fig. 13.13). In addition to elevated HDL-C, HRT was associated with increases in mean TG and reductions in LDL-C and fibrinogen levels. This study confirms the beneficial effect of estrogen on primary CAD event rate in postmenopausal women. Whether HRT exerts a beneficial effect in women with CAD will be determined by the results of an ongoing secondary prevention trial.

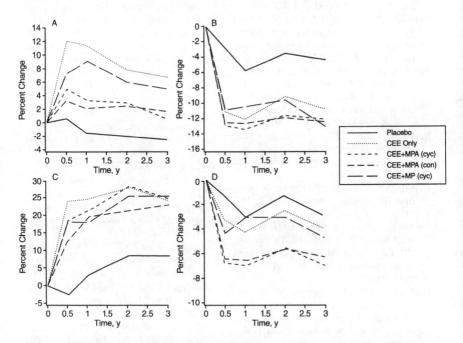

Figure 13.13. Mean percent change from baseline by treatment arm for HDL cholesterol (A), LDL cholesterol (B), triglycerides (C), and total cholesterol (D). CEE = conjugated equine estrogen, MPA = medroxyprogesterone acetate, MP = micronized progesterone. From Writing Group for the PEPI Trial. Effects of estrogen or estrogen/progestin regimens on heart disease risk factors in postmenopausal women: The postmenopausal estrogen/progestin interventions (PEPI) trial. JAMA 1995;273:199–208. Reproduced with permission. Copyright © 1995, American Medical Association.

Suggested Readings

American Heart Association. Heart and stroke facts. Dallas: American Heart Association, 1992.

Ayanian JZ, Epstein AM. Differences in the use of procedures between women and men hospitalized for coronary heart disease. N Engl J Med 1991;325:221–225.

Bass KM, Newschaffer CJ, Klag MJ, Bush TL. Plasma lipoprotein levels as predictors of cardiovascular death in women. Arch Intern Med 1993;153:2209–2216.

Bell MR, Holmes DR Jr, Berger PB, Garratt KN, Bailey KR, Gersh BJ. The changing in-hospital mortality of women undergoing percutaneous transluminal coronary angioplasty. JAMA 1993;269:2091–2095.

Bush TL, Fried LP, Barrett-Connor E. Cholesterol, lipoproteins, and coronary heart disease in women. Clin Chem 1988;34:B60–B70.

Castelli WP. The triglyceride issue: A view from Framingham. Am Heart J 1986; 112:432–437.

Colditz GA, Bonita R, Stampfer MJ, Willett WC, Rosner B, Speizer FE, Hennekens CH. Cigarette smoking and risk of stroke in middle-aged women. N Engl J Med 1988;318:937–41.

Colditz GA, Willett WC, Stampfer MJ, Rosner B, Speizer FE, Hennekens CH. Menopause and the risk of coronary heart disease in women. N Engl J Med 1987; 316:1105–1110.

Cosgrove DM, Loop FD, Lytle BW, et al. Determinants of 10-year survival after primary myocardial revascularization. Ann Surg 1985;202:480–490.

Cosgrove DM. Coronary artery surgery in women. Cardiovas Rev Rep. 1994;Sept: 54–59.

Cowley MJ, Mullin SM, Kelsey SF, et al. Sex differences in early and long-term results of coronary angioplasty in the NHLBI PTCA Registry. Circulation 1985;71 :90–97.

Cupples LA, D'Agostino RB. Some risk factors related to the annual incidence of cardiovascular disease and death using pooled repeated biennial measurements: Framingham Heart Study, 30-year follow-up. In: Kannel WB, Wolf PA, Farrison RJ, eds. The Framingham Heart Study: An Epidemiological Investigation of Cardiovascular Disease. US National Heart, Lung, and Blood Institute. NIH Publication No. 87-2703, 1987, Section 34.

Ettinger B. Hormone replacement therapy and coronary heart disease. Obstet Gynecol Clin North Am 1990;17:741–757.

Eysmann SB, Douglas PS. Reperfusion and revascularization strategies for coronary artery disease in women. JAMA 1992 ;268:1903–1907.

Fisher LD, Kennedy JW, Davis KB, et al. Association of sex, physical size, and operative mortality after coronary artery bypass in the Coronary Artery Surgery Study (CASS). J Thorac Cardiovasc Surg 1982;84:334–341.

Folsom AR, Kaye SA, Sellers TA, et al. Body fat distribution and 5-year risk of death in older women. JAMA 1993;269:483–487.

Greenland P, Reicher-Reiss H, Goldbourt U, et al. In-hospital and 1-year mortality in 1,524 women after myocardial infarction. Circulation 1991;83:484–491.

Gruppo Italiano Per Lo Studio Della Sopravvivenza Nell'Infarto Miocardico: GISSI-2. A factorial randomized trial of alteplase versus streptokinase and heparin versus no heparin among 12,490 patients with acute myocardial infarction. Lancet 1990;336:65–71.

Gurwitz JH, Col NF, Avorn J. The exclusion of the elderly and women from clinical trials in acute myocardial infarction. JAMA 1992;268:1417–1422.

Higgenbotham MB, Morris KG, Coleman E, et al. Sex-related differences in normal cardiac response to upright exercise. Circulation 1984;70:357–366.

Higgins M, Thom T. Cardiovascular disease in women as a public health problem. In: Wenger NK, Speroff L, Packard B, eds. Cardiovascular health and disease in women. Greenwich: Le Jacq Communications, Inc, 1993:15–19.

Holm K, Penckofer S. Cardiovascular risk factors in women. J Myocard Ischemia 1992;4:25–46.

ISIS-2 (Second International Study of Infarct Survival) Collaborative Group. Randomized trial of intravenous streptokinase, oral aspirin, both, or neither among 17,187 cases of suspected acute myocardial infarction: ISIS-2. Lancet 1988;2:349–360.

Kannel WB. Nutrition and the occurrence and prevention of cardiovascular disease in the elderly. Nutr Rev 1988;46:68–78.

Kannel WB, Wilson PWF. Risk factors that attenuate the female coronary disease advantage. Arch Intern Med 1995;155: 57–61.

Kelsey SF, James M, Holubkov AL, Holubkov R, Cowley MJ, Detre KM, Investigators from the NHLBI Percutaneous Transluminal Coronary Angioplasty Registry. Results of percutaneous transluminal coronary angioplasty in women. Circulation 1993;87: 720–727.

Khan SS, Nessim S, Gray R, et al. Increased mortality of women in coronary artery bypass surgery: Evidence for referral bias. Ann Intern Med 1990;112:561–567.

Manson JE, Stampfer MJ, Colditz GA, et al. A prospective study of aspirin use and primary prevention of cardiovascular disease in women. JAMA 1991;266:521–527.

Maynard C, Althouse R, Cerqueira M, et al. Underutilization of thrombolytic therapy in eligible women with acute myocardial infarction. Am J Cardiol 1991;68: 529–539.

Maynard C, Litwin PE, Martin JS, et al. Gender differences in the treatment and outcome of acute myocardial infarction: Results from the Myocardial Infarction Triage and Intervention Registry. Arch Intern Med 1992;152:972–976.

National Center for Health Statistics: Health, United States, 1990. Hyattsville, MD: US Public Health Service, 1991.

National Center for Health Statistics: Vital statistics of the United States, vol II, Mortality, part B. HDDS Public Health Service Pub. No. (PHS) 90–1102. Washington, DC, US Government Printing Office, 1990.

Pratt CM, Francis MJ, Divine GW, Young JB. Exercise testing in women with chest pain. Are there additional exercise characteristics that predict true positive test results? Chest 1989;95:139–44.

Rosenberg L, Kaufman DW, Helmrich SP, Miller DR, Stolley PD, Shapiro S. Myocardial infarction and cigarette smoking in women younger than 50 years of age. JAMA 1985;253:2965–2969.

Steingart RM, Packer M, Hamm P, et al. Sex differences in the management of coronary artery disease. N Engl J Med 1991;325:226–230.

Sullivan JM, Vander Zwaag R, Hughes JP, et al. Estrogen replacement and coronary artery disease. Effect on survival in postmenopausal women. Arch Intern Med 1990;150:2557–2562.

Topol EJ, Califf RM, Vandormael M, et al., and the Thrombolysis and Angioplasty in Myocardial Infarction-6 Study Group. A randomized trial of late reperfusion therapy for acute myocardial infarction. Circulation 1992;85:2090–2099.

Weiner DA, Ryan TJ, McCabe CH, et al. Correlations among history of angina, ST-segment response and prevalence of coronary-artery disease in the Coronary Artery Surgery Study (CASS). N Engl J Med 1979;301:230–235.

Wenger NK. Gender, coronary artery disease, and coronary bypass surgery. Ann Intern Med 1990;112:557–583.

White HD, Barbash GI, Modan M, et al., for the Investigators of the International Tissue Plasminogen Activator/Streptokinase Mortality Study. Circulation 1993;88[part 1]:2097–2103.

Willett WC, Manson JE, Stampfer MJ, et al. Weight, weight change, and coronary heart disease in women. Risk within the 'normal' weight range. JAMA 1995;273: 461–465.

Writing Group for the PEPI Trial. Effects of estrogen or estrogen/progestin regimens on heart disease risk factors in postmenopausal women: The postmenopausal estrogen/progestin interventions (PEPI) trial. JAMA 1995;273:199–208.

14/ Special Populations

AFRICAN-AMERICANS

African-Americans, representing 12% of the U.S. population, have experienced declines in cardiovascular events analogous to Caucasians. Although CAD death rates among young and middle-aged African-Americans are higher than in Caucasians, the trend reverses in later years (Fig. 14.1). Among all age groups, sudden cardiac death is more common in African-Americans (Fig. 14.2).

One possibility in attempting to explain race-related differences in CAD rates may be disparity in health care. Indeed, Ayanian and coworkers found higher rates of revascularization procedures in Caucasian patients (Fig. 14.3). Surveying nearly 34,000 patients discharged from the Department of Veterans Affairs, Peterson and colleagues concurred that African-Americans received 33% fewer cardiac procedures (e.g., coronary arteriography) following acute MI and were 64% less likely to have a CABG or PTCA performed (see also Whittle et al.). African-Americans

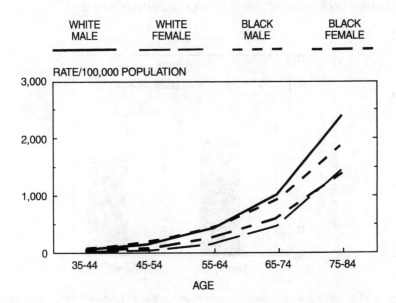

Figure 14.1. Death rates for CHD by age, race, and sex: United States, 1987. From Goldberg RJ. Coronary heart disease: Epidemiology and risk factors. In: Ockene IS, Ockene JK, eds. Prevention of Coronary Heart Disease. Boston: Little, Brown and Company, 1992; Chapter 1. Reproduced with permission.

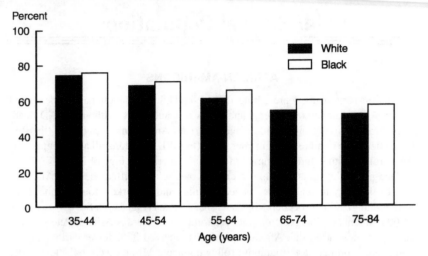

Figure 14.2. Percentage of men dying of ischemic heart disease whose place of death was coded as out of hospital or in emergency room by race and age: 40 states, 1985. From Gillum RF. Sudden coronary death in the United States: 1980–1985. Circulation 1989;79:756–765. Reproduced with permission. Copyright © 1989, American Heart Association.

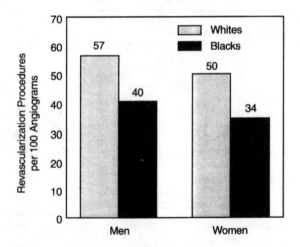

Figure 14.3. Rates of revascularization procedures within 90 days after coronary angiography by race and sex among Medicare Part A enrollees 65 to 74 years of age during 1987. From Ayanian JZ, Udvarhelyi IS, Gatsonis CA, et al. Racial differences in the use of revascularization procedures after coronary angiography. JAMA 1993;269:2642–2646. Reproduced with permission. Copyright © 1993, American Medical Association.

were also more likely to survive 1 month post-MI, perhaps reflecting the enhanced effect of thrombolytic therapy (see Sane et al.) independent of whether surgical revascularization or medical therapy was instituted (see also Maynard et al.). Unfortunately, neither CAD severity nor left ventricular function were evaluated in these two large observational studies and it is possible that nonsignificant CAD or moderate CAD with preserved ventricular function may have precluded recommendations for revascularization in African-American patients. Alternatively, more African-Americans may have decided against surgery as previously documented in the Coronary Artery Surgery Study (CASS) registry.

In evaluating Medicare admissions, Kahn and associates found that while black or poor patients fared worse in overall medical care (e.g., mean process score), they were also more likely to be hospitalized in urban teaching hospitals, where superior medical treatment was provided (Fig. 14.4). Hence, there were no significant differences overall in health care stratified by either race or poverty status. Similarly, in the 30-year follow-up of the Charleston Heart Study, the black:white CAD mortality rate ratios were not different (Table 14.1) (see Keil et al., 1993).

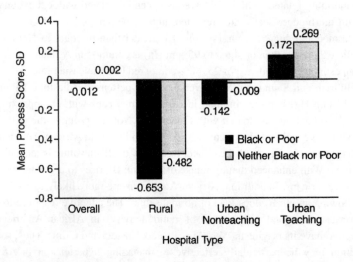

Figure 14.4. Mean process scores (in standard deviation units) by hospital type for patients who are black or poor as compared with others. From Kahn KL, Pearson ML, Harrison ER, Desmond KA, Rogers WH, Rubenstein LV. Health care for black and poor hospitalized Medicare patients. JAMA 1994;271:1169–1174. Reproduced with permission. Copyright © 1994, American Medical Association.

Table 14.1. Age-Adjusted Rates of Mortality from Coronary Heart Disease and from Any Cause*

Group	Coronary Heart Disease		Any Cause	
	Rate (95% CI)	No. Affected/ Total	Rate (95% CI)	No. Affected/ Total
White men	5.2 (4.1–6.3)	138/634	15.3 (13.1–17.5)	384/634
Black men	4.6 (3.0–6.2)	56/319	18.9 (15.5–22.3)	210/319
White women	2.1 (1.6–2.6)	99/714	7.3 (6.4–8.3)	315/714
Black women	3.2 (2.3–4.0)	67/437	12.7 (10.6–14.8)	251/437

*Mortality rates are expressed per 1000 person-years. CI=confidence interval.
Reprinted by permission of The New England Journal of Medicine from Keil JE, Sutherland SE, Knapp RG, Lackland DT, Gazes PC, Tyroler HA. Mortality rates and risk factors for coronary disease in black as compared with white men and women. N Engl J Med 1993;329:73–78, Copyright 1993, Massachusetts Medical Society.

Certain cardiac risk factors (e.g., hypertension, cigarette smoking, diabetes mellitus) are more prevalent in African-Americans. Klag and associates reported a 2 mm Hg increase in systolic and diastolic blood pressure (BP) for each standard deviation increase in skin darkness, as measured by a reflectometer. Elevations in CAD mortality related to high BP have also been associated with educational status with the highest death rates reported among the least educated (Table 14.2). Mild to moderate hypertension (systolic BP greater than or equal to 160 mm Hg, diastolic BP greater than or equal to 95 mm Hg) is common in African-Americans, with an estimated prevalence of 25–30% compared to a Caucasian rate of 17–20% (see Hildreth and Saunders). Moreover, severe hypertension (diastolic BP greater than 115 mm Hg) is more common in African-Americans with an approximately sixfold increased rate compared with Caucasians. Not surprisingly, the prevalence of hypertensive and end-stage renal disease is also higher in African-Americans.

It has been postulated that the greater frequency of BP elevation is related to salt sensitivity. With enhanced dietary intake of sodium, BP rises to a greater extent in African-Americans. In addition, African-Americans are more likely to retain sodium following an intravenous load of normal saline. The adaptive response to sodium conservation (and suppression of renin activity) in African-Americans is believed to have its origins in West Africa (see Blaustein and Grim). Thus, sodium restriction may be particularly effective in managing hypertension in African-Americans. Moreover, dietary potassium and calcium supplementation may have a salutary effect on BP in these salt-sensitive individuals, owing in part to impeding renal arteriolar narrowing and reducing parathyroid hormone mediated vasoconstriction (see also Chapter 7).

Table 14.2. Five-Year All-Cause Mortality by Educational Class and Race in the HDFP Referred Care Group

Referred care group	< High School Education			High school graduate			> High school education			All		
	n	Deaths	Rate/100	n	Deaths	Rate/100	n	Deaths	Rate/100	n	Deaths	Rate/100
All	2535	273	9.04*	1557	87	6.27	1242	49	4.52	5334	409	7.67
Whites	858	80	7.06†	1113	61	5.64	1008	36	3.81	2979	177	5.59
Blacks	1677	193	11.73†	444	26	6.94	234	13	5.54	2355	232	10.54

Adjustment is to distribution in the whole study. In this and subsequent tables with age-sex-race adjustment, the adjusted rates are based on 16 cells (4 age groups, 2 sexes, 2 races). In some cells with few persons, there may be no deaths, and this could influence final adjusted rates disproportionately.
*Age-sex-race-adjusted.
†Age-sex-adjusted
From Hypertension Detection and Follow-Up Program Cooperative Group. Educational level and 5-year all-cause mortality in the hypertension detection and follow-up program. Hypertension 1987;9:641–646.

Importantly, effective management (dietary and/or pharmacologic) of hypertension is effective in retarding deleterious consequences such as nephrosclerosis in both Caucasians and African-Americans (see Flack et al.). In the Hypertension Detection and Follow-up Program, there was a 20–30% reduction in CAD event rate with treatment of elevated BP.

Cigarette smoking is more prevalent among African-Americans than any other subset of Americans (see Chapter 9). In a survey of smoking and quitting patterns among African-Americans, Orleans and colleagues found that while the majority were light smokers (one-half pack or less per day), the brands they chose were often high in tar, nicotine, and menthol. The reduced effectiveness in smoking cessation efforts compared to Caucasians have in part been attributed to low participation in smoking cessation behavioral programs (see Novotny et al.). African-Americans are also more likely to gain weight after smoking cessation (see Williamson et al.).

Diabetes mellitus (DM) is another important cardiovascular risk factor in African-Americans, in whom the mortality rate is enhanced twofold compared with Caucasians. The prevalence of DM is higher in middle-aged (45–65 years) African-Americans, most notably in women, as quantified in the National Health and Nutritional Examination Survey (NHANES) (Table 14.3) (see Flegal et al.). Moreover, among those diagnosed with NIDDM, insulin use was highest among African-Americans (37.2%) and lowest in Cubans (16.7%) (Fig. 14.5) (see Harris).

Nonetheless, the devastating sequelae of DM (e.g., macro- and microvascular complications) are higher in African-Americans. Renal nephropathy and end stage renal disease are markedly higher among African-Americans than in Caucasians and mortality rates from DM have increased in African-American men. Studies have been undertaken to examine whether genetic markers may be useful in evaluating susceptibility to insulin sensitivity. Indeed, Banerji and colleagues reported differences at the HLA-DQ locus in chromosome 6 between insulin-resistant and insulin-sensitive African-American subjects.

Obesity is twice as common in African-Americans than in Caucasians. Kumanyika reported significant weight gains in black women upon entering middle-age (Table 14.4). Abdominal adiposity has been shown to be significantly asso-

Table 14.3 Prevalence (%) of Diabetes Mellitus

Age (years)	African-American		Caucasian	
	Male	Female	Male	Female
20–44	1.8	2.6	0.5	1.3
45–74	8.5	11.4	6.0	5.8

Data from Flegal KM, Ezzati TM, Harris MI, et al. Prevalence of diabetes in Mexican Americans, Cubans, and Puerto Ricans from the Hispanic Health and Nutrition Examination Survey, 1982–1984. Diabetes Care 1991;14:628–638.

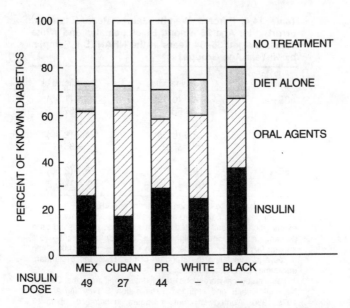

Figure 14.5. Percentage distribution of Hispanics, whites, and blacks with diagnosed NIDDM in the U.S. population aged 20–74 years by type of treatment for diabetes. Daily insulin dose (U) is presented for Hispanics. MEX=Mexican American, PR=Puerto Rican. From Harris MI. Epidemiological correlates of NIDDM in hispanics, whites, and blacks in the U.S. population. Diabetes Care 1991;14(Suppl 3):639–648. Reproduced with permission.

ciated with arteriographic CAD in African-American women (see Clark et al.). While abdominal or central adiposity associated with insulin resistance and hypertension (e.g., Syndrome X) have been confirmed in Caucasian populations, studies in African-Americans have been divergent. For example, O'Brien and colleagues reported that obesity was not the culprit for the higher prevalence of NIDDM observed in middle-aged black men (see also Falkner et al.; Chaiken et al.).

Total cholesterol levels are similar between African-Americans (men=200 mg/dL, women=205 mg/dL) and Caucasians (men=205 mg/dL, women=205 mg/dL) aged 20–74 according to NHANES, (see Johnson et al.). The prevalence of elevated TC (greater than 240 mg/dL) was detected in 16% of African-Americans compared with 19% of Caucasians (see Sempos et al.). Mean levels of LDL-C, HDL-C and TG are shown in Table 14.5. In addition to HDL-C, Lp(a) levels are also higher in African-Americans, compared with Caucasians (see Chapter 11). Whether these lipoprotein alterations impact on CAD rate has not been addressed

Table 14.4. Percent Weight Gain† (Mean (Standard Error)) after Age 25 Among Black Females and White Females Aged 35–64 Years in the NHANES II Sample, by 10-Year Age Groups‡

Age group (years)	White females	Black females
35–44	14.6 (0.69)* (n = 633)	23.5 (1.95) (n = 87)
45–54	18.5 (0.85) (n = 563)	21.3 (2.30) (n = 85)
55–64	19.8 (0.67)* (n = 1,040)	28.7 (2.30) (n = 114)

*t test of black-white difference significant at p <0.0001.
†Weight gain was calculated as the difference between weight at examination and self-reported weight at age 25, expressed as a percentage of reported weight at age 25. Sample weights were applied in calculating means. Design effects were not taken into account in calculating the standard errors. Thus, these standard errors may be underestimates.
‡These analyses were done using data tapes from the Second National Health and Nutrition Examination Survey (NHANES), 1976–1980. Women who were pregnant, lactating, or up to 12 months postpartum at interview and women with a weight/height index ($kg/m^{1.5}$) above the 99th percentile were excluded from these calculations.
From Kumanyika S. Obesity in black women. Epidemiologic Reviews 1987;9:31–50. Reproduced with permission.

Table 14.5 Mean Serum LDL-C, HDL-C, and TG in the United States 1988–1991 (mg/dL)

	LDL-C	HDL-C	TG
African-Americans			
Men	126	53	105
Women	126	58	95
Caucasians			
Men	132	46	149
Women	126	55	129

Data from Johnson CL, Rifkind BM, Sempos CT, et al. Declining serum total cholesterol levels among U.S. adults. The National Health and Nutrition Examination Surveys. JAMA 1993;269:3002–3008.

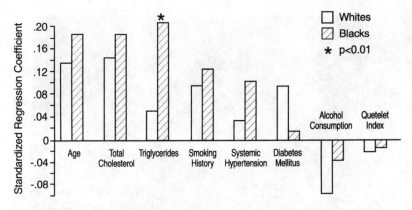

Figure 14.6. Standardized multiple linear regression coefficients related to coronary artery occlusion in males. Models were fit separately for each race. From Freedman DS, Gruchow HW, Manley JC, Anderson AJ, Sobocinski KA, Barboriak JJ. Black/white differences in risk factors for arteriographically documented coronary artery disease in men. Am J Cardiol 1988;62:214–219. Reproduced with permission.

in prospective, randomized, controlled trials. Despite reduced mean TG levels in African-Americans, Freedman and associates recently reported an independent association between TG and arteriographic CAD in black men (Fig. 14.6).

Low socioeconomic status (SES) has provided another basis for racial disparity and elevated CAD rates in young and middle-aged African-Americans. While only 1 in 10 Caucasian families live below the poverty level, the number of economically disadvantaged African-Americans is threefold higher. Associated with low SES are reduced opportunities for educational advancement, lower prioritization for overall health care and preventive measures which further contribute to higher CAD rates. More intensive efforts focused on educating the inner city community are warranted. To this end, the National Heart, Lung, and Blood Institute recently established a task force designed to identify, implement and support further research in this very important area (see Lenfant).

CHILDHOOD, ADOLESCENCE, AND EARLY ADULTHOOD

Although atherosclerosis and its devastating sequelae are often not manifest until midlife, the process is initiated at a young age. As outlined in Chapter 2, fatty streaking in the aorta is a ubiquitous process, occurring in all societies (Fig. 14.7). Autopsies performed in infants who died before their first birthday evidenced aortic fatty streaking in approximately 40% (see Woolf) and, by age 3 years, in all sub-

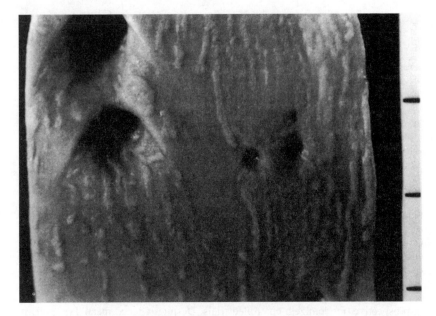

Figure 14.7. Aorta of a 19-year-old white man showing fatty streaking in the thoracic portion of the vessel. The mouth of the intercostal artery shown displays a marked concentration of streaks proximal to the ostium with relative sparing of the actual flow divider. From Woolf N. The morphology of atherosclerotic lesions. In: Crawford T, ed. Pathology of Atherosclerosis. London: Butterworth Scientific, 1982:47–82. Reproduced with permission.

jects. Despite the uniform presence of fatty streaking in children, surface involvement is small. By puberty, however, up to 25% of the aortic surface area may be covered with lipid.

Studies from the Pathological Determinants of Atherosclerosis in Youth (PDAY) have disclosed that the lower abdominal aorta is more likely to be laden with lipid deposits than either the midabdominal or thoracic aorta, a finding that simulates atherosclerotic predilection in adults (see Wissler et al.). Coronary fatty streaking on the other hand, begins during adolescence. By the third decade of life, 90% of individuals display evidence of coronary streaking in at least one of the major epicardial vessels. The significance of these findings was brought to light in a landmark study by Enos and colleagues. Autopsy data from young soldiers killed in Korea (mean age 22 years), disclosed that while coronary lesions were present in the majority of soldiers (77.3%), 15% had significant CAD (at least one vessel with 50% or greater reduction in coronary luminal diameter) (Table 14.6).

Table 14.6. Percentage of Cases Showing Varying Amounts of Luminal Narrowing

Amount of Luminal Narrowing	% of Cases
"Fibrous" thickening or streaking causing insignificant luminal narrowing.	35.0
Plaques causing luminal narrowing over	
10%	13.3
20%	6.3
30%	3.7
40%	3.0
50%	3.0
60%	1.7
70%	1.0
80%.	1.3
90%	5.3
Plaques causing complete occlusion of one or more vessels	3.0

From Enos WF, Holmes RH, Beyer J. Coronary disease among United States soldiers killed in action in Korea. Preliminary report. JAMA 1953;152:1090–1093.

Atherosclerotic progression demonstrates racial divergence. Compared to young Caucasians (aged 10 to 25 years), African-Americans exhibit a 1.5-fold greater degree of aortic fatty streaking and surface involvement which persists after adjustment of conventional cardiac risk factors, including lipids and lipoproteins, BP, and obesity (see Freedman et al., 1988) (Fig. 14.8). This contrasts with the higher prevalence of fibrous plaques in Caucasians compared with African-American adults suggesting that there may be racial divergence in atherosclerotic progression rate. It has been proposed that these differences have resulted in part from physicochemical alterations of fatty streaks in Caucasians (e.g., greater extracellular lipid), thereby facilitating atherosclerotic progression to more complicated lesions.

Cardiovascular Risk Factors

Epidemiologic studies have examined the relevance and prognostic implications of cardiovascular risk factors in the young. In addition to immutable factors (e.g., positive family history), potentially modifiable risk factors include cigarette smoking, hyperlipidemia, hypertension, and obesity/sedentary lifestyle.

CIGARETTE SMOKING

At present there are more than 3 million adolescent smokers in the United States, with approximately 3,000 new smokers added daily. Nearly 75% of smokers develop an addiction by age 18. While the overall prevalence of cigarette smoking has decreased during the past several decades (see Chapter 9), the rates have increased in younger segments of our society. Initiation of cigarette smoking is often predicated on one or more factors (Table 14.7). Among the most important factors are peer pressure, family income (e.g., low SES), and advertising campaigns (e.g., Old Joe the Camel). The influence of cigarette advertising was recently assessed in children aged 3 to 6 years. The recognition rate of Old Joe the Camel was 30% in 3-year-old children. The alarming percentage of 6-year-olds recognizing the logo (91.3%) was similar to recognition of the Mickey Mouse logo (Fig. 14.9). As Marlboro and Camel are perceived by teenagers (aged 12 to 17 years) as the two most heavily advertised (70%) smoking brands, it is not surprising that these brands were the most purchased in a sample of younger individuals residing in California

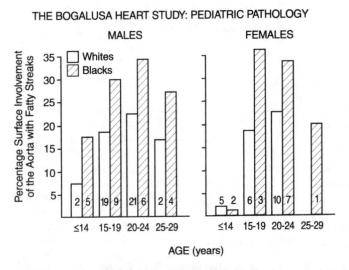

THE BOGALUSA HEART STUDY: PEDIATRIC PATHOLOGY

Figure 14.8. Black-white differences in aortic surface involvement with fatty streaks. Values represent median levels within each race, sex, and age group. The two black girls in the youngest age group were 3 and 5 years of age. From Freedman DS, Newman WP III, Tracy RE, et al. Black-white differences in aortic fatty streaks in adolescence and early adulthood: The Bogalusa Heart Study. Circulation 1988;77:856–864. Reproduced with permission. Circulation. Copyright © 1988 American Heart Association.

Table 14.7. Factors Associated with Cigarette Smoking

Friends smoking
Siblings smoking
Parents' education level
Smoker's image
Exemplars
Independence
Rebelliousness

From Mittelmark MB, Murray DM, Luepker RV, Pechacek TF, Pirie PL, Pallonen UE. Predicting experimentation with cigarettes: The childhood antecedents of smoking study (CASS). Am J Public Health, 77:206–208, 1987. Reproduced with permission.

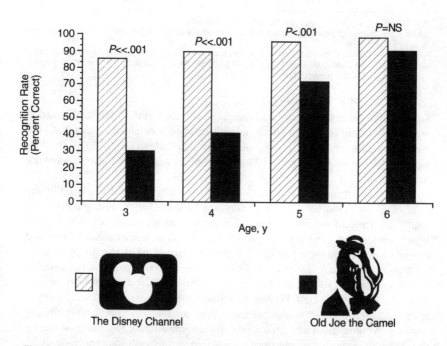

Figure 14.9. Logo recognition rates for The Disney Channel and Old Joe by subject age. From Fischer PM, Schwartz MP, Richards JW Jr, Goldstein AO, Rojas TH. Brand logo recognition by children aged 3 to 6 years. Mickey Mouse and Old Joe the Camel. JAMA 1991;266:3145–3148. Reproduced with permission. Copyright © 1991, American Medical Association.

Table 14.8. Brands Purchased by Smokers in California

Age, y†	Brand Purchased, %*			Sample Size, n
	Marlboro	Camel	Other	
Males				
12–17	55.4 ± 12.6	24.5 ± 8.0	18.0 ± 13.4	131
18–24	71.3 ± 5.1	12.7 ± 3.6	16.0 ± 4.5	567
25–29	61.7 ± 7.6	13.8 ± 6.9	24.5 ± 5.8	470
30–44	47.7 ± 2.9	10.5 ± 2.1	41.8 ± 3.3	1579
≥45	21.1 ± 2.7	8.1 ± 2.8	70.8 ± 3.3	1316
Females				
12–17	63.3 ± 15.7	21.7 ± 13.7	13.4 ± 9.6	102
18–24	69.4 ± 7.1	5.5 ± 3.2	25.1 ± 7.3	461
25–29	49.5 ± 7.2	3.6 ± 2.5	46.9 ± 8.3	467
30–44	33.0 ± 4.0	2.3 ± 0.9	64.7 ± 4.2	1500
≥45	12.7 ± 3.1	2.2 ± 1.2	85.1 ± 3.6	1594

*Numbers given are percentages ± 95% confidence intervals.
†In the youngest age group of both sexes, a small percentage did not purchase cigarettes but obtained them by other means.
From Pierce JP, Gilpin E, Burns DM, et al. Does tobacco advertising target young people to start smoking? Evidence from California. JAMA 1991;266:3154–3158. Reproduced with permission. Copyright © 1991, American Medical Association.

(Table 14.8). An equally celebrated campaign launched in the 1960s and aimed at initiating smoking in 10- to 17-year-old girls resulted in heightened sales that were most prominent among those who never attended college (Fig. 14.10). In 1990 alone, RJ Reynolds spent nearly 100 million dollars to promote cigarette smoking in adolescents.

It has been estimated that more than 1 billion dollars is spent yearly on illegal sales of tobacco to minors. The most common locations for cigarette purchases by youths are convenience stores, gas stations, and vending machines. Adoption of legislation restricting the sale of cigarettes to minors has been examined. Jason and coworkers examined the effect of cigarette sale restrictions in a small community in Illinois. A monetary fine of up to $500 was imposed on any merchant convicted of selling cigarettes to a minor. The minor was charged $25 if caught with tobacco products. During a 2-year follow-up period, cigarette sales to minors were virtually eliminated. It is hoped that recent legislation introduced to Congress prohibiting smoking in public areas and authorizing stricter regulation of tobacco products by the FDA will impact on young smokers and impede this vexatious epidemic.

FAMILY HISTORY

There is incontrovertible evidence that a parental history of premature CAD markedly enhances the likelihood of early atherogenesis in their progeny. If a first-

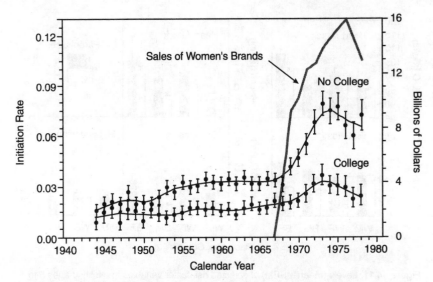

Figure 14.10. Left ordinate, trends in initiation rates for 10- to 17-year-old girls during each calendar year for those who ultimately did and did not attend college. Right ordinate, combined sales in billions of dollars for Virginia Slims, Silva Thins, and Eve cigarettes. From Pierce JP, Lee L, Gilpin E. Smoking initiation by adolescent girls, 1944 through 1988. JAMA 1994;271:608–611. Reproduced with permission. Copyright © 1994, American Medical Association.

degree relative has CAD, the risk is enhanced by approximately 15%. Compared to the general population, that risk is doubled if the biologic family member is younger than 55 years at the time of diagnosis. If two first-degree family members develop premature CAD, the risk exceeds 50%. Elevations in CAD rates are influenced by genes and environmental factors. Specific genetic markers that are associated with an increased risk of CAD include the lymphocyte antigen locus (diabetes mellitus), the Apo AI-CIII-AIV gene complex (familial low HDL-C) and the LDL-C receptor gene (familial hypercholesterolemia).

Several studies have examined the relationship between parental cardiovascular disease/CAD risk factors and associated CAD risk factors in children and young adults. Parental hypertension has also been found to correlate with increases in left ventricular mass in the offspring (see Nielsen and Oxhøj). Among children aged 5 to 17 years whose parents were diabetic, Bao et al. reported a higher prevalence of hyperglycemia in African-Americans and obesity in African-American females (Fig. 14.11). In young adult children aged 18 to 31 years whose parents suffered an

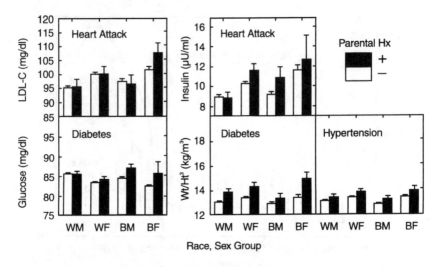

Figure 14.11. Levels (mean ± SEM) of selected risk factor variables in offspring ages 5 to 17 years by parental history (Hx) of disease, race, and sex. WM=white males, WF=white females, BW=black males, BF=black females, LDL-C=LDL cholesterol. From Bao W, Srinivasan SR, Wattigney WA, Berenson GS. The relation of parental cardiovascular disease to risk factors in children and young adults. The Bogalusa Heart Study. Circulation 1995;91:365–371. Reproduced with permission. Circulation. Copyright © 1995 American Heart Association.

MI, LDL-C levels were higher in Caucasians and insulin levels higher in African-Americans. As with the younger age group, parental DM was associated with hyperglycemia and obesity, being most prominent in African-American females (Fig. 14.12). Among offspring whose fathers suffered an MI, LDL-C and apo B concentrations were higher and apo AI concentrations lower compared to children without paternal CAD (see Freedman et al., 1986). Associations between parental CAD and risk factors in the progeny have also been reported in the Coronary Artery Development in Young Adults (CARDIA) Study (see Burke et al.).

HYPERLIPIDEMIA

Autopsy data obtained from the Bogalusa Heart Study have disclosed an important correlation between early aortic lesion development and concentrations of LDL-C and TC. Newman and associates also found a similar positive correlation between coronary lesions and VLDL-C concentrations (Fig. 14.13). Age-related levels of lipids and lipoproteins are shown in Table 14.9. Although elevated levels of TC and LDL-C in childhood do not necessarily translate into hyperlipidemia dur-

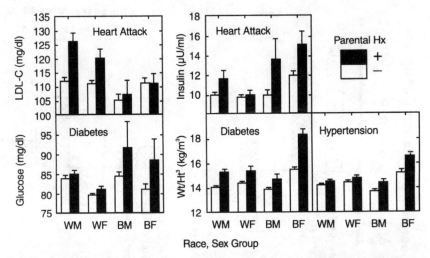

Figure 14.12. Levels (mean ± SEM) of selected risk factor variables in offspring ages 18 to 31 years by parental history (Hx) of disease, race, and sex. WM=white males, WF=white females, BW=black males, BF=black females, LDL-C=LDL cholesterol. From Bao W, Srinivasan SR, Wattigney WA, Berenson GS. The relation of parental cardiovascular disease to risk factors in children and young adults. The Bogalusa Heart Study. Circulation 1995;91:365–371. Reproduced with permission. Circulation. Copyright © 1995 American Heart Association.

ing adulthood, the National Cholesterol Education Program recommends screening TC measurements with associated parental hypercholesterolemia (greater than 240 mg/dL).

Classification of TC and LDL-C is outlined in Table 14.10. If there is a family history of premature CAD, or screening TC exceeds 200 mg/dL, lipoprotein analysis is recommended. Borderline elevations in TC are repeated and if the level is equal to or greater than 170 mg/dL, a complete lipoprotein profile should be obtained. An American Heart Association Step I diet that restricts cholesterol (less than 300 mg/day), total fat (less than 30% of calories), and saturated fat (less than 10% of calories) is recommended when LDL-C is greater than 130 mg/dL. A U.S. multicenter trial recently assessed the effect of dietary restriction in hyperlipidemic children with physiological/psychobehavioral correlates (see DISC Study).

After a 6 to 12 month dietary trial, pharmacologic therapy is recommended in children over 10 years of age under the following two conditions: (1) LDL-C levels greater than or equal to 190 mg/dL in the absence of a family history of premature CAD, (2) LDL-C greater than or equal to 160 mg/dL in the presence of a family history of premature CAD or two or more risk factors identified in the child/

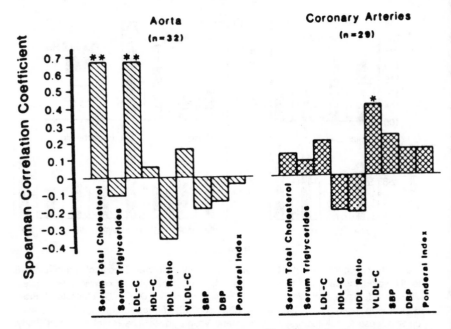

Figure 14.13. Associations between the percentage of fatty-streak involvement and risk-factor values. Reprinted by permission of The New England Journal of Medicine from Newman WP III, Freedman DS, Voors AW, Gard PD, Srinivasan SR, Cresanta JL. Relation of serum lipoprotein levels and systolic blood pressure to early atherosclerosis. The Bogalusa Heart Study. N Engl J Med 1986;314:138–144, Copyright © 1986, Massachusetts Medical Society.

adolescent. The only lipid-lowering medications with proven efficacy and safety in this age group are the bile acid sequestrants. The dose recommended for these agents is outlined in Table 14.11 (see Farah et al.). Nicotinic acid has also been used in children and adolescents with heterozygous familial hypercholesterolemia. Other agents including the HMG-CoA reductase inhibitors have, as of this writing, not been approved for use in children or adolescents.

HYPERTENSION

Blood pressure increases during childhood. Upon evaluating children ranging in age from 9 to 18 years in Muscatine, Iowa, Schieken and colleagues found that elevated BP correlated with increased left ventricular wall mass. Importantly, left ven-

Table 14.9. Percentiles of Total Cholesterol, LDL, HDL, and Triglycerides in Children and Adolescents

Percentile	10th	25th	50th	75th	90th
	Total Cholesterol (mg/dL)				
Boys					
Age					
0–4	129	141	156	176	192
5–9	134	147	164	180	197
10–14	131	144	160	178	196
15–19	124	136	150	170	188
Girls					
Age					
0–4	124	143	161	177	195
5–9	138	150	168	184	201
10–14	135	148	163	179	196
15–19	131	144	160	177	197
	LDL (mg/dL)				
Boys					
Age					
5–9	71	82	93	106	121
10–14	74	83	97	112	126
15–19	70	82	96	112	127
Girls					
Age					
5–9	75	91	101	118	129
10–14	75	83	97	113	130
15–19	67	80	96	114	133
	HDL (mg/dL)				
Boys					
Age					
5–9	43	50	56	65	72
10–14	41	47	57	63	73
15–19	35	40	47	54	61
Girls					
Age					
5–9	39	48	54	63	69
10–14	41	46	54	60	66
15–19	39	44	53	63	70

Table 14.9. *continued*

Percentile	10th	25th	50th	75th	90th
		Triglycerides (mg/dL)			
Boys					
Age					
0–4	34	41	53	69	87
5–9	34	41	53	67	88
10–14	38	46	61	80	105
15–19	44	56	71	94	124
Girls					
Age					
0–4	39	46	61	79	99
5–9	37	45	57	73	93
10–14	45	56	72	93	117
15–19	45	55	70	90	117

Data from the Lipid Research Clinics Prevalence Study in North America. National Heart, Lung, and Blood Institute. The Lipid Research Clinics Population Studies Data Book: Volume I-The Prevalence Study. Bethesda, MD: U.S. Department of Health and Human Services, Public Health Service, National Institutes of Health, NIH Pub. No. 80,1527, July 1980.

Table 14.10. Classification of Total and LDL-Cholesterol Levels in Children and Adolescents from Families With Hypercholesterolemia or Premature Cardiovascular Disease

Category	Total Cholesterol (mg/dL)	LDL-Cholesterol (mg/dL)
Acceptable	<170	<110
Borderline	170–199	110–129
High	≥200	≥130

From National Cholesterol Education Program. Report of the expert panel on blood cholesterol levels in children and adolescents. U.S. Department of Health and Human Services, NIH Publication No. 91,2732. September 1991.

tricular mass, elevated BP responses during exercise, and childhood obesity are predictors of elevated BP. Moreover, there is an approximately 25% increased risk of elevated BP in children with a parental history of HTN (see Berenson et al.). In the Minneapolis Children's Blood Pressure Study, Munger and coworkers found BP correlations between mothers and their children, suggesting shared environmental factors. Racial differences in BP do not become apparent until adolescence, when HTN begins to emerge prominently in African-Americans.

Based on the recommendations of the Second Task Force on Blood Pressure Control in Children, it has been recommended that all individuals over the age of 3

Table 14.11. Initial Dosage Schedule for Treatment of Familial Hypercholesterolemic Children and Adolescents with a Bile Acid Sequestrant*

Daily Doses of Bile Acid Sequestrant†	Total Cholesterol (TC) and Low Density Lipoprotein Cholesterol (LDL-C) Levels after Diet (mg/dL)	
	TC	LDL-C
1	<245	<195
2	245–300	195–235
3	301–345	236–280
4	>345	

*These are generally recommended doses and may require adjustment based on the patient's response.

†One dose is the equivalent of a 9 g packet of cholestyramine (containing 4 g cholestyramine and 5 g filler), one bar of cholestyramine, or 5 g of colestipol.

Reproduced from National Cholesterol Education Program. Report of the Expert Panel on Blood Cholesterol Levels in Children and Adolescents. U.S. Department of Health and Human Services, NIH Publication No. 91, 2732. September 1991. Data from Farah JR, Kwiterovich PO Jr, Neill CA. Dose effect relation of cholestyramine in children and young adults with familial hypercholesterolemia. Lancet 1977;1:59–63.

years have BP measurements obtained. Table 14.12 lists the range of elevated BPs in children and adolescents. The most common causes of elevated BP are shown in Table 14.13. Initial therapy involves hygienic measures, including weight loss through dietary modification and aerobic exercise. Weight loss has been shown to reduce elevated BP in children. Although the amount of sodium restriction needed to impact on BP in childhood and adolescence has not been established, the Task Force advocates a limit of 85 to 100 mEq of sodium or 5 to 6 grams of sodium chloride daily in conjunction with foods high in potassium (see also Chapter 7).

The pharmacologic treatment of elevated BP is limited to systolic and/or diastolic BP exceeding the 90th percentile. The various antihypertensive agents and doses are shown in Table 14.14 and should be used following the stepped-care approach (Fig. 14.14). Hypertensive adolescent girls should be advised not to use oral contraceptives and to sparingly utilize nonsteroidal anti-inflammatory agents for dysmenorrhea.

OBESITY/SEDENTARY LIFESTYLE

Childhood obesity is a very common problem with a prevalence rate of 15% by the age of 5 years. During adolescence, the number rises to 25%, approximating the adult rate. It is axiomatic that childhood obesity leads to adult obesity. Unless

Table 14.12. High Normal (90th Percentile) and High (≥95th Percentile) Values of Systolic and Diastolic Blood Pressures in Children*

Age (years)	High normal blood pressure (mm Hg)		High blood pressure (mm Hg)	
	Systolic	Diastolic	Systolic	Diastolic
≤2	106	69	≥112	≥74
3–5	109	69	≥116	≥76
6–9	115	74	≥122	≥78
10–12	122	78	≥126	≥82
13–15	129	82	≥136	≥86
16–18	136	84	≥142	≥92

*Values are similar for males and females.

From Task Force on Blood Pressure Control in Children. Report of the Second Task Force on Blood Pressure Control in Children—1987. Pediatrics 1987;79:1–25. Reproduced by permission of Pediatrics, Vol 79, Copyright © 1987.

Table 14.13. Commonest Causes by Age Group of Chronic Sustained Hypertension in Children and Adolescents Seen in Clinical Populations*

Age Group	Cause
Newborn infants	Renal artery thrombosis, renal artery stenosis, congenital renal malformations, coarctation of the aorta, bronchopulmonary dysplasia
Infancy–6 yr	Renal parenchymal diseases,† coarctation of the aorta, renal artery stenosis
6–10 yr	Renal artery stenosis, renal parenchymal diseases, primary hypertension
Adolescence	Primary hypertension, renal parenchymal diseases

*No good population data are available for estimating the true prevalence of these conditions.
†Includes renal structural and inflammatory lesions, as well as tumors.
From Task Force on Blood Pressure Control in Children. Report of the Second Task Force on Blood Pressure Control in Children—1987. Pediatrics 1987;79:1–25. Reproduced by permission of Pediatrics, Vol 79, Copyright © 1987.

weight loss occurs by the end of adolescence, less than four out of every 100 obese teenagers will eventually become thin adults. Obesity is most prevalent among female Caucasians. Indeed, early atherogenesis may be enhanced by the attendant higher risk of DM, HTN, and hyperlipidemia. Using triceps skin-fold thickness as an indicator of adiposity, Freedman and coworkers found positive correlations with TC, LDL-C, TG, and an inverse association with HDL-C (Fig. 14.15).

Table 14.14. Antihypertensive Medications*

	Dose	No. of Times/Day	Route
Diuretics			
Hydrochlorothiazide (Hydrodiuril, Esidrix)	1–2 mg/kg	2	Oral
Chlorthalidone (Hygroton)	0.5–2 mg/kg	1	Oral
Furosemide (Lasix)	0.5–2 mg/kg	2	Oral, intravenous
Spironolactone (Aldactone)	1–2 mg/kg	2	Oral
Triamterene (Dyrenium)	1–2 mg/kg	2	Oral
Adrenergic inhibitors			
β-adrenergic antagonists			
Metoprolol (Lopressor)	1–4 mg/kg	2	Oral
Atenolol (Tenormin)	1–2 mg/kg	1	Oral
Propranolol (Inderal)	1–3 mg/kg	3	Oral
Central adrenergic inhibitors			
Methyldopa (Aldomet)	5–10 mg/kg	2	Oral
Clonidine (Catapres)	0.05–0.40 mg	2	Oral
Guanabenz (Wytensin)	0.03–0.08 mg	2	Oral
α_1-Adrenergic antagonist			
Prazosin hydrochloride (Minipress)	0.5–7 mg	3	Oral
Vasodilators			
Hydralazine (Apresoline)	1–5 mg/kg	2 or 3	Oral, intramuscular, IV (drip)
Minoxidil (Loniten)	0.1–1.0 mg/kg	2	Oral
Diazoxide (Hyperstat)†	3–5 mg/kg/dose		IV (bolus)
Nitroprusside (Nipride)†	1–8 μg/kg/min		IV (drip)
Angiotensin-converting enzyme inhibitor			
Captopril			
<6 mo of age	0.05–0.5 mg/kg	3	
>6 mo of age	0.5–2.0 mg/kg	3	Oral

*Not to exceed usual adult dosage with all drugs.
†Primary use is in hypertensive emergencies.
From Task Force on Blood Pressure Control in Children. Report of the Second Task Force on Blood Pressure Control in Children—1987. Pediatrics 1987;79:1–25. Reproduced by permission of Pediatrics, Vol 79, © 1987.

As obesity may be perpetuated by a sedentary lifestyle, The Council on Cardiovascular Disease in the Young, issued a statement regarding physical fitness in children. They suggested a curriculum that provides guidelines for regular conditioning (see Riopel et al.). Specific sports recommended for grade and junior high school students include soccer, basketball, volleyball, and swimming. With epiphyses fusure (during high school) more competitive sports may be pursued. Barring injury, athletic endeavors during this formative period should spearhead a lifelong effort to offset CAD risk.

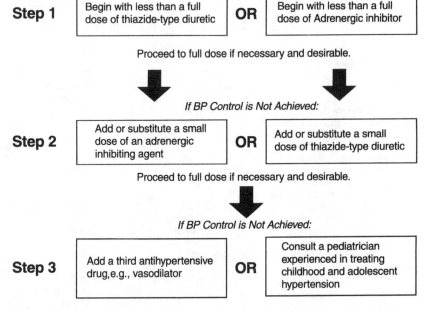

Step 1

| Begin with less than a full dose of thiazide-type diuretic | **OR** | Begin with less than a full dose of Adrenergic inhibitor |

Proceed to full dose if necessary and desirable.

If BP Control is Not Achieved:

Step 2

| Add or substitute a small dose of an adrenergic inhibiting agent | **OR** | Add or substitute a small dose of thiazide-type diuretic |

Proceed to full dose if necessary and desirable.

If BP Control is Not Achieved:

Step 3

| Add a third antihypertensive drug,e.g., vasodilator | **OR** | Consult a pediatrician experienced in treating childhood and adolescent hypertension |

Figure 14.14. Stepped-care approach to antihypertensive drug therapy. From Task Force on Blood Pressure Control in Children. Report of the second task force on blood pressure control in children—1987. Pediatrics 1987;79:1–25. Reproduced by permission of Pediatrics, Vol 79, Copyright © 1987.

GERIATRICS

The prevalence of CAD in the elderly (aged 65 and older) is greater than 25% and cardiovascular disease accounts for the preponderance of deaths. Compared with younger individuals, the risk of an acute MI is nearly threefold greater among senior citizens. The same CAD risk factors reported in young and middle-aged adults are also applicable in the aged. Because the risk of cardiovascular death exceeds 80% in patients with preexisting CAD, aggressive efforts to modify CAD risk factors should be emphasized.

Cigarette Smoking

Elderly subjects who continue to smoke experience significantly higher rates of MI and cardiovascular death (Fig. 14.16) (see also Hermanson et al.). Importantly, the adage "It is never too late to quit smoking" is applicable to the aged, as data from CASS demonstrated reductions in CAD event rate for this subgroup.

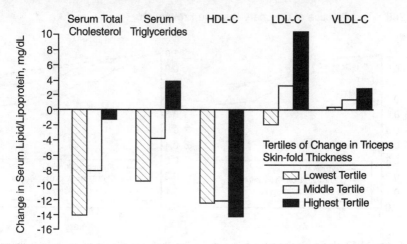

Figure 14.15. Relationship of changes in triceps skin-fold thickness to changes in serum lipid and lipoprotein levels in children over a five-year period. Mean changes in serum lipid and lipoprotein levels within tertiles of triceps skin-fold thickness change are shown. Mean levels of triceps skin-fold thickness change within tertiles are −0.6 mm, 4.2 mm, and 10.7 mm. HDL-C=high-density lipoprotein cholesterol; LDL-C=low-density lipoprotein cholesterol; and VLDL-C=very low-density lipoprotein cholesterol. From Freedman DS, Burke GL, Harsha DW, et al. Relationship of changes in obesity to serum lipid and lipoprotein changes in childhood and adolescence. JAMA 1985;254:515–520. Reproduced with permission. Copyright © 1985, American Medical Association.

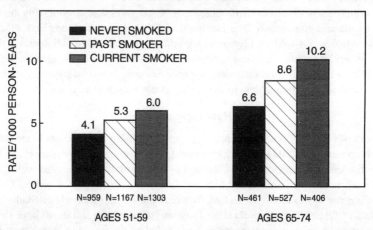

Figure 14.16. CHD incidence by smoking status in middle-aged and elderly men. From Benfante R, Reed D, Frank J. Does cigarette smoking have an independent effect on coronary heart disease incidence in the elderly? Am J Public Health 1991;81:897–899. Reproduced with permission.

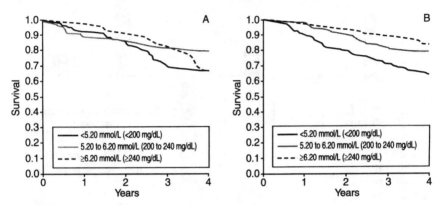

Figure 14.17. Kaplan-Meier survival curves for the study sample, stratified by total serum cholesterol level in men (**A**) and women (**B**). From Krumholz HM, Seeman TE, Merrill SS, et al. Lack of association between cholesterol and coronary heart disease mortality and morbidity and all-cause mortality in persons older than 70 years. JAMA 1994;272:1335–1340. Reproduced with permission. Copyright © 1994, American Medical Association.

Diabetes

The prevalence of DM increases with age with nearly 20% of U.S. octogenarians afflicted. As emphasized in Chapter 8, CAD rates are considerably higher among diabetic individuals. The incidence of CAD is higher among both elderly diabetic males (1.4-fold) and females (2.1-fold) compared with nondiabetics. Other cardiovascular events (e.g., stroke, congestive heart failure) are also increased, particularly in elderly female diabetics. Aggressive management of hyperglycemia is often advocated, although data in the elderly is not presently available.

Hyperlipidemia

Serum cholesterol is an independent predictor of cardiovascular death in the elderly with preexisting CAD (see Pekkanen et al.). Moreover, aggressive management of hyperlipidemia reduces cardiovascular and overall mortality in the aged with CAD (see the Scandinavian Simvastatin Survival Study). In elderly subjects without CAD, however, the association is muddled. Whereas the Framingham Heart Study (see Castelli et al.) and The Honolulu Heart Program (see Benfante and Reed) have yielded positive associations, other studies have failed to disclose any correlation. For example, in one of the largest studies to date, nearly 1,000 elderly subjects (older than 70 years) were followed for 4 years. Results found that elevated TC or TC:HDL-C ratio was not associated with increased CAD or total mortality rates (Fig. 14.17).

Table 14.15. Potential Drug Interactions with Lipid-Lowering Agents

Lipid-lowering agents	Interacting drug	Potential side effect(s)
Niacin	Nitroglycerin Antihypertensive agents: - Beta blockers - Alpha agonists - Diuretics - ACE inhibitors - Vasodilators	Possible additive vasodilating effect Postural hypotension
	Insulin Oral hypoglycemics	Changes in blood glucose may require modification in diet and/or hypoglycemic therapy
Cholestyramine	Digoxin l-thyroxine Penicillin G Phenobarbital Phenylbutazone Propranolol Tetracyclines Thiazides Warfarin	Delayed or reduced absorption
Lovastatin	Azathioprine Clofibrate Cyclosporine Gemfibrozil Immune globulin Nicotinic acid Warfarin	Myopathy and/or elevated CPK Increased PT and/or clinically evident bleeding
Gemfibrozil	Cyclosporine Lovastatin	Myopathy and/or elevated CPK Increased PT and/or clinically evident bleeding

From Miller M, Gottlieb SO. Preventive maintenance of the aging heart. Geriatrics 1991;46:22–30. Reproduced with permission.

From the aforementioned, it appears justified to aggressively treat hyperlipidemia in subjects with established CAD, irrespective of age. As such, it is also important to recognize that elderly subjects with CAD will be receiving other medications. One must therefore be cognizant of potential drug interactions when lipid-lowering medications are selected (Table 14.15). In elderly subjects without symptomatic CAD, there are presently no formal recommendations for the use of lipid-lowering therapy. Rather, dietary and other hygienic measures are suggested.

Table 14.16. Prevalence of Hypertension (Systolic BP>160 mm Hg or Diastolic BP>95 mm Hg, or both) Compared in a Younger and Older Age Group

	Age (35–44 yrs)	Age (65–74 yrs)
Black women	29%	59%
Black men	39%	50%
White women	10%	42%
White Men	18%	35%

From Weber MA, Neutel JM, Cheung DG. Hypertension in the aged: A pathophysiologic basis for treatment. Am J Cardiol 1989;63:25H–32H. Reproduced with permission.

Hypertension

The prevalence of elevated BP increases with age (Table 14.16) (see Weber et al.). In the Framingham Heart Study, the incidence of CAD with isolated systolic hypertension (the most common form of hypertension in the elderly) was highest with increasing age (Fig. 14.18). Of perhaps greater consequence is the prognostic significance of left ventricular hypertrophy (Fig. 14.19). With combined elevations in systolic and diastolic BP (e.g., BP greater than or equal to 160/95), the risk of CAD is tripled in men and doubled in women over 65 years of age. Moreover, stroke risk is tripled in both sexes and the rate of congestive heart failure is quadrupled in men and doubled in women.

Beard and colleagues recently reviewed the results of six published trials of treatment of mild hypertension including the Australian trial, the European Working Party trial of hypertension in the elderly (EWPHE), Coope and Warrender's trial of treatment of hypertension in elderly patients, the Systolic Hypertension in the Elderly Program (SHEP), the Swedish Trial in Old Patients (STOP) with hypertension, and the Medical Research Council (MRC) trial of hypertension in older adults (Table 14.17). There was a general trend toward reduction in cardiovascular events, including significant reductions in cardiac and stroke deaths in many of the studies (Table 14.18). The data from these studies suggest an aggressive approach for treating elderly subjects (tested to age 80 years) with elevated systolic (greater than 160 mm Hg) with or without diastolic (greater than 90 mm Hg) hypertension.

Aggressive lowering of diastolic BP has been greeted with trepidation in view of the purported "J curve" phenomenon (see Chapter 7). However, in the SHEP study, diastolic pressures were safely lowered to less than 70 mm Hg without an increase in CAD events. In patients with diastolic hypertension or combined systolic and diastolic hypertension, diastolic BP should be reduced to approximately 80–85 mm Hg.

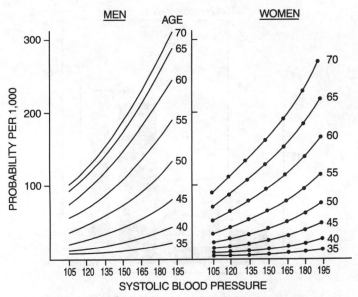

Figure 14.18. Risk of coronary heart disease among nonsmoking men and women with low-risk cholesterol (CHOL.) levels not intolerant to glucose and with no electrocardiogram-left ventricular hypertrophy (ECG-LVH). From Castelli WP, Wilson PWF, Levy D, Anderson K. Cardiovascular risk factors in the elderly. Am J Cardiol 1989;63:12H–19H. Reproduced with permission.

Sedentary Lifestyle

Sedentary lifestyle appears to influence CAD rate in the elderly. In their study of Harvard Alumni, Paffenbarger and associates found that sedentary men aged 65 to 74 had a twofold increased risk of CAD events compared to active men who expended 2,000 or more kcal per week. Similar results were observed in 65-to-69-year-old men who participated in the Honolulu Heart Program. Following adjustment of other cardiovascular risk factors, sedentary lifestyle remained an independent predictor of CAD in this age group (see Donahue et al.). Post-MI elderly patients may also benefit from a supervised cardiac rehabilitation and exercise training program (see Lavie et al.).

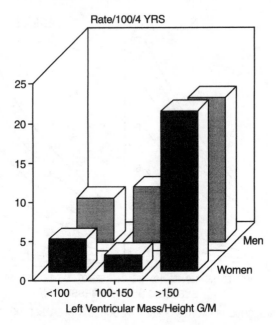

Figure 14.19. Left ventricular mass/height by echocardiography, as a risk factor for coronary heart disease. Adapted from Levy D, Garrison RJ, Savage DD, et al. Left ventricular mass and incidence of coronary heart disease in an elderly cohort: The Framingham Heart Study. Ann Intern Med 1989;110:101–107. Reproduced with permission.

Cardioprotective Agents (see also Chapter 10)

ACE INHIBITORS

As reported in the Survival and Ventricular Enlargement (SAVE) Trial, the use of the angiotensin converting enzyme inhibitor, captopril (25 to 50 mg three times daily), post-MI, was found to reduce cardiovascular and all-cause mortality. Similar cardiovascular benefits were observed in both young subjects and the elderly (older than 70 years), who comprised 15% of the study population (see Pfeffer et al.). Unless contraindicated, elderly post-MI subjects with compromised ventricular function (left ventricular ejection fraction less than 40%) should receive ACE inhibitor therapy.

ASPIRIN

In the Physician's Health Study, 325 mg of aspirin administered every other day was shown to reduce the risk of MI in subjects older than 60 years by approximately

Table 14.17 Entry Criteria, Blood Pressure at Entry, Goal Pressure, and Achieved Pressures (mm Hg) in Six Trials of Treating Hypertension in the Elderly

	Australian	EWPHE	Coope and Warrender	SHEP	STOP-Hypertension	MRC
No. of patients	582	840	884	4736	1627	4396
Age range (years)	60–69	60–97	60–79	70–>80	70–84	65–74
Blood pressure entry criteria:						
Systolic	<200	160–239	190–230	160–219	180–230 or <180	160–209
Diastolic	95–109	90–119	105–120	<90	90–120 or 105–120	<115
Mean blood pressure at entry	165/101	182/101	197/100	170/77	195/102	185/91
Blood pressure goal:						
Systolic			<170	<160/↓ 20*	<160	<160/<150*
Diastolic	<90<80**	<90	<105		95	
Treatment:						
Initial	Chlorthalidone	Hydrochlorothiazide + triamterine	Atenolol	Chlorthalidone	(1) Hydrochlorothiazide + amiloride (2) Or atenolol or metoprolol or pindolol	(1) Hydrochlorothiazide + amiloride (2) Atenolol
Add on	Various	Methyldopa	Bendrofluazide Methyldopa	Atenolol	(1) Atenolol or metoprolol or pindolol (2) Hydrochlorothiazide + amiloride	(1) Atenolol (2) Hydrochlorothiazide
Blood pressure obtained:						
Treatment group	143/87	149/85	162/77	144/68	167/87	152/79
Placebo group	155/94	172/94	180/88	155/71	186/96	167/85

*Depending on entry systolic pressure.   ***Initial goal <90 mm Hg, reduced to <80 mm Hg after two years.
From Beard, K, Bulpitt C, Mascie-Taylor H, O'Malley, K, Sever, P, Webb, S. Management of elderly patients with sustained hypertension. Br Med J 1992;304:412–416.

Table 14.18 Percentage Change in Event Rates, Six Trials.

	Australian	EWPHE	Coope and Warrender	SHEP	STOP-Hypertension	MRC
Non-fatal events:						
Stroke	-37	-35	-27	-37*	-38*	-30
Myocardial infarction	+18	NR	+11	-33*	-16	NR
All cardiac	-10	-9	-26	-40*	NR	-13
All cardiovascular	-26	-36*	-26	-36*	NR	-25*
Fatal events:						
Stroke	-1	-32	-70*	-29	-73*	-12
Cardiac	-75†	-38*	+1	-20†	-25‡	-22‡
All cardiovascular	+13	+21	NR	+5	NR	+5
Total deaths	-23	-9	-3	-13	-43*	-3
All events:						
Stroke	-34	-36*	-42*	-36*	-47*	-25*
Cardiac	-19	-20	-15	-27*	-13‡	-19‡
Cardiovascular	-24	-34*	-23*	-32*	-40*	-17*

NR=Not reported. *p<0.05. †Ischemic heart disease. ‡Myocardial infarction.

50% (Table 14.19). Despite the lack of randomized controlled data in secondary prevention, extrapolation from younger subjects suggests that aspirin, unless contraindicated, should be employed in the elderly.

β–BLOCKERS

Several randomized studies have demonstrated the cardioprotective effect of β-blockers in postinfarction elderly patients. In the β-Blocker Heart Attack Trial (BHAT), elderly subjects (60 to 69 years) receiving propranolol vs placebo experienced a greater reduction in death rate (33.3%) compared with younger subjects (30 to 59 years) (18.9%). The beneficial effect was also observed for a longer period of time in the elderly (36 months) compared with younger participants (6 months).

In a recent review of several trials, Forman and associates concluded that the use of β-blockade post-MI in the elderly reduces mortality by 40%. Unfortunately, many physicians might be wary of the use of β-blockers in this subgroup because of the concern of more severe or intolerable side-effects. However, in the BHAT study, there was no age disparity in side effect incidence. Thus, barring contraindications, β-blockade should be considered part of the post-MI regimen in the elderly.

Table 14.19. Risk of MI with Aspirin Use Versus Placebo: Physicians' Health Study

Age	Number of MIs/Total number of patients (%)		Relative risk
	Aspirin group	Placebo group	
40–49	27/4,527 (0.6)	24/4,524 (0.5)	1.12
50–59	51/3,725 (1.4)	87/3,725 (2.3)	0.58
60–69	39/2,045 (1.9)	84/2,045 (4.1)	0.46
70–84	22/740 (3.0)	44/740 (6.0)	0.49

From Miller M, Gottlieb SO. Preventive maintenance of the aging heart. Geriatrics 1991;46:22–30. (Adapted by permission of The New England Journal of Medicine from Steering Committee of the Physician's Health Study Research Group. Final report on the aspirin component of the ongoing Physician's Health Study, N Engl J Med 1989;321:129, Copyright © 1989, Massachusetts Medical Society.)

Suggested Readings

African-Americans

Ayanian JZ, Udvarhelyi IS; Gatsonis CA, et al. Racial differences in the use of revascularization procedures after coronary angiography. JAMA 1993;269:2642–2646.

Banerji MA, Norin AJ, Chaiken RL, Lebovitz HE. HLA-DQ associations distinguish insulin-resistant and insulin-sensitive variants of NIDDM in black Americans. Diabetes Care 1993;16:429–433.

Blaustein MP, Grim CE. The pathogenesis of hypertension: Black-white differences. In: Saunders E, Brest AN, eds. Cardiovascular diseases in blacks. Philadelphia: F.A. Davis Company, 1991:97–114.

Chaiken RL, Banerji MA, Huey H, Lebovitz HE. Do blacks with NIDDM have an insulin-resistance syndrome? Diabetes 1993;42:444–449.

Clark LT, Karve MM, Rones KT, Chang-DeMoranville B, et al. Obesity, distribution of body fat and coronary artery disease in black women. Am J Cardiol 1994;73:895–896.

Council on Ethical and Judicial Affairs. Black-white disparities in health care. JAMA 1990;263:2344–2346.

Falkner B, Hulman S, Kushner H. Insulin-stimulated glucose utilization and borderline hypertension in young adult blacks. Hypertension 1993;22:18–25.

Flack JM, Neaton JD, Daniels B, Esunge P. Ethnicity and renal disease: Lessons from the multiple risk factor intervention trial and the treatment of mild hypertension study. Am J Kidney Dis 1993;21:31–40.

Flegal KM, Ezzati TM, Harris MI, et al. Prevalence of diabetes in Mexican Americans, Cubans, and Puerto Ricans from the Hispanic Health and Nutrition Examination Survey, 1982–1984. Diabetes Care 1991;14:628–638.

Ford E, Cooper R, Castaner A, Simmons B, Mar M. Coronary arteriography and coronary bypass survey among whites and other racial groups relative to hospital-based incidence rates for coronary artery disease: Findings from NHDS. Am J Public Health 1989;79:437–440.

Freedman DS, Gruchow HW, Manley JC, Anderson AJ, Sobocinski KA, Barboriak JJ. Black/white differences in risk factors for arteriographically documented coronary artery disease in men. Am J Cardiol 1988;62:214–219.

Freedman DS, Strogatz DS, Eaker E, Joesoef MR, DeStefano F. Differences between black and white men in correlates of high density lipoprotein cholesterol. Am J Epidemiol 1990;132:656–669.

Gillum RF. Cardiovascular disease in the United States: An epidemiologic overview. In: Saunders E, Brest AN, eds. Cardiovascular diseases in blacks. Philadelphia: F.A. Davis Company, 1991: 3–16.

Goldberg RJ. Coronary heart disease: Epidemiology and risk factors. In: Ockene IS, Ockene JK eds. Prevention of coronary heart disease. Boston: Little, Brown and Company, 1992.

Harris MI. Epidemiological correlates of NIDDM in hispanics, whites, and blacks in the U.S. population. Diabetes Care 1991; 14:639–648.

Hildreth C, Saunders E. Hypertension in blacks: Clinical overview. In: Saunders E, Brest AN, eds. Cardiovascular diseases in blacks. Philadelphia: F.A. Davis Company, 1991:85–96.

Hypertension Detection and Follow-up Program Cooperative Group. Five-year findings of the hypertension detection and follow-up program. II. Mortality by race-sex and age. JAMA 1979;242:2572–2577.

Hypertension Detection and Follow-Up Program Cooperative Group. Educational level and 5-year all-cause mortality in the hypertension detection and follow-up program. Hypertension 1987;9:641–646.

Johnson CL, Rifkind BM, Sempos CT, et al. Declining serum total cholesterol levels among US adults. The National Health and Nutrition Examination Surveys. JAMA 1993;269:3002–3008.

Kahn KL, Pearson ML, Harrison ER, Desmond KA, Rogers WH, Rubenstein LV. Health care for black and poor hospitalized medicare patients. JAMA 1994; 271:1169–1174.

Keil JE, Sutherland SE, Knapp RG, Lackland DT, Gazes PC, Tyroler HA. Mortality rates and risk factors for coronary disease in black as compared with white men and women. N Engl J Med 1993;329:73–78.

Keil JE, Sutherland SE, Knapp RG, Tyroler HA. Does equal socioeconomic status in black and white men equal risk of mortality? Am J Public Health 1992;82: 1133–1136.

Klag MJ, Whelton PK, Coresh J, Grim CE, Kuller LH. The association of skin color with blood pressure in US blacks with low socioeconomic status. JAMA 1991;265: 599–602.

Kumanyika S. Obesity in black women. Epidemiologic Reviews 1987;9:31–50.

Lenfant C. Report of the NHLBI Working Group on research in coronary heart disease in blacks. Circulation 1994;90: 1613–1623.

Maynard C, Fisher LD, Passamani ER. Survival of black persons compared with white persons in the Coronary Artery Surgery Study (CASS). Am J Cardiol 1987;60:513–518.

Murray RF Jr. Skin color and blood pressure. Genetics or environment? JAMA 1991; 265:639–640.

Novotny TE, Warner KE, Kendrick JS, Remington PL. Smoking by blacks and whites: Socioeconomic and demographic differences. Am J Public Health 1988; 78:1187–1189.

O'Brien TR, Flanders WD, Decoufle P, Boyle CA, DeStefano F, Teutsch S. Are racial differences in the prevalence of diabetes in adults explained by differences in obesity? JAMA 1989;262:1485–1488.

Orleans CT, Schoenback VJ, Salmon MA, et al. A survey of smoking and quitting patterns among black Americans. Am J Public Health 1989;79:176–181.

Peterson ED, Wright SM, Daley J, Thibault GE. Racial variation in cardiac procedure use and survival following acute myocardial infarction in the Department of Veterans Affairs. JAMA 1994;271:1175–1180.

Sane DC, Stump DC, Topol EJ, Sigmon KN, Clair WK, Kereiakes DJ. Racial differences in responses to thrombolytic therapy with recombinant tissue-type plasminogen activator. Circulation 1991;83:170–175.

Sempos CT, Cleeman JI, Carroll MD, Johnson CL, Bachorik PS, Gordon DJ. Prevalence of high blood cholesterol among US adults. JAMA 1993;269:3009–3014.

U.S. Department of Health and Human Services. Morbidity and mortality chartbook on cardiovascular, lung and blood diseases 1990. National Institutes of Health: National Heart, Lung and Blood Institute, 1990.

Whittle J, Conigliaro J, Good CB, Lofgren RP. Racial differences in the use of invasive cardiovascular procedures in the Department of Veterans Affairs Medical System. N Engl J Med 1993;329:621–627.

Williamson DF, Madans J, Anda RF, Kleinman JC, Giovino GA, Byers T. Smoking cessation and severity of weight gain in a national cohort. N Engl J Med 1991; 324:739–745.

Childhood

Bao W, Srinivasan SR, Wattigney WA, Berenson GS. The relation of parental cardiovascular disease to risk factors in children and young adults. The Bogalusa Heart Study. Circulation 1995;91:365–371.

Beaty TH, Neel JV, Fajans SS. Identifying risk factors for diabetes in first degree relatives of non-insulin dependent diabetic patients. Am J Epidemiol 1982;115:380–97.

Berenson GS, Srinivasan SR, Nicklas TA, Webber LS. Cardiovascular risk factors in children and early prevention of heart disease. Clin Chem 1988;34:B115–B122.

Burke GL, Savage PJ, Sprafka JM, et al. Relation of risk factor levels in young adulthood to parental history of disease. The CARDIA Study. Circulation 1991;84:1176–1187.

Burns TL, Moll PP, Lauer RM. The relation between ponderosity and coronary risk factors in children and their relatives. The Muscatine Ponderosity Family Study. Am J Epidemiol 1989;129:973–987.

Dennison BA, Kikuchi DA, Srinivasan SR, Webber LS, Berenson GS. Parental history of cardiovascular disease as an indication for screening for lipoprotein abnormalities in children. J Pediatr 1989;115:186–194.

Enos WF, Holmes RH, Beyer J. Coronary disease among United States soldiers killed in action in Korea. Preliminary report. JAMA 1953;152:1090–1093.

Farah JR, Kwiterovich PO Jr, Neill CA. Dose effect relation of cholestyramine in children and young adults with familial hypercholesterolemia. Lancet 1977;1:59–63.

Fischer PM, Schwartz MP, Richards JW Jr, Goldstein AO, Rojas TH. Brand logo recognition by children aged 3 to 6 years. Mickey Mouse and Old Joe the Camel. JAMA 1991;266:3145–3148.

Flegal KM, Ezzati TM, Harris MI, et al. Prevalence of diabetes in Mexican-Americans, Cubans, and Puerto Ricans from the Hispanic Health and Nutrition Examination Survey, 1982–1984. Diabetes Care 1991;14:628–638.

Freedman DS, Newman WP III, Tracy RE, et al. Black-white differences in aortic fatty streaks in adolescence and early adulthood: The Bogalusa Heart Study. Circulation 1988;77:856–864.

Freedman DS, Srinivasan SR, Shear CL, Franklin FA, Webber LS, Berenson GS. The relation of apolipoproteins A-I and B in children to parental myocardial infarction. N Engl J Med 1986;315:721–726.

Freedman DS, Burke GL, Harsha DW, et al. Relationship of changes in obesity to serum lipid and lipoprotein changes in childhood and adolescence. JAMA 1985;254:515–520.

Jason LA, Ji PY, Anes MD, Birkhead SH. Active enforcement of cigarette control laws in the prevention of cigarette sales to minors. JAMA 1991;266:3159–3161.

Lauer RM, Clarke WR. Childhood risk factors for high adult blood pressure: The Muscatine Study. Pediatrics 1984;84:633–641.

Mahoney LT, Schieken RM, Clarke WR, Lauer RM. Left ventricular mass and exercise responses predict future blood pressure. The Muscatine Study. Hypertension 1988;12:206–213.

Mittelmark MD, Murray DM, Leupker RV, Pechacek TF, Pirie PL, Pallonen UE. Predicting experimentation with cigarettes. The childhood antecedents of smoking study (CASS). Am J Public Health 1987;77:206–208.

Munger RG, Prineas RJ, Gomez-Marin O. Persistent elevation of blood pressure among children with a family history of hypertension: The Minneapolis Children's Blood Pressure Study. J Hypertens 1988;6:647–653.

National Cholesterol Education Program. Report of the expert panel on blood cholesterol levels in children and adolescents. U.S. Department of Health and Human Services, NIH Publication No. 91,2732. September 1991.

National Heart, Lung, and Blood Institute. The Lipid Research Clinics Population Studies

Data Book: Volume I-The Prevalence Study. Bethesda, MD: U.S. Department of Health and Human Services, Public Health Service, National Institutes of Health, NIH Pub. No. 80,1527, July 1980.

Newman WP III, Freedman DS, Voors AW, Gard PD, Srinivasan SR, Cresanta JL. Relation of serum lipoprotein levels and systolic blood pressure to early atherosclerosis. The Bogalusa Heart Study. N Engl J Med 1986;314:138–144.

Nielsen JR, Oxhøj H. Echocardiographic variables in progeny of hypertensive and normotensive parents. Acta Med Scand 1988;S693(217):61–64.

Pierce JP, Lee L, Gilpin E. Smoking initiation by adolescent girls, 1944 through 1988. JAMA 1994;271:608–611.

Pierce JP, Gilpin E, Burns DM, et al. Does tobacco advertising target young people to start smoking? JAMA 1991;266:3154–3158.

Pirie PL, Murray DM, Luepker RV. Smoking prevalence in a cohort of adolescents, including absentees, dropouts, and transfers. Am J Public Health 1988;78: 176–178.

Price JH, Desmond SM, Ruppert ES, Stelzer CM. Pediatricians' perceptions and practices regarding childhood obesity. Am J Prev Med 1989;2:95–103.

Riopel DA, Boerth RC, Coates TJ, Hennekens CH, Miller WW, Weidman WH. Coronary risk factor modification in children: Exercise. Circulation 1986;74:1189A–1191A.

Sallis JF, Patterson TL, Buono MJ, Nader PR. Relation of cardiovascular fitness and physical activity to cardiovascular disease risk factors in children and adults. Am J Epidemiol 1988;127:933–941.

Schieken RM, Clarke WR, Lauer RM. Left ventricular hypertrophy in children with blood pressures in the upper quintile of the distribution. The Muscatine Study. Hypertension 1981;3:669–675.

Shear CL, Webber LS, Freedman DS, Srinivasan SR, Berenson GS. The relationship between parental history of vascular disease and cardiovascular disease risk factors in children: The Bogalusa Heart Study. Am J Epidemiol 1985;122: 762–771.

Strazzullo P, Cappuccio FP, Trevisan M, et al. Leisure time physical activity and blood pressure in schoolchildren. Am J Epidemiol 1988;127:726–733.

Task Force on Blood Pressure Control in Children. Report of the Second Task Force on blood pressure in children—1987. Pediatrics 1987;79:1–25.

Wattigney WA, Harsha DW, Srinivasan SR, Webber LS, Berenson GS. Increasing impact of obesity on serum lipids and lipoproteins in young adults. The Bogalusa Heart Study. Arch Intern Med 1991; 151:2017–2022.

Wissler RW. New insights into the pathogenesis of atherosclerosis as revealed by Pathobiological Determinants of Atherosclerosis in Youth. Atherosclerosis 1994;108(Suppl):S3–S20.

Woolf N. The morphology of atherosclerotic lesions. In: Crawford T, ed. Pathology of Atherosclerosis. London: Butterworth Scientific, 1982:47–82.

Writing Group for the DISC Collaborative Research Group. Efficacy and safety of lowering dietary intake of fat and cholesterol in children with elevated low-density lipoprotein cholesterol: The Dietary Intervention Study in Children (DISC). JAMA 1995;273:1429–1435.

Geriatrics

β-Blocker Heart Attack Trial Research Group. A randomized trial of propranolol in patients with acute myocardial infarction. JAMA 1982;247:1707–1714.

Beard K, Bulpitt C, Mascie-Taylor H, O'Malley K, Sever P, Webb S. Management of elderly patients with sustained hypertension. Br Med J 1992;304:412–416.

Benfante R, Reed D, Frank J. Does cigarette smoking have an independent effect on coronary heart disease incidence in the elderly? Am J Public Health 1991;81: 897–899.

Benfante R, Reed D. Is elevated serum cholesterol level a risk factor for coronary heart disease in the elderly? JAMA 1990;263: 393–396.

Castelli WP, Wilson PWF, Levy D, Anderson K. Cardiovascular risk factors in the elderly. Am J Cardiol 1989;63:12H–19H.

Donahue RP, Abbott RD, Reed DM, Yano K. Physical activity and coronary heart disease in middle-aged and elderly men: The Honolulu Heart Program. Am J Public Health 1988;78:683–685.

Fletcher AE, Bulpitt CJ. How far should blood pressure be lowered? N Engl J Med 1992;326:251–254.

Forman DE, Gutiérrez Bernal JL, Wei JY. Management of acute myocardial infarction in the very elderly. Am J Med 1992;93:315–326.

Hermanson B, Omenn GS, Kronmal RA, et al. Beneficial six-year outcome of smoking cessation in older men and women with coronary artery disease. N Engl J Med 1988;319:1365–1369.

Krumholz HM, Seeman TE, Merrill SS, et al. Lack of association between cholesterol and coronary heart disease mortality and morbidity and all-cause mortality in persons older than 70 years. JAMA 1994;272:1335–1340.

Lavie CJ, Milani RV, Littman AB. Benefits of cardiac rehabilitation and exercise training in secondary coronary prevention in the elderly. J Am Coll Cardiol 1993;22: 678–683.

Levy D, Garrison RJ, Savage DD, et al. Left ventricular mass and incidence of coronary heart disease in an elderly cohort: The Framingham Heart Study. Ann Intern Med 1989;110:101–107.

Manolio TA, Furberg CD. Age as a predictor of outcome: What role does it play? Am J Med 1992;92:1–6.

Miller M, Gottlieb SO. Preventive maintenance of the aging heart. Geriatrics 1991; 46:22–30.

Paffenbarger RS Jr, Hyde RT, Wing AL, Hsieh C-C. Physical activity, all-cause mortality, and longevity of college alumni. N Engl J Med 1986;314:605–613.

Pekkanen J, Linn S, Heiss G, et al. Ten-year mortality from cardiovascular disease in relation to cholesterol level among men with and without preexisting cardiovascular disease. N Engl J Med 1990; 322:1700–1707.

Pfeffer MA, Braunwald E, Moyé LA, et al. Effect of captopril on mortality and morbidity in patients with left ventricular dysfunction after myocardial infarction: Results of the survival and ventricular enlargement trial. N Engl J Med 1992; 327:669–677.

Scandinavian Simvastatin Survival Study Group. Randomised trial of cholesterol lowering in 4444 patients with coronary heart disease: The Scandinavian Simvastatin Survival Study (4S). Lancet 1994; 344:1383–1389.

Steering Committee of the Physicians' Health Study Research Group. Final report on the aspirin component of the ongoing Physicians' Health Study. N Engl J Med 1989;321:129–135.

Weber MA, Neutel JM, Cheung DG. Hypertension in the aged: A pathophysiologic basis for treatment. Am J Cardiol 1989;63:25H–32H.

Index